Fundamentals of Anaesthesia and Acute Medicine

Cardiovascular Physiology

Second edition

Edited by

Hans-Joachim Priebe

Professor of Anaesthesia, University Hospital, Freiburg, Germany

and

Karl Skarvan

Professor of Anaesthesia, University of Basel, Switzerland

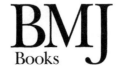

BMJ Books is an imprint of the BMJ Publishing Group
www.bmjbooks.com

First published in 1995
by the BMJ Publishing Group, BMA House, Tavistock Square,
London WC1H 9JR

Second edition published in 2000

British Library Cataloguing in Publication Data
A catalogue record for this book is available
from the British Library

ISBN 0-7279-1427-8

Typeset in Great Britain by
Apek Digital Imaging, Nailsea, North Somerset
Printed and bound in Great Britain by J.W. Arrowsmith Ltd, Bristol

Contents

FUNDAMENTALS OF ANAESTHESIA AND ACUTE MEDICINE

Series editors

Ronald M Jones, Professor of Anaesthetics, St Mary's Hospital Medical School, London, UK
Alan R Aitkenhead, Professor of Anaesthetics, University of Nottingham, UK
Pierre Foëx, Nuffield Professor of Anaesthetics, University of Oxford, UK

Titles already available:

Cardiovascular Physiology (second edition)
Edited by Hans Joachim Priebe and Karl Skarvan

Clinical Cardiovascular Medicine in Anaesthesia
Edited by Pierre Coriat

Intensive Care Medicine
Edited by Julian Bion

Management of Acute and Chronic Pain
Edited by Narinder Rawal

Neuro-Anaesthetic Practice
Edited by H Van Aken

Neuromuscular Transmission
Edited by Leo HDJ Booij

Paediatric Intensive Care
Edited by Alan Duncan

Forthcoming:

Pharmacology of the Critically Ill
Edited by Maire Shelly and Gilbert Park

Anaesthesia for Obstetrics and Gynaecology
Edited by Robin Russell

Contributors

John Atlee III, MD
Professor of Anesthesiology
Department of Anesthesiology, Medical College of Wisconsin, Milwaukee,
USA

James E Baumgardner, PhD, MD
Assistant Professor of Anesthesia and Bioengineering
Department of Anesthesia, University of Pennsylvania, Philadelphia, USA

Wolfgang Buhre, MD
Department of Anaesthesia, Georg-August Universität, Göttingen,
Germany

Andreas Hoeft, PhD, MD
Professor of Anaesthesia and Chairman
Department of Anaesthesia, Rheinische Friedrich-Wilhelms Universität
Bonn, Germany

Nguyen D Kien, PhD
Professor of Anesthesiology
Department of Anesthesiology, School of Medicine, University of
California, Davis, USA

Alex L Loeb, PhD
Assistant Professor of Anesthesia and Pharmacology
Department of Anesthesia, University of Pennsylvania, Philadelphia, USA

David E Longnecker, MD
Robert Dunning Dripps Professor and Chairman
Department of Anesthesia, University of Pennsylvania, Philadelphia, USA

David K Menon, MD, FRCP, FRCA
Lecturer in Anaesthesia, University of Cambridge
Director, Neurosciences Critical Care Unit, Department of Anaesthesia,
Addenbrooke's Hospital, Cambridge, UK

Niraj Nijhawan, MD, MS
Assistant Professor of Anesthesiology
Zablocki Veterans Administration Medical Center, Milwaukee, Wisconsin, USA

Hans-Joachim Priebe, MD, FRCA
Professor of Anesthesiology
University Hospital, Freiburg, Germany

John A Reitan, MD
Professor of Anesthesiology
Department of Anesthesiology, School of Medicine, University of California, Davis, USA

Karl Skarvan, MD
Professor of Anaesthesia
Department of Anaesthesia, University Hospital, Basel, Switzerland

Keith Sykes, MB BChir, FRCA
Emeritus Professor, Nuffield Department of Anaesthetics, University of Oxford, UK

Anne B Taegtmeyer, BM BCh
Clinical Research Fellow
Cardiothoracic Surgery Division, National Heart and Lung Institute, Imperial College of Science, Technology and Medicine, London, UK

Heinrich Taegtmeyer, MD, DPhil
Professor of Medicine
Department of Internal Medicine, Division of Cardiology, University of Texas – Houston Medical School, Houston, USA

David C Warltier, PhD, MD
Professor of Anesthesiology, Cardiology and Medicine and
Vice-Chairman of Research
Department of Anesthesiology, Medical College of Wisconsin, Milwaukee, USA

Foreword

The pace of change within the biological sciences continues to increase and nowhere is this more apparent than in the specialties of anaesthesia, acute medicine, and intensive care. Although many practitioners continue to rely on comprehensive but bulky texts for reference, the accelerating rate of biomedical advances makes this source of information increasingly likely to be dated, even if the latest edition is used. The series *Fundamentals of anaesthesia and acute medicine* aims to bring to the reader up to date and authoritative reviews of the principal clinical topics which make up the specialties. Each volume will cover the fundamentals of the topic in a comprehensive manner but will also emphasise recent developments or controversial issues.

International differences in the practice of anaesthesia and intensive care are now much less than in the past, and the editors of each volume have commissioned chapters from acknowledged authorities throughout the world to assemble contributions of the highest possible calibre. Three volumes will appear annually and, as the pace and extent of clinically significant advances varies among the individual topics, new editions will be commissioned to ensure that practitioners will be in a position to keep abreast of the important developments within the specialties.

Not only does the pace of advance in biomedical science serve to justify the appearance of an international series of this nature but the current awareness of the need for more formal continuing education also underlines the timeliness of its appearance. The editors would welcome feedback from readers about the series, which is aimed at both established practitioners and trainees preparing for degrees and diplomas in anaesthesia and intensive care.

RONALD M JONES
ALAN R AITKENHEAD
PIERRE FOËX

Preface

In the few years since the first edition of *Cardiovascular Physiology*, knowledge in this field has again expanded tremendously. This second edition is therefore written to keep the reader updated on progress in this area, and to further improve his/her understanding of basic cardiovascular physiology.

The understanding of basic cardiovascular physiology is more important than ever. The patient population is becoming progressively more elderly and infirm. Even the old and sick undergo increasingly complex and stressful procedures.

More effective prehospital trauma care improves initial survival of previously fatal injuries, but for subsequent long-term survival the cardiovascular system is challenged to the maximum. New guidelines on perioperative cardiac evaluation restrict the extent of preoperative testing. The concept of "same day surgery" limits the time available for preoperative optimisation of cardiovascular performance. Minimally invasive surgical techniques decrease tissue trauma, but they can impose an additional burden on the cardiovascular system.

Furthermore, current medical practice encourages restriction of blood transfusion and acceptance of low haemoglobin concentrations which often requires an increase in cardiac work to maintain oxygen delivery. Early postoperative extubation and rapid hospital discharge can pose additional stress on the cardiovascular system.

Not surprisingly, therefore, cardiovascular complications remain the dominant cause of overall perioperative morbidity and mortality. For all of these and many others a solid understanding of cardiovascular physiology remains a prerequisite for optimum patient care.

All chapters have been completely revised and updated. We gratefully acknowledge the contributions of all authors. Without their work and expertise, this monograph would not have been possible.

HANS-JOACHIM PRIEBE
KARL SKARVAN

1: Cardiac cellular physiology and metabolism

HEINRICH TAEGTMEYER, ANNE B TAEGTMEYER

New horizons

Cardiac cellular physiology and metabolism have long been considered areas of interest to only a small group of basic scientists. Although, in the past, clinicians have laid the foundations for much of the work in this area,[1 2] their research was descriptive and its clinical use limited to the detection of coronary artery disease by the release of lactate or alanine from the ischaemic myocardium.[3–5] When, it was shown (by isotopic methods) that lactate release occurred in the presence of net lactate extraction by the normal human heart,[6] it appeared that the potential for invasive assessment of cardiac metabolism to detect coronary artery or other forms of heart disease could not be fulfilled.

A number of technical advances in the diagnosis and treatment of heart disease have reawakened the interest in cardiac cell metabolism by clinical investigators and basic scientists alike. The most dramatic recent examples include reports on enhanced myocardial function in transgenic mice overexpressing the β_2-adrenergic receptor,[7] highly efficient gene transfer into adult ventricular myocytes,[8] the grafting of fetal myocytes into adult host myocardium,[9] and the transfer of autologous myoblasts into damaged myocardium.[10]

It seems, however, that the ultimate success of gene therapy for the failing heart continues to be constrained by the inadequate understanding of the underlying pathophysiological events. New insights into cellular physiology and pathophysiology have come from the use of positron labelled metabolic tracers or tracer analogues, which are used for non-invasive assessment of regional myocardial blood flow and metabolism as a tool to differentiate between reversible and irreversible myocardial ischaemia.[11–13] Other examples also include the use of tomographic nuclear magnetic resonance (NMR) spectroscopy for the early detection of contractile dysfunction in the pressure overloaded left ventricle.[14] Cellular mechanisms of adaptations to ischaemia, reperfusion, and reperfusion injury have come into focus when it became possible to reverse the deleterious effects of compromised

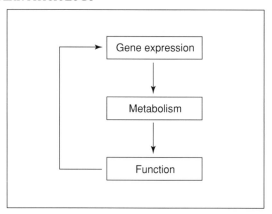

Fig 1.1 Metabolism as link between gene expression and contractile function of the heart. The heart acutely adapts to changes in function by changing its metabolic rates. Chronic changes in function alter the expression of metabolic genes.[16]

or absent blood flow.[15] Recently, we found that ventricular unloading reproduces the fetal pattern of gene expression also found in the hypertrophied heart.[16] The induction of a fetal gene response provides a molecular basis for the functional improvement of the failing heart after treatments such as the left ventricular assist device (LVAD) which allow the heart to "rest".

We now recognise that the precise and rapid regulation of energy substrate metabolism allows the heart to adapt to changes in workload from one beat to the next. We also recognise that metabolism forms the essential link between gene expression, on the one hand, and contractile function of the heart, on the other (Fig 1.1).

The message is clear: modern management of patients with overt or latent cardiac dysfunction includes physiological approaches that only a decade ago were unimaginable. It is therefore appropriate to review some of the salient concepts of cellular function and energy transfer in heart muscle and relate them to specific clinical situations, which are addressed in the second part of this chapter. The interested reader may also wish to refer to the recent monograph "Energy metabolism of the heart: from basic concepts to clinical applications" for more detailed information.[17]

Principles of energy transfer in heart muscle

Heart muscle possesses a complex, yet very efficient system of energy transfer. At the centre of this system is a network of enzyme catalysed reactions. Although bewildering at first glance, the purpose of this network is easy to understand, and a number of simple principles on function and

Salient features of heart muscle

- Consumer and provider of energy
- High rate of energy turnover
- Metabolic omnivore
- Depends on O_2 for energy production
- Only limited endogenous food reserves
- Wide range of adaptations

metabolism of the heart are worth remembering. These are listed in the box and discussed below.

The heart, like any organ of the mammalian body, consists of a number of different components, all of which are in a constant state of flux. These include:

- interactive proteins
- purine bases
- energy providing intermediates
- membranes
- ions
- signal molecules.

In addition, heart muscle has retained its ability to adapt to environmental changes by altering the synthesis and/or degradation rates of specific proteins or, acutely, by changing the flux through metabolic pathways in order to maintain its state of equilibrium. Only the most severe environmental changes, such as those induced by an interruption of O_2 supply, result in a cessation of energy production and consequent heart muscle failure, which in turn causes a collapse of the blood circulation.

Heart muscle is both a consumer and a provider of energy. The heart consumes energy locked in the chemical bonds of fuels through their controlled combustion, and converts chemical energy into physical energy. The predominant form of physical energy of the heart consists of pump work. In this respect, the heart can be considered to be a transducer (that is, a device that receives energy from one system and transmits it to another). As a result of its ability to convert chemical energy into mechanical energy, the heart also provides energy in the form of substrates and O_2 both for itself and to the rest of the body. In this context, two important concepts emerge:

1 The heart is a "hot spot" of metabolic activity because ATP (the chemical energy available for conversion to mechanical energy at the contractile site) must be continuously resynthesised from its breakdown products

ADP and P_i (inorganic phosphate). The greater the work output, the higher the rate of ATP turnover.

2 When the heart's ability to convert chemical into mechanical energy is impaired (for whatever reason), the consequences result in functional and metabolic abnormalities in the rest of the body. These abnormalities are commonly referred to as "heart failure".

There is no organ in the human body that is not affected by an impairment of energy transfer in the heart.

The role of ATP as the main provider of chemical energy for various cell functions was first postulated by Lipmann[18] when he drew attention to the biological importance of the ATP–ADP couple. The rate of ATP turnover in the heart is far greater than in other organs of the mammalian body, and it is often underestimated. A simple calculation, based on measurements of myocardial O_2 consumption, indicates that in the course of 24 hours the human heart produces (and uses) 5 kg ATP; in other words, more than 10 times its own weight and more than 1000 times the amount of ATP stored in the heart and readily available for hydrolysis at any one instant in time.[19] Although the human heart accounts for only 0·5% of the total body weight, it claims 10% of the body's O_2 consumption. Lastly, it is important to remember that the *rate of energy turnover*, and not the tissue content of ATP, is the determinant of myocardial energy metabolism.[20–22]

As the heart meets the bulk of its energy needs by oxidative phosphorylation of ADP, it is not surprising that heart muscle cells are also richly endowed with mitochondria, the cell organelles that contain the enzymes of oxidative metabolism. There is a close correlation of mitochondrial volume fraction, heart rate, and total body O_2 consumption.[23] Not only are cardiac mitochondria abundant in number, they also contain a far larger number of cristae (the morphological sites of the respiratory chain enzymes) than mitochondria in other organs such as the liver, brain, or skeletal muscle.[24]

Finally, energy metabolism of the heart must also be considered in the context of energy transfer in biological systems in general. Knowledge of the vast array of metabolic pathways in the cell is often regarded with apprehension by students of biochemistry. The complexities of pathways become comprehensible when one considers the following three general principles:

1 The first law of thermodynamics
2 The second law of thermodynamics
3 The principle of moiety conservation.

Understanding these three principles also makes it easier to comprehend the clinical relevance of altered myocardial metabolism in the setting of myocardial ischaemia, infarction, or reperfusion.

Thermodynamic aspects of energy transfer in biological systems

Energy transfer in biological systems obeys the first and second law of thermodynamics. These two laws state that, within a closed system, energy can be converted only from one form into another, and that a process will occur spontaneously only if it is associated with an increase in disorder (or entropy) of the system. In short: nothing comes from nothing.

Energy is captured through the process of photosynthesis. The captured energy is, in turn, released through the reactions of intermediary metabolism to produce reducing equivalents, which combine with molecular O_2 to from H_2O (see below). Most dehydrogenase reactions are also linked to decarboxylation reactions (for example, pyruvate dehydrogenase, isocitrate dehydrogenase, and 2-oxoglutarate dehydrogenase) resulting in the liberation of carbon dioxide. Carbon dioxide and water are, in turn, the substrate for photosynthesis. The description of this simple energy cycle emphasises the fact that, in the biological environment, molecules are recycled.

Metabolic pathways and moiety conserved cycles

It is a characteristic property of all living cells, including heart muscle, to provide an environment in which complex chemical reactions can proceed quickly at relatively low temperatures and low substrate concentrations. The efficient transfer of energy occurs via enzyme catalysed metabolic pathways, at the centre of which are moiety conserved cycles (that is, a cycle in which the concentration of the participating intermediaries neither increases nor decreases). Moiety conserved cycles permit multiple use of given resources and are most likely to result from evolutionary selection.[25 26]

A metabolic pathway is defined as a series of enzyme catalysed reactions that starts with a flux generating step, usually a reaction catalysed by a non-equilibrium reaction or transport of the metabolite across a membrane, and ends with the removal of a product (for details see the literature[27 28]).

Biochemists distinguish between the *control* and *regulation* of metabolism, because these determine energy transfer in the cell.[26] In heart muscle, control of a metabolic pathway means that a change in the level of a control factor (for example, work load, hormones or drugs, substrate concentration, coronary flow, or O_2 availability) will change the rate of substrate flux. In contrast, regulation of a metabolic pathway means that flux of a substrate in a metabolic pathway is dictated by the activity of enzymes, regulators of enzymes, cofactors, and signal transduction pathways.

Many, but not all, of the regulators of energy transfer pathways are part of *moiety conserved cycles*. The largest moiety conserved cycle is in fact the circulation itself, where erythrocytes and plasma serve as a vehicle for the transport of O_2 and substrates and the removal of CO_2 and metabolic end

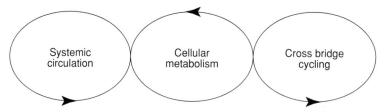

Fig 1.2 Energy transfer in heart muscle: efficient energy transfer occurs in moiety conserved cycles. (See text for further details.)

products. The hydrolysis of ATP through cross bridge cycling inside the myocardial cell itself is also a moiety conserved cycle; it acts:

• to decrease the proton gradient
• to increase the oxidation of NADH
• to increase flux through the citric acid cycle
• to increase acetyl-CoA utilisation
• to increase substrate consumption.

A convenient way of viewing energy transfer in heart muscle is as a "three-ring-circus", consisting of systemic circulation, cellular metabolism, and cross bridge cycling (Fig 1.2). The cycles interact, just like cog-wheels, in such a way that an increase in the rotation rate of one cycle causes a concurrent increase in the rotation rate of the other two (Fig 1.3). Thus an increase in cross bridge cycling leads to an increase in cellular metabolism and systemic circulation, which in turn provides the larger substrate load required by the metabolism cycle to maintain the new level of functioning. Conversely, it has been pointed out that, in animals with long circulation times, less substrate and less oxygen are delivered to the cell, and as both limit the rate of the metabolic reaction, the speed of the cycles is slow. In animals with short circulation times, all the needed components of the

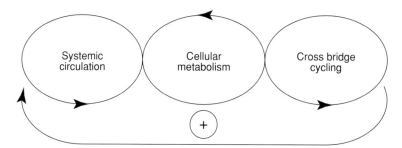

Fig 1.3 Interaction of cycles involved in energy transfer: feedback control of cycles is illustrated by the example of increased contractile activity. (See text for further details.)

reactions are delivered to the site in a continuous rapid stream and reactions occur almost explosively.[29]

Another example of a moiety conserved cycle is one that governs intracellular calcium homoeostasis. According to Barry and Bridge,[30] calcium homoeostasis in cardiac myocytes is of functional importance for at least three reasons:

1 The resting cytosolic calcium concentration ($[Ca^{2+}]$) of less than 0.2 μmol/l necessary to allow the contractile elements to relax during diastole must be maintained against a 5000-fold gradient across the sarcolemma ($[Ca^{2+}] > 1$ mmol/l).

2 Excitation–contraction coupling involves a complex interaction of membrane electric elements mediated by specific ion channels. This results in Ca^{2+} influx, which triggers the release of large amounts of Ca^{2+} from the sarcoplasmic reticulum via Ca^{2+} specific release channels[31] and subsequent extrusion of Ca^{2+}. To maintain steady state homoeostasis in this cycle the amount of Ca^{2+} entering the cell with each contraction must be extruded before the next contraction. Likewise, the large amount of Ca^{2+} released from the sarcoplasmic reticulum must be pumped back into the storage compartment. As a net result, only small amounts of Ca^{2+} enter and leave the cell with each cardiac cycle.

3 The force of contraction in cardiac myocytes is modulated by variations in the magnitude of the Ca^{2+} transient. Hormones or drugs that modify Ca^{2+} homoeostasis may significantly alter the force of contraction. In addition, cytosolic Ca^{2+} may be taken up into the mitochondria. Although the mitochondrial Ca^{2+} stores are only indirectly related to the contraction–relaxation cycle, Ca^{2+} ions are regulators of a number of intramitochondrial enzymes that are activated by Ca^{2+}.[32]

Thus Ca^{2+} ions form a link between utilisation and production of ATP. Although this hypothesis has not yet been proven,[33] Denton and McCormack[34] have proposed that the main role of the Ca^{2+} transporting system within the inner mitochondrial membrane should be viewed primarily as a means by which changes in the cytosolic $[Ca^{2+}]$ could be relayed into mitochondria and hence influence the activity of the intramitochondrial Ca^{2+} sensitive dehydrogenases. As Ca^{2+} is the only second messenger for hormones that is transferred across the inner mitochondrial membrane, an important feature of this hypothesis is a suggested mechanism by which mitochondrial oxidative metabolism and, hence, ATP supply could be stimulated to meet increased demands for ATP that are associated with the stimulation of the processes promoted by increases in cytosolic Ca^{2+}.[32] The same authors suggest that, when the Ca^{2+} dependent mechanism for activating oxidative metabolism is available (that is, via the Ca^{2+} sensitive enzymes in the mitochondrial matrix), then it is the preferred mechanism for promoting the overall process of oxidative phosphorylation.[32]

The sliding filament model of contraction represents another example of a moiety conserved cycle. The molecular mechanisms involved in the sliding filament model of cross bridge formation between actin and myosin have recently been elucidated.[35] The essence of the sliding filament model is that the myosin head binds to the actin filament in one orientation, rotates to a second orientation, and then detaches. The cycle is driven in one direction by coupling these transitions to the steps of ATP hydrolysis. Elucidation of the structure of myosin and a model for the actomyosin complex during contraction, including the description of an ATP binding pocket, have advanced our understanding of the molecular design of muscle motors.

One important consequence of energy transfer through moiety conserved cycles is that the loss of a moiety in any one of the cycles may lead to a loss of energy transfer within the cell. The following are examples of such losses:

1 The loss of contractile proteins (such as when degradation exceeds synthesis), for example, in certain forms of dilated cardiomyopathy or chronic myocardial ischaemia.
2 The loss of oxaloacetate from the citric acid cycle through either side reactions, such as transamination, or the inhibition of one or more of the cycle enzymes.

Depletion of a moiety is recovered through its resynthesis from precursors via a series of reactions termed 'anaplerosis'. Hans Kornberg has defined anaplerosis as the replenishment of a depleted cycle by an intermediate precursor.[36] A case in point is the contractile dysfunction of the isolated working rat heart perfused with acetoacetate, which is completely reversed by the addition of glucose as a second substrate.[37] The cause for the contractile dysfunction is an inhibition of the enzyme 2-oxoglutarate dehydrogenase as a result of sequestration of free coenzyme A,[38 39] resulting in a shortage of oxaloacetate for the citrate synthase reaction.[40] The cause of normalisation of contractile function with the addition of glucose is the carboxylation of pyruvate through the NADP dependent malic enzyme reaction.[41]

As ischaemia also depletes the citric acid cycle of its intermediates, especially succinate,[42] it is tempting to speculate that the increased glucose and/or lactate requirement in postischaemic myocardium[43-45] may be a reflection of the increased need for replenishment of the depleted cycle.

A second important consequence of energy transfer through moiety conserved cycles is the effective *recycling of moieties*. These moieties not only involve larger carbon molecules, such as glucose and fatty acids, but also the smaller organic acids of the citric acid cycle, and especially recycling of CO_2 and H_2O. Without the recycling of H_2O, ATP production in the citric acid cycle would be 60% less than it is with its recycling of H_2O (6 versus 15 moles ATP per mole pyruvate oxidised). As Ephraim Racker wrote:[46]

> Mitochondria cleave water without the drama of sunlight and chlorophyll. They perform this task, unnoticed by textbooks, in the quiet and unobtrusive manner characteristic of Hans Krebs and his cycle.

It stands to reason that, under certain circumstances, the *excess of a moiety* may also lead to contractile dysfunction of the heart. This occurs for example in ischaemia, reperfusion, and myocardial stunning, where the cells and their organelles may be flooded with Ca^{2+},[47–49] oxygen derived free radicals,[50–53] and protons,[54 55] resulting in cell swelling, osmotic stress, and membrane damage.[56]

Catabolism of substrates

In the heart, the direction of most enzyme catalysed reactions is catabolic, that is, substrates with high potential energy are broken down to products with low potential energy. Synthetic, or anabolic, reactions such as those serving protein, glycogen, or triglyceride synthesis are quantitatively of lesser importance, but ultimately they serve to improve the efficiency of energy production in heart muscle. Thus, heart muscle is endowed with an efficient system of energy transfer, which liberates energy locked in chemical bonds through the generation of reducing equivalents and their reaction with molecular O_2 in the respiratory chain. It should be stated once more that the main purpose of intermediary metabolism in normal heart muscle is the production of reducing equivalents for ATP synthesis by oxidative phosphorylation of ADP.

As proposed by Lehninger,[57] it is convenient to group the breakdown of substrates into three stages:

1 The first stage consists of the breakdown of substrates to acetyl-CoA.
2 The second stage is the oxidation of acetyl-CoA in the citric acid cycle.
3 The third stage is the reaction of reducing equivalents with molecular O_2 in the respiratory chain, where electron transfer is coupled to rephosphorylation of ADP to ATP.

As ATP production is tightly coupled to ATP utilisation, so is substrate oxidation tightly coupled to cardiac work.[37 58–62] It appears that, in the presence of adequate substrate supply, the maximal rate of oxidation of substrate is determined by the capacity of the 2-oxoglutarate dehydrogenase reaction in the citric acid cycle.[63] The exact mechanism by which respiration is coupled to energy expenditure in vivo is not, however, known.[64] The *efficiency* of oxidative phosphorylation for energy production is, however, well established – 1 mole of glucose, when oxidised, yields 36 moles of ATP, whereas the same amount of glucose yields only 2 moles of ATP when metabolised to lactate under anaerobic conditions:

$$1 \text{ mol glucose} \xrightarrow[\text{(Aerobic)}]{\text{Oxidation}} 36 \text{ mol ATP}$$

$$1 \text{ mol glucose} \xrightarrow[\text{(Anaerobic)}]{\text{Metabolism to lactate}} 2 \text{ mol ATP}$$

On a mole for mole basis, the energy yield from the oxidation of long chain fatty acids is even greater than that from glucose or lactate.

Nutrition of the heart and myocardial protein turnover

The recent interest in healthy nutrition for the heart has almost exclusively focused on cholesterol because of its role in the development of coronary artery disease. There is little appreciation of the fact that, in terms of general descriptors of energy metabolism, heart muscle functions not simply as a conformer in response to substrate availability,[65] but that substrate utilisation is controlled by the physiological demands on the system. Likewise, there is little appreciation of the fact that the heart stores endogenous substrates such as glycogen and triglycerides, and it does so in response to changes in the dietary state.[66 67] In contrast to skeletal muscle, starvation increases the tissue content of both glycogen and triglycerides in heart muscle, an observation consistent with a biologist's definition of true "hibernation".

Another fact that is not appreciated is that the heart continuously synthesises and degrades its own constituent proteins,[68] a process that is significantly slowed down by myocardial ischaemia.[69 70] Although protein turnover is perhaps the most difficult metabolic process to study in the heart in vivo, and although it appears that each protein has its own characteristic half life,[71] recent estimates indicate that 4·8% of myocardial protein is synthesised each day,[72] that is, the mammalian heart regenerates itself completely over a period of three weeks. As the net muscle mass is a function of both synthesis and degradation, hypertrophy may be the result of either increased rates of protein synthesis or decreased rates of protein degradation. Although acute volume overload of the myocardium leads to an increase in synthesis, it appears that chronic volume overload leads to suppression of protein degradation.[72] The pathways linking mechanical signals to changes in cardiac myocyte degradation rates are not known,[73] and the unravelling of mechanisms involved in myocardial protein degradation continue to pose a challenge to cellular and molecular biologists.

10

Substrate competition

As a result of the omnivorous nature of the heart, glucose, lactate, fatty acids, ketone bodies, and, under certain circumstances, amino acids are all converted to acetyl-CoA and so compete to be the fuel of respiration (Fig 1.4). The relative predominance of one fuel over another depends on the arterial substrate concentration (which, in the case of fatty acids, ketone bodies, and lactate, can vary greatly – Table 1.1), hormonal influences, workload, and O_2 supply. Likewise, the utilisation of specific substrates by the heart varies with the physiological state of its environment. When Bing[1] cannulated the coronary sinus and measured aorta–coronary sinus differences in substrate concentrations across the heart, he observed a proportional relationship between substrate concentration in the blood and substrate uptake by the heart for all substrates investigated, that is, glucose,

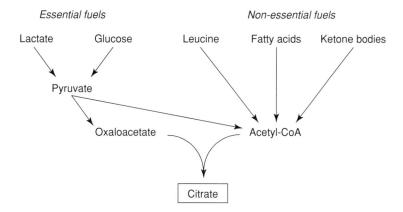

Fig 1.4 Essential and non-essential fuels for cardiac energy production. Note that glucose, lactate, and pyruvate provide both substrates for the citrate synthase reaction – acetyl-CoA and oxaloacetate. Carboxylation of pyruvate leading to the formation of oxaloacetate is an anaplerotic pathway. The importance of anaplerosis in the normal contractile function of the heart has recently been elucidated.[41]

Table 1.1 Metabolite concentrations in human plasma under various conditions

	Glucose (μmol/l)	Lactate (μmol/l)	Free fatty acids (μmol/l)	Ketone bodies (μmol/l)
Rest (postabsorptive)	5·0	0·5	0·1	0·1
Running (90 min)	5·0	5·0	1·7	1·8
Fasting	4·5	1·0	1·6	4·5
Diabetic ketoacidosis	30·0	1·0	1·7	10·0

Reproduced by permission from Taegtmeyer H. *Basic Res Cardiol* 1984;**79**:322–36.

lactate, fatty acids, ketone bodies, and amino acids. Subsequent work by Keul et al.[2] has established that the contribution of fuels to the fuel of respiration for the heart depends on the physiological state of the whole body, which can vary greatly. The data from Keul's work are of interest, because they show glucose uptake to be relatively constant (16–31%), whereas the uptake of fatty acids plus ketone bodies and the uptake of lactate vary considerably (from 25% to 63%, and from 5% to 61%, respectively). This observation is of relevance with respect to fatty acids and ketone bodies. Although fatty acid oxidation can be almost completely suppressed when lactate and pyruvate are abundant, there is a consistent rate of carbohydrate use. The need for glucose or lactate is most probably the result of the need for pyruvate carboxylation and the anaplerosis of the citric acid cycle. In keeping with this hypothesis we have shown that lactate (40 mmol/l) suppresses glucose uptake by the isolated working rat heart by 90%, whereas β-hydroxybutyrate at the same concentration suppresses glucose uptake by only 64%.[74] Collectively these findings suggest that the fuels for cardiac energy metabolism can be grouped (Fig 1.4) into *essential fuels*, which provide both acetyl-CoA and oxaloacetate:

- glucose
- lactate
- pyruvate
- certain amino acids

and *non-essential fuels*, which provide only acetyl-CoA:

- fatty acids of all chain lengths
- ketone bodies
- leucine.

Fatty acids are the preferred fuel for respiration in the fasted state,[75] but, even when fatty acid or ketone body concentrations are high, a certain amount of glucose continues to be oxidised.[37 76] Conversely, high lactate concentrations, such as those observed with strenuous exercise, can provide almost all[77] or the bulk of the fuel for respiration.[76]

Even amino acids, when present in very high concentrations, can become a fuel for respiration in heart muscle.[1] In this respect, the heart is not different from the body as a whole. When an omnivorous animal consumes a normal meal containing protein, carbohydrate, and fat, the degradation of any excess amino acids (that is, amino acids not needed for growth and replacement) takes precedence over the degradation of carbohydrates and fats.[78] This phenomenon results from strict control of amino acid metabolism by their K_m values (the Michaelis constant – the concentration of substrate required for half maximal velocity of an enzyme catalysed reaction) and reveals an *important principle of metabolic control*. As dietary protein or amino acids cannot be stored in major quantities, the amino acids from intestinal digestion are distributed unchanged in blood plasma and tissues. By contrast, products of carbohydrate and fat digestion can be stored rapidly as either glycogen or triglycerides. As this storage process begins immediately, fluctuations in plasma glucose and fatty acid levels are moderate and transient compared with fluctuations in amino acid levels. The increased amino acid concentrations in blood and tissues after a meal automatically cause an increased rate of amino acid degradation, because the K_m values of the enzymes initiating amino acid degradation are in general high and exceed the concentration of amino acids in the tissues.

In summary, many factors contribute to the selection of energy providing fuels for the heart. According to Krebs,[78] they may be classified under three main categories:

1 Concentration of the direct fuel in the tissue.
2 The presence, in the tissue, of the enzymes required for the degradation.
3 The kinetic properties of the key enzymes, especially of those that initiate the release of energy.

Each of these three main factors is, in turn, very complex and depends on a variety of components. The entry of fuels into the cell, as well as synthesis and degradation of stored fuel reserves, is controlled by hormones such as insulin and epinephrine (adrenaline) as well as by other environmental factors, with cAMP (cyclic adenosine $3':5'$-monophosphate) and a cascade of intracellular signals acting as second messengers. Among the kinetic properties of the key enzymes, the important ones are the K_m values (see above) and the inhibition and activation of enzymes by tissue constituents, which exercise either feedback inhibition or allosteric control through allosteric effectors or covalent modification. When the workload of the heart is raised acutely, these factors act together to trigger the preferential oxidation of glycogen,[79 80] thereby ensuring immediate availability of energy for contraction. In short: the heart functions best when it oxidises several substrates simultaneously.

Clinical relevance of myocardial metabolism

Altered energy metabolism is the cause of many clinical forms of heart disease (summarised in the box). In a review on myocardial metabolism, Lionel Opie[81 82] referred to a "decline and resurgence of myocardial metabolism". We have identified three areas of clinical relevance:

1 Tracing of metabolic pathways for the diagnosis of ischaemia and other forms of heart disease.

Clinical forms of heart disease caused by altered energy metabolism

Myocardial ischaemia
Latent ischaemia
Hibernation
Myocardial infarction
Reperfusion/reperfusion injury
Stunning/postischaemic dysfunction
Preconditioning/stress response

Cardiomyopathies
Dilated cardiomyopathies
Systolic dysfunction
Hormonal or nutritional deficiencies

Hypertrophy
Adaptation
Maladaptation
Diastolic/systolic dysfunction

2 "Metabolic mechanisms of heart disease", where contractile failure represents the end result of profound metabolic derangements.
3 Metabolic support for the failing heart includes replenishment of cofactors or intermediary metabolites in certain forms of dilated cardiomyopathy with resultant improvement in contractile performance, and support for the failing heart after prolonged periods of ischaemia as occurs in hypothermic ischaemic arrest.[81] [82]

Tracing metabolic pathways in the intact heart

A detailed knowledge of the pathways of individual substrates for energy production is usually not required by the clinician diagnosing or treating patients with heart disease. Metabolism comes under scrutiny, however, when coronary arteries are not (or are no longer) obstructed and yet the heart fails to contract, for example, as occurs in cardiomyopathies or in reperfused myocardium after complete coronary occlusion. More importantly, substrate metabolism has come into focus through the development of new, non-destructive imaging techniques such as NMR spectroscopy and positron emission tomography (PET), which permit the assessment of regional metabolic processes in the in vitro and in vivo beating heart.[13] [21] [83–91] Although NMR spectroscopy is able to detect derangements in energy rich phosphate metabolism before the development of contractile dysfunction,[14] PET imaging allows us to detect reversibly ischaemic, viable myocardium.[92–94]

NMR spectroscopy

The basis of NMR spectroscopy is that, even though all nuclei of atoms have an overall positive charge, some also have a "spin" which gives them a magnetic moment.[95] A powerful magnetic field orients the nuclear spins and, hence, establishes their different energy states. Transitions between adjacent energy states are induced by the application of an oscillating magnetic (or radiofrequency) field. The device that provides the radiofrequency field is also used to detect the result and signal or resonance (hence, the name radiofrequency coil or probe). Biologically important nuclei with a spin are ^1H, ^2H, ^{13}C, ^{15}N, ^{17}O, ^{31}P, ^{23}Na, ^{39}K, ^{87}Rb, and ^{19}F. Selective enrichment of low abundance nuclei (for example, ^{13}C) leads to an increase in their sensitivity.

Natural abundance NMR spectroscopy is most commonly used in the form of ^{31}P NMR spectroscopy, which yields distinct, quantitative resonance peaks for monophosphate esters, inorganic phosphates, phosphocreatine, and ATP. Analysis of energy rich phosphates in the beating heart in vivo by NMR spectroscopy of ^{31}P supports the view that, over a relatively wide range, the tissue content of ATP does not correlate with the rate of energy use as measured by the rate of ATP turnover, that is, O_2 consumption or contractile performance of the heart.[21] The recent introduction of a tomographic (spatial stacked plot) analysis of ^{31}P NMR spectra has added a new dimension to the analysis of energy rich phosphates in vivo. When this technique was applied to a group of patients with left ventricular hypertrophy caused by aortic stenosis and/or insufficiency, heart failure was characterised by a decline in the phosphocreatine:ATP ratio.[14] The adaptation of isotopomer analysis of ^{13}C natural abundance or labelled compounds permits the analysis of flux through specific pathways, especially the citric acid cycle and glycogen turnover, through the acquisition of serial spectra.[84 89–91] A main advantage of NMR spectroscopy is the specificity of the technique, which allows tracing of the flux of specific metabolites into and out of metabolic pools. The isotopomeric enrichment of glutamate as an index for flux through the citric acid cycle is an example.

Positron emission tomography

The tracing of metabolic pathways with short lived, positron emitting tracers has so far been more successful in its clinical application than NMR spectroscopy, mainly because there is technology that makes it possible to assess regional differences of metabolic activity of the heart by visual inspection and quantitative analysis of radioactivity in "regions of interest".[13 96] Two types of approaches can be distinguished:

1 *Uptake and retention* of a tracer analogue such as fluorodeoxyglucose (FDG).

15

2 *Uptake and clearance* of tracers such as ^{11}C-labelled fatty acids, where the rapid phase of clearance from the tissue represents either β-oxidation and oxidation in the citric acid cycle (in the case of long chain fatty acids), or oxidation in the citric acid cycle alone (in the case of acetate).

Whereas the uptake and retention of FDG is linear with time and follows zero order kinetics, the clearance of labelled fatty acids is biexponential,[97–99] suggesting both rapid and slow turnover pools for both long and short chain fatty acids. Relative size and slope of each of the exponential components of the ^{11}C time–activity curve relate to oxidation and release from storage of the labelled compound. Both FDG and ^{11}C-labelled fatty acids have been used clinically to assess substrate metabolism in normal and ischaemic myocardium.

The argument of whether enhanced glucose uptake (assessed with FDG) or residual oxidative capacity (assessed by the early, rapid clearance phase of [^{11}C]acetate) constitutes the gold standard for reversible tissue injury in ischaemic, reperfused, or "hibernating" myocardium has not been settled. The clinical utility of a perfusion–metabolism mismatch is, however, clear: preserved metabolic activity in the absence of significant coronary flow (manifested by the retention of FDG and the absent uptake of the flow marker ^{13}NH$_3$, respectively) is strongly suggestive of myocardium that has the potential to resume normal contractile function (and hence oxidative metabolism) once blood flow and O$_2$ supply have been restored. It appears that the usefulness of imaging regional metabolic activity in heart muscle is limited, because the same functional information can be obtained with less expensive, more direct methods such as the assessment of contractile reserve.

Metabolic adaptation and deadaptation: the cellular consequences of ischaemia and reperfusion

Heart muscle regulates its energy supply by regulating coronary blood flow in accordance with the energy needs of the cell. For example, under resting conditions, coronary flow is about 1 ml/min per g wet weight in humans, and it increases in proportion to myocardial oxygen consumption; that is, when oxygen consumption doubles, coronary flow doubles, and so on. Conversely, a reduction in coronary flow results in a reduction in myocardial oxygen delivery and a consequent reduction in contractile force. In clinical practice, this relationship manifests itself as stress induced asynergy or "hibernating myocardium".

The earliest forms of ischaemia, defined as lack of oxygen supply resulting from inadequate blood flow, occur in patients who are unable to increase coronary flow in response to increased energy demands. As resting coronary flow is normal in this setting, this form of ischaemia is sometimes referred to as "normal flow" ischaemia. By contrast, when coronary flow is

16

reduced at rest, the term "low flow ischaemia" has been used. The extreme form of ischaemia is, of course, reached by the complete occlusion of a coronary artery with subsequent necrosis of the tissue supplied. Thus, there is a continuum of ischaemia, with mild, "normal flow" ischaemia at one end of the spectrum and the extreme situation of myocardial infarction at the other.

Ischaemia affects myocardial energy metabolism by slowing down aerobic metabolism of substrates, reducing the tissue content of phospho-creatine and adenine nucleotides, and first increasing and then slowing down anaerobic metabolism of substrates. Just as there is a continuum of relative restriction of oxygen delivery, one might expect a continuum of metabolic responses to ischaemia. With "normal flow" ischaemia, heart muscle is still capable of oxidising fatty acids and glucose under resting conditions. As coronary blood flow decreases, the relative contribution of glucose to the residual oxidative metabolism increases, and oxidation of glucose may account for a greater percentage of aerobic ATP production.[100] Increased uptake of a glucose analogue by ischaemic myocardium has also been found when the energy demand for the heart was increased by pacing or exercise.[6 101] There is increased lactate release from the stressed myocardium[6 102] and increased glucose uptake, especially when fatty acid levels are low.[103] Possible reasons for increased glucose uptake with stress and ischaemia are as follows:

1 Glucose makes better use of the limited amount of O_2 available to the myocyte. If blood supply is mildly reduced, the heart switches from fatty acids to glucose as the preferred fuel for respiration.
2 Glycolysis yields a small amount of ATP through substrate level phosphorylation in the cytosol, independent of the availability of O_2 (2 mol ATP/mol glucose, whereas 36 mol ATP are produced per mol glucose oxidised).
3 Glucose transport is enhanced in oxygen deprived tissue. Thus, more glucose enters the cell, and glucose is preferred over fatty acids as a substrate for energy production.

The regulation of intermediary metabolism of glucose, fatty acids, and amino acids during ischaemia is complex and requires further discussion with respect to accumulation of intermediary metabolites and reversibility of ischaemic tissue damage. When oxygen becomes rate limiting for energy production, flux through the electron transport system of the respiratory chain slows down and the ratio of the reduced form of nicotinamide adenine dinucleotide (NADH) to the oxidised form (NAD$^+$) (that is, [NADH] : [NAD$^+$]) increases. This reduced state reflects a lack of ATP production by oxidative phosphorylation, which is accompanied by a loss of contractile function.

17

The exact biochemical mechanisms responsible for the rapid loss of contractile function are not yet known with certainty. There are those who implicate the loss of ATP[104] and others who implicate the accumulation of potentially toxic intermediary products such as hydrogen ions (H$^+$)[105 106] or lactate.[107] Kübler and Katz[108] thought it unlikely that decreased ATP supplies for energy consuming reactions in the myocardial cell cause the observed decrease in myocardial contractility, because of the low K_m for ATP at the substrate binding sites of energy consuming reactions in the heart. In other words, at prevailing concentrations of ATP in the ischaemic, non-contracting tissue, enzymes such as myosin ATPase should still operate at near maximal velocity. Instead, Kübler and Katz[108] speculated that small changes in ATP may already exert modulatory effects on ion fluxes, and the large amount of inorganic phosphate may form insoluble precipitates of calcium phosphate that trap calcium in the sarcoplasmic reticulum and mitochondria. Another possible explanation for the discrepancy between ATP content and ATP conversion into useful energy for the heart is the trapping, or "compartmentation", of ATP in a compartment that is not accessible to the enzymes of the contractile apparatus or ion pumps (for example, mitochondria).

Examining the acute effects of ischaemia on phosphocreatine and ATP, Gudbjarnason et al[109] found that breakdown of phosphocreatine was more rapid than that of ATP. The kinetic heterogeneity of ATP and phospho-creatine depletion seems to indicate an inhibition of transfer of ATP from mitochondria to the cytosol, and it has been speculated that the reduction in regeneration of cytosolic ATP causes the early cessation of contractile activity in ischaemic myocardium. It is reasonable to state that the actual biochemical mechanism for contractile failure in the ischaemic and infarcted myocardium continues to remain elusive. Recent experimental work has emphasised the phenomenon of ischaemic preconditioning[110] and the role of stress proteins in myocardial protection.[111] With the exception of glutamate, glucose is the only substrate yielding ATP by anaerobic substrate level phosphorylation.[17] Glucose uptake is increased with low flow ischaemia both in vitro[112] and in vivo,[113] as a result of translocation of glucose transporters to the plasma membrane. Addition of insulin further enhances glucose uptake and glycogen.[112] Thus, the effects of ischaemia are additive.

Metabolic support of the acutely ischaemic myocardium

The use of glucose, insulin, and potassium (GIK) as inotropic metabolic support for the acutely ischaemic, reperfused myocardium is controversial and has largely been abandoned on the basis of theoretical[114] and experimental[107] argument. Likewise, the use of GIK in the setting of acute myocardial infarction, first proposed by Sodi-Pallares and his co-workers in Mexico (1962) and further developed by Rackley and his co-workers in the

USA[115-117] has not generally been accepted because of inconclusive evidence in earlier clinical trials.[118] In spite of substantial experimental evidence in support of beneficial effects of substrate manipulation especially promoting glucose metabolism in myocardial ischaemia,[119-122] the concept of metabolic support for the failing ischaemic (or postischaemic) myocardium was relegated to the antics of medical therapy.

Glycogen loading of rat hearts 90 min before hypothermic ischaemic arrest significantly improves ischaemia tolerance, as evidenced by a return of normal left ventricular function after 12 h of ischaemia (instead of 3 h in controls).[123] In contrast, glycogen depletion before ischaemia failed to improve left ventricular function of rabbit heart after hypothermic ischaemic arrest.[124] There is a correlation between glycogen content, on the one hand, and the tissue content of energy rich phosphates and recovery of function with reperfusion, on the other, although the mechanism for the protective effect of GIK is still unknown.

The effect of glycogen loading on recovery of function and associated biochemical parameters after a brief (15 min) period of normothermic ischaemia and reperfusion in rat hearts[125 126] showed that glycogen loaded hearts recovered faster than their controls, used more glucose, maintained normal energy rich phosphate levels, and lost a significantly smaller amount of marker proteins (myoglobin, lactate dehydrogenase, citrate synthase) with reperfusion. Although these studies are largely descriptive, they point to a physiological role for glycogen, which complements its role as endogenous substrate but is still elusive to a mechanistic analysis.

Although there are no prospective, controlled, clinical studies that examine the efficacy of GIK in patients with refractory left ventricular failure after cardiopulmonary bypass and hypothermic ischaemic arrest for aortocoronary bypass surgery, a small randomised clinical trial on 22 patients examined the efficacy of GIK (for the protocol see Table 1.2) for up to 48 h.[127] The results were so striking (a 50% increase in cardiac index, a 30% decrease in the requirement for inotropic drugs, and a 75% decrease in 30 day mortality) that surgeons at the Texas Heart Institute now use GIK

Table 1.2 Glucose–insulin–potassium (GIK) for metabolic support of the postischaemic failing heart

D-Glucose	500 g
Regular insulin	80 U
KCl	100 mmol
In 1000 ml H₂0, infusion rate 1 ml/kg per h; requires indwelling catheter	

Protocol: blood for glucose and K^+ before, and at 1, 6, 12, 24, and 48 h after initiation of treatment. Supplemental insulin only if blood glucose exceeds 300 mg% and/or K+ exceeds 5.3 mmol/l

Exclusion criteria: creatinine > 3 mg/dl, bilirubin > 3 mg/dl

From Gradinak et al.[127]

routinely in the management of postoperative refractory left ventricular failure of different aetiologies. In addition, protocols of preoperative glycogen loading are being developed for the ex vivo preservation of a donor heart for cardiac transplantation and for high risk patients with compromised left ventricular function (left ventricular ejection fraction $<30\%$ before surgery). To a large extent, these protocols are now employed on an empirical basis with good success, but unfortunately lack the benefit of rigorous scientific scrutiny.

An important, but little appreciated, intervention for reducing mortality in acute myocardial infarction is the concept of metabolic support with intravenous GIK. A recent meter analysis by Fath-Ordoubadi and Beatt[128] revealed that GIK reduced in-hospital mortality of myocardial infarction by 28–48%. This magnitude of reduction in mortality is comparable to that achieved with thrombolytic therapy[129] and supports the concept that metabolic protection of ischaemic myocardium is as important as reperfusion itself.[130]

Conclusions

The heart is both a consumer and a provider of energy. Energy transfer in heart muscle is highly efficient and occurs through a series of moiety conserved cycles. New methods developed over the past decade have resulted in a better understanding of the physiology of myocardial cell function, and gene therapy for the correction of cellular defects is looming on the horizon. The ultimate success of new treatment modalities is, however, still constrained by an inadequate understanding of the underlying pathophysiological events. These recent developments point to a need for the re-examination of the concept and application of metabolic treatment for the failing myocardium in defined clinical settings, such as reperfusion after an acute ischaemic event, controlled hypothermic ischaemic arrest, or acute myocardial infarction.

Acknowledgements

We thank Rachel Ralston for her help in preparing the manuscript for publication. The authors' laboratory is supported by grants from the US Public Health Service, National Institutes of Health (R01-HL 43113) and the American Heart Association, National Center.

1 Bing RJ. The metabolism of the heart. *Harvey Lect* 1955;**50**:27–70.
2 Keul J, Doll E, Steim H, Homburger H, Kern H, Reindell H. Über den Stoffwechsel des menschlichen Herzens I. *Pflügers Arch Ges Physiol* 1965;**282**:1–27.

3 Gorlin R, Brachfeld N, Messer JV, Turner JD. Physiologic and biochemical aspects of disordered coronary circulation. *Ann Intern Med* 1959;**51**:698–706.

4 Krasnow N, Neill WA, Messer JV, Gorlin R. Myocardial lactate and pyruvate metabolism. *J Clin Invest* 1962;**41**:2075–85.

5 Mudge GH, Mills RM, Taegtmeyer H, Gorlin R, Lesch M. Alterations of myocardial amino acid metabolism in chronic ischaemic heart disease. *J Clin Invest* 1976;**58**:1185–92.

6 Gertz EW, Wisneski JA, Neese RA, Bristow JD, Searle GL, Hanlon JT. Myocardial lactate metabolism:Evidence of lactate release during net chemical extraction in man. *Circulation* 1981;**63**:1273–9.

7 Milano CA, Allen LF, Rockman HA, et al. Enhanced myocardial function in transgenic mice overexpressing the β_2-adrenergic receptor. *Science* 1994;**264**:582–6.

8 Kirshenbaum LS, MacLellan WR, Mazur W, French BA, Schneider MD. Highly efficient gene transfer into adult ventricular myocytes by recombinant adenovirus. *J Clin Invest* 1993;**92**:381–7.

9 Soonpaa MH, Koh GY, Klug MG, Field LJ. Formation of nascent intercalated disks between grafted fetal cardiomyocytes and host myocardium. *Science* 1994;**264**:98–101.

10 Taylor DA, Atkins BZ, Hungspreugs P, et al. Regenerating functional myocardium: improved performance after skeletal myoblast transplantation. *Nature Med* 1998;**4**:929–33.

11 Schelbert HR, Schwaiger M. Positron emission tomography studies of the heart. In: Phelps M, Mazziota J, Schelbert H, eds, *Positron emission tomography and autoradiography: principles and applications for the brain and the heart*. New York: Raven Press, 1986:581–661.

12 Bergmann SR. Clinical applications of assessments of myocardial substrate utilization with positron emission tomography. *Mol Cell Biochem* 1989;**88**:201–8.

13 Schwaiger M, Hicks R. The clinical role of metabolic imaging of the heart by positron emission tomography. *J Nucl Med* 1991;**32**:565–78.

14 Conway MA, Allis J, Duwerkerk R, Niioua T, Rajagopalan B, Radda GK. Low phosphocreatine/ATP ratio detected in vivo in the failing hypertrophied human myocardium using ^{31}P magnetic resonance spectroscopy. *Lancet* 1991;**338**:973–6.

15 Kloner RA, Przyklenk K. Understanding the jargon: a glossary of terms used (and misused) in the study of ischaemia and reperfusion. *Cardiovasc Res* 1993;**27**:162–6.

16 Depre C, Shipley GL, Chen W, et al. Unloaded heart in vivo replicates fetal gene expression of cardiac hypertrophy. *Nature Med* 1998;**4**:1269–75.

17 Taegtmeyer H. Energy metabolism of the heart: From basic concepts to clinical applications. *Curr Prob Cardiol* 1994;**19**:57–116.

18 Lipmann F. Metabolic generation and utilization of phosphate bond energy. *Adv Enzymol* 1941;**1**:99–165.

19 Taegtmeyer H. Cardiac preconditioning does not require myocardial stunning. *Ann Thorac Surg* 1993;**55**:400.

20 Taegtmeyer H, Russell RR, Silvestain AL, Shafer D. Depressed function and energy metabolism of hearts from spontaneously diabetic BB/W rats. *J Mol Cell Cardiol* 1985;**17**:44.

21 Balaban RS, Kontor HL, Katz LA, Briggs RW. Relation between work and phosphate metabolite in the in vivo paced mammalian heart. *Science* 1986;**232**:1121–3.

22 Kupriyanov VV, Lakomkin VL, Kapelko VI, Steinschneider AY, Ruuge EK, Saks VA. Dissociation of adenosine triphosphate levels and contractile function in isovolumic hearts perfused with 2-deoxyglucose. *J Mol Cell Cardiol* 1987;**19**:729–40.

23 Barth E, Stämmler G, Speiser B, Schaper J. Ultrastructural quantitation of mitochondria and myofilaments in cardiac muscle from 10 different animal species including man. *J Mol Cell Cardiol* 1992;**24**:669–81.

24 McNutt NS, Fawcett DW. Myocardial ultrastructure. In: Langer G, Brady A, eds, *The mammalian myocardium*, New York: John Wiley & Sons, 1974:1–49.

25 Baldwin JE, Krebs HA. The evolution of metabolic cycles. *Nature* 1981;**291**:381–2.

26 Brown GC. Control of respiration and ATP synthesis in mammalian mitochondria and cells. *Biochem J* 1992;**284**:1–13.

27 Newsholme EA, Start C. Regulation in Metabolism. London: John Wiley & Sons, 1973: 349 PP.
28 Newsholme EA, Leech AR. *Biochemistry for the medical sciences* Chichester: John Wiley, 1983:952 PP.
29 Coulson RA, Hernandez T, Herbert JD. Metabolic rate, enzyme kinetics in vivo. *Comp Biochem Physiol* 1977;**56A**:251–62.
30 Barry WH, Bridge JHB. Intracellular calcium homeostasis in cardiac myocytes. *Circulation* 1993;**87**:1806–15.
31 Fabiato A. Calcium induced release of calcium from the cardiac sarcoplasmic reticulum. *Am J Physiol* 1983;**245**:C1-14.
32 McCormack JG, Halestrap AP, Denton RM. Role of calcium ions in reperfusion of mammalian intramitochondrial metabolism. *Physiol Rev* 1990;**70**:391–425.
33 Lehninger AL, Reynafarie B, Vercesi A. Transport and accumulation of calcium in mitochondria. *Ann NY Acad Sci* 1978;**307**:160–76.
34 Denton RM, McCormack JG. On the role of the calcium transport cycle in the heart and other mammalian mitochondria. *FEBS Lett* 1980;**119**:1–8.
35 Rayment I, Holden HM, Whittacker M, et al. Structure of actin–myosin complex and its implications for muscle contraction. *Science* 1993;**261**:58–65.
36 Kornberg HL. Anaplerotic sequences and their role in metabolism. *Essays Biochem* 1966;**2**:1–31.
37 Taegtmeyer H, Hems R, Krebs HA. Utilization of energy providing substrates in the isolated working rat heart. *Biochem J* 1980;**186**:701–11.
38 Taegtmeyer H. On the inability of ketone bodies to serve as the only energy providing substrate for rat heart at physiological work load. *Basic Res Cardiol* 1983;**78**:435-50.
39 Russell RR, Taegtmeyer H. Coenzyme A sequestration in rat hearts oxidizing ketone bodies. *J Clin Invest* 1992;**89**:968–73.
40 Russell RR, Taegtmeyer H. Changes in citric acid cycle flux and anaplerosis antedate the functional decline in isolated rat hearts utilizing acetoacetate. *J Clin Invest* 1991;**87**:384–90.
41 Russell RR, Taegtmeyer H. Pyruvate carboxylation prevents the decline in contractile function of rat hearts oxidizing acetoacetate. *Am J Physiol* 1991;**261**:H1756-62.
42 Taegtmeyer H. Metabolic responses to cardiac hypoxia:Increased production of succinate by rabbit papillary muscles. *Circ Res* 1978;**43**:808–15.
43 Schwaiger M, Schelbert H, Ellison D, et al. Sustained regional abnormalities in cardiac metabolism after transient ischemia in the chronic dog model. *J Am Coll Cardiol* 1985;**6**:337–47.
44 Schwaiger M, Neese RA, Araujo L, et al. Sustained nonoxidative glucose utilization and depletion of glycogen in reperfused canine myocardium. *J Am Coll Cardiol* 1989;**13**:745–54.
45 Czernin J, Porenta G, Brunken R, et al. Regional blood flow, oxidative metabolism, and glucose utilization in patients with recent myocardial infarction. *Circulation* 1993;**88**:884–95.
46 Racker E. Energy cycles in health and disease. *Curr Top Cell Regul* 1981;**18**:361–75.
47 Steenbergen C, Murphy E, Levy L, London RE. Elevation in cytosolic free calcium concentration early in myocardial ischemia in perfused rat heart. *Circ Res* 1987;**60**:700–7.
48 Tani M, Neely JR. Role of intracellular Na^+ in Ca^{2+} overload and depressed recovery of ventricular function of reperfused ischemic rat hearts. Possible involvement of H^+-Na^+ and Na^+-Ca^{2+}. *Circ Res* 1989;**65**:1045–56.
49 Marban E, Kitakaze M, Koretsune Y, Yue DT, Chacko VP, Pike MM. Quantification of $[Ca^{2+}]_i$ in perfused hearts. Critical evaluation of the 5F-BAPTA and nuclear magnetic response method as applied to the study of ischemia and reperfusion. *Circ Res* 1990;**66**:1255–67.
50 Rao PS, Cohen MV, Mueller HS. Production of free radicals and lipid peroxides in early experimental myocardial ischemia. *J Mol Cell Cardiol* 1983;**15**:713–16.
51 Kloner RA, Przyklenk K, Whittacker P. Deleterious effects of oxygen radicals in ischemia/reperfusion. Resolved and unresolved issues. *Circulation* 1989;**80**:1115–27.

52 Ferrari R, Alfieri O, Curello S, et al. Occurrence of oxidative stress during reperfusion in human heart. *Circulation* 1990;**81**:201–11.

53 Bolli R. Mechanism of myocardial "stunning". *Circulation* 1990;**82**:723–38.

54 Klein HH, Puschmann S, Schaper J, Schaper W. The mechanism of the tetrazolium reaction in identifying experimental infarction. *Virchow's Arch (A)* 1983;**393**:287–97.

55 Dennis SC, Gevers W, Opie LH. Protons in ischemia:Where do they come from, where do they go to? *J Mol Cell Cardiol* 1991;**23**:1077–86.

56 Jennings RB, Reimer KA, Steenbergen C. Myocardial ischemia revisited. The osmolar load, membrane damage, and reperfusion. *J Mol Cell Cardiol* 1986;**18**:769–80.

57 Lehninger AL. *Biochemistry*, 1st edn. New York: Worth Publishers, 1970:1013 PP.

58 Winterstein H. Ueber die Sauerstoffatmung des isolierten Säugetierherzens. *Z Allg Physiol* 1904;**4**:333–59.

59 Rohde E. Über den Einfluss der mechanischen Bedingungen auf die Tätigkeit und den Sauerstoffverbrauch des Warmblüterherzens. *Naunyn-Schmiedeberg's Arch Ges Exp Path Pharmakol* 1912;**68**:401–10.

60 Evans CL. The effect of glucose on the gaseous metabolism of the isolated mammalian heart. *J Physiol (Lond)* 1914;**47**:407–18.

61 Neely JR, Liebermeister H, Battersby EJ, Morgan HE. Effect of pressure development on oxygen consumption by isolated rat heart. *Am J Physiol* 1967;**212**:804–14.

62 Nguyên VTB, Mossberg KA, Tewson TJ, et al. Temporal analysis of myocardial glucose metabolism by ^{18}F–2-deoxy–2-fluoro-D-glucose. *Am J Physiol* 1990;**259**:H1022-31.

63 Cooney GJ, Taegtmeyer H, Newsholme EA. Tricarboxylic acid cycle flux and enzyme activities in the isolated working rat heart. *Biochem J* 1981;**200**:701–3.

64 Balaban RS. Regulation of oxidative phosphorylation in the mammalian cell. *Am J Physiol* 1990;**258**:C377-89.

65 Jones BP, Shan X, Park Y. Coordinated multisite regulation of cellular energy metabolism. *Annu Rev Nutr* 1992;**12**:327–43.

66 Evans, G. The glycogen content of the rat heart. *J Physiol (Lond)* 1934;**82**:468–80.

67 Denton RM, Randle PJ. Concentrations of glycerides and phospholipids in rat heart and gastrocnemius muscles. *Biochem J* 1967;**104**:416–22.

68 Gevers W. Protein metabolism of the heart. *J Mol Cell Cardiol* 1984;**16**:3–32.

69 Lesch M, Taegtmeyer H, Peterson MB, Vernick R. Studies on the mechanism of the inhibition of myocardial protein synthesis during oxygen deprivation. *Am J Physiol* 1976;**230**:120–6.

70 Taegtmeyer H, Lesch M. *Altered protein and amino acid metabolism in myocardial hypoxia and ischemia.* Amsterdam: Elsevier/North Holland, 1980:347–60.

71 Morgan HE, Rannels DE, McKee EE. Protein metabolism of the heart. In: Berne, R, ed, *Handbook of physiology: the cardiovascular system: the heart.* Washington, DC: American Physiology Society, 1979:845–71.

72 Magid NM, Borer JS, Young MS, Wallerson DC, Demonteiro C. Suppression of protein degradation in progressive cardiac hypertrophy of chronic aortic regurgitation. *Circulation* 1993;**87**:1249–57.

73 Samarel AM. Hemodynamic overloaded the regulation of myofibrillar protein degradation. *Circulation* 1993;**87**:1418–20.

74 Taegtmeyer H, Doenst T, Mommessin JI, Guthrie PH, Williams CM. Further evidence for the importance of anaplerosis in the isolated working rat heart: A tracer kinetic study with [^{18}F] fluoro–2-deoxyglucose (FDG). *Circulation* 1993;**88**:I–284 (Abstract).

75 Rothlin ME, Bing RJ. Extraction and release of individual free fatty acids by the heart and fat deposits. *J Clin Invest* 1961;**40**:1380–5.

76 Keul J, Doll E, Keppler D. *Energy metabolism of human muscle.* Basel: S Karger, 1972:313 PP.

77 Drake AJ, Haines JR, Noble MM. Preferential uptake of lactate by the normal myocardium in dogs. *Cardiovasc Res* 1980;**14**:65–72.

78 Krebs HA, Williamson DH, Bates MW, Page MA, Hawkins RA. The role of ketone bodies in caloric homeostasis. In: Weber, G, ed, *Advances in enzyme regulations*, vol. 9. New York: Pergamon Press, 1971:387–409.

79 Goodwin GW, Ahmad F, Doenst T, Taegtmeyer H. Energy provision from glycogen, glucose and fatty acids upon adrenergic stimulation of isolated working rat heart. *Am J Physiol* 1998;**274**:H1239-47.

80 Goodwin GW, Taylor CS, Taegtmeyer H. Regulation of energy metabolism of the heart during acute increase in heart work. *J Biol Chem* 1998;**273**:29530-9.

81 Opie LH. Cardiac metabolism–emergence, decline, and resurgence. Part I. *Cardiovasc Res* 1992;**26**:721-33.

82 Opie LH. Cardiac metabolism – emergence, decline, and resurgence. Part II. *Cardiovasc Res* 1992;**26**:817-30.

83 Gadian DG, Hoult DI, Radda GK, Seeley PJ, Chance B, Barlow C. Phosphorous nuclear magnetic resonance studies in normoxic and ischemic cardiac tissue. *Proc Natl Acad Sci USA* 1976;**73**:291-332.

84 Weiss ES, Hoffman EJ, Phelps ME, et al. External detection and visualization of myocardial ischemia with ^{11}C substrates in vitro and in vivo. *Circ Res* 1976;**39**:24-32.

85 Jacobus WE, Taylor G, Hollis DP, Nunnally RL. Phosphorous nuclear magnetic resonance of perfused working rat hearts. *Nature* 1977;**265**:756-8.

86 Ingwall JS. Phosphorous nuclear magnetic resonance spectroscopy of cardiac and skeletal muscles. *Am J Physiol* 1982;**242**:H729-44.

87 Bottomley PA. Noninvasive study of high energy phosphate metabolism in human heart by depth-resolved ^{31}P NMR spectroscopy. *Science* 1985;**229**:769-72.

88 Schelbert HR. Assessment of myocardial metabolism by PET: A sophisticated dream or clinical reality? *Eur J Nucl Med* 1986;**12**:570-5.

89 McMillin-Wood JB. Biochemical approaches in metabolism: application to positron emission tomography. *Circulation* 1985;**72**:IV145-50.

90 Taegtmeyer H, Mossberg KA, Nguyen VTB. Positron labelled tracers: A window for the assessment of energy metabolism in heart and skeletal muscle. *Acta Radiol* 1991;**376**:40-44.

91 Lewandowski ED. Nuclear magnetic resonance evaluation of metabolic and respiratory support of work load in intact rabbit hearts. *Circ Res* 1992;**70**:576-82.

92 Tillisch J, Brunken R, Marshall R, et al. Prediction of reversibility of cardiac wall motion abnormalities predicted by positron tomography, [18]fluoro-deoxyglucose, and [13]NH₃. *N Engl J Med* 1986;**314**:884-8.

93 Gould KL, Yoshida K, Haynie M, Hess MJ, Mullani NA, Smalling RW. Myocardial metabolism of fluoro-deoxyglucose compared to cell membrane integrity for the potassium analogue R6–82 for assessing viability and infarct size in man by PET. *J Nucl Med* 1991;**32**:1-9.

94 Yoshida K, Gould KL. Quantitative relation of myocardial infarct size and myocardial viability by positron emission tomography of left ventricular ejection fraction and 3-year mortality with and without revascularization. *J Am Coll Cardiol* 1993;**22**:984-97.

95 Radda GU. Control, bioenergetics, and adaptation in health and disease: noninvasive biochemistry from nuclear magnetic resonance. *FASEB J* 1992;**6**:3032-8.

96 Bergman RN. Toward physiological understanding of glucose tolerance. *Diabetes* 1989;**38**:1512-27.

97 Schelbert H, Henze E, Sochor H. Effects of substrate availability on myocardial ^{11}C palmitate kinetics by positron emission tomography in normal subjects and patients with ventricular dysfunction. *Am Heart J* 1986;**111**:1055-65.

98 Brown MA, Marshall DR, Sobel BE, Bergmann SR. Delineation of myocardial oxygen utilization with carbon–11 labelled acetate. *Circulation* 1987;**76**:687-96.

99 Buxton DB, Schwaiger M, Nguyen NA, Phelps ME, Schelbert HR. Radiolabelled acetate as a tracer of myocardial tricarboxylic acid cycle flux. *Circ Res* 1988;**63**:628-34.

100 Opie LH, Owen P, Thomas M, Samson R. Coronary sinus lactate measurements in assessment of myocardial ischemia: Comparison with changes in lactate/pyruvate and ß-hydroxybutyrate/acetoacetate ratios and with release of hydrogen, phosphate, and potassium from the heart. *Am J Cardiol* 1973;**32**:295-305.

101 Schelbert HR. The Heart. In: Ell P, Homan B, eds, *Computed emission tomography.* Oxford: Oxford University Press, 1982:91-133.

102 Gertz EW, Wisneski JA, Neese R. Myocardial lactate extraction: Multidetermined metabolic function. *Circulation* 1980;**61**:256-61.

103 Wisneski JA, Gertz EW, Neese RA, Gruenke LD, Morris DL, Craig JC. Metabolic fate of extracted glucose in normal human myocardium. *J Clin Invest* 1985;**76**:1819–27.

104 Hearse DJ. Myocardial enzyme leakage. *J Mol Med* 1977;**2**:185–200.

105 Katz AM, Hecht HH. The early "pump" failure of the ischemic heart. *Am J Med* 1969;**47**:497–502.

106 Williamson JR, Shaffer SW, Ford C, Safer B. Contribution of tissue acidosis to ischemic injury in the perfused rat heart. *Circulation* 1976;**53**:3–14.

107 Neely JR, Grotyohann LW. Role of glycolytic products in damage to myocardium: Dissociation of adenosine triphosphate levels and recovery of function of reperfused canine myocardium. *Circ Res* 1984;**55**:816–24.

108 Kübler W, Katz AM. Mechanism of early "pump" failure of the ischemic heart: Possible role of adenosine triphosphate depletion and inorganic phosphate accumulation. *Am J Cardiol* 1977;**40**:467–71.

109 Gudbjarnason S, Mathes P, Ravens KG. Functional compartmentation of ATP and creatine phosphate in heart muscle. *J Mol Cell Cardiol* 1970;**1**:325–39.

110 Murry CE, Jennings RB, Reimer KA. Preconditioning with ischemia: a delay of lethal cell injury in ischemic myocardium. *Circulation* 1986;**74**:1124–36.

111 Marber MS. Stress proteins and myocardial protection. *Clin Sci* 1994;**86**:375–81.

112 Chen TM, Goodwin GW, Guthrie PH, Taegtmeyer H. Effects of insulin on glucose uptake by rat hearts during and after coronary flow reduction. *Am J Physiol* 1997;**273**:H2170-7.

113 Young LH, Renfu Y, Russell R, et al. Low-flow ischemia leads to translocation of canine heart GLUT–4 and GLUT–1 glucose transporters to the sarcolemma in vivo. *Circulation* 1997;**95**:415–22.

114 Neely JR, Morgan HE. Relationship between carbohydrate and lipid metabolism and the energy balance of heart muscle. *Annu Rev Physiol* 1974;**36**:413–39.

115 Rogers WJ, Stanley AW, Breing JB, et al. Reduction of hospital mortality rate of acute myocardial infarction with glucose-insulin-potassium infusion. *Am Heart J* 1976;**92**:441–54.

116 Rackley CE, Russell RO, Rogers WJ, Papapierto SE. Clinical experience with glucose-insulin-potassium therapy in acute myocardial infarction. *Am Heart J* 1981;**102**:1038–49.

117 Whitlow PL, Rogers WJ, Smith LR, et al. Enhancement of left ventricular function by glucose-insulin-potassium infusion in acute myocardial infarction. *Am J Cardiol* 1982;**49**:811–20.

118 Medical Research Council Working Party. Potassium, glucose, and insulin treatment for acute myocardial infarction. *Lancet* 1968;**ii**:1355–60.

119 Opie LH. The glucose hypothesis:Relation to acute myocardial ischemia. *J Mol Cell Cardiol* 1970;**1**:107–15.

120 Hearse DJ, Chain EB. The role of glucose in the survival and "recovery" of the anoxic isolated perfused rat heart. *Biochem J* 1972;**128**:1125–33.

121 Opie LH, Bruyneel K, Owen P. Effects of glucose, insulin, potassium infusion and tissue metabolic changes within first hour of myocardial infarction in the baboon. *Circulation* 1975;**52**:49–57.

122 Apstein CS, Gravino FN, Haudenschild CC. Determinants of a protective effect of glucose and insulin on the ischemic myocardium. Effects on contractile function, diastolic compliance, metabolism, and ultrastructure during ischemia and reperfusion. *Circ Res* 1983;**52**:515–26.

123 McElroy DD, Walker WE, Taegtmeyer H. Glycogen loading improves left ventricular function of the rabbit heart after hypothermic ischemic arrest. *J Appl Cardiol* 1989;**4**:455–65.

124 Lagerstrom CF, Walker WE, Taegtmeyer H. Failure of glycogen depletion to improve left ventricular function of the rabbit heart after hypothermic ischemic arrest. *Circ Res* 1988;**63**:81–6.

125 Schneider CA, Nguyêñ VTB, Taegtmeyer H. Feeding and fasting determine postischemic glucose utilization in isolated working rat hearts. *Am J Physiol* 1991;**260**:H542-8.

126 Schneider CA, Taegtmeyer H. Fasting in vivo delays myocardial cell damage after brief periods of ischemia in the isolated working rat heart. *Circ Res* 1991;**68**:1045–50.

127 Gradinak S, Coleman GM, Taegtmeyer H, Sweeney MS, Frazier OH. Improved cardiac function with glucose-insulin-potassium after coronary bypass surgery. *Ann Thorac Surg* 1989;**48**:484–9.
128 Fath-Ordoubadi F, Beatt KJ. Glucose-insulin-potassium therapy for treatment of acute myocardial infarction. An overview of randomized placebo-controlled trials. *Circulation* 1997;**96**:1152–6.
129 Apstein CS, Taegtmeyer H. Glucose-insulin-potassium in acute myocardial infarction. The time has come for a large prospective trial. *Circulation* 1997;**96**:1074–7.
130 Taegtmeyer H. Metabolic support for the postischaemic heart. *Lancet* 1995;**345**:1552–5.

2: Ventricular performance

KARL SKARVAN

Preservation of optimal cardiovascular function represents one of the foremost goals of anaesthetic management during the perioperative period. Only rarely does the heart work under such challenging and rapidly varying conditions as during this time. Acute changes in ventricular loading, gas exchange, intrathoracic pressure, autonomic nervous tone, and blood properties, as well as the effects of anaesthetic and other drugs, and various released mediators, all put a formidable stress on the heart. This may give rise to perioperative cardiac morbidity even in patients with normal hearts, although patients with limited cardiac reserve are, of course, at much higher risk and require a great deal of the anaesthetist's attention. Hence, a proper understanding of ventricular function is a prerequisite to correct evaluation and optimisation of cardiac function in the perioperative period. With regard to the predominant role of the left ventricle in haemodynamic function, this chapter focuses on the normal performance of the left ventricle and its determinants.

Ventricle as a muscle

The fundamental properties of the myocardium have been thoroughly studied in isolated animal and human heart muscle preparations. The resting length of the unstressed muscle strip represents the starting point for the following considerations (Fig 2.1). The resting length can be increased by attaching a small weight to one end of the muscle strip. This weight will stretch the muscle to a longer resting length in proportion to the attached weight, as well as in proportion to the elastic properties of the muscle. This distending force or weight (expressed in grams) is called the preload of the muscle. The preload, which is related to the resting length of the sarcomeres of the myocardium, has an important impact on the next contraction of the muscle.[1] When the muscle is prevented from shortening (isometric contraction), the active force developed during contraction is directly proportional to its preload. When the muscle is allowed to shorten (isotonic contraction), both the extent and velocity of shortening will increase in proportion to the preload. This dependence of contraction

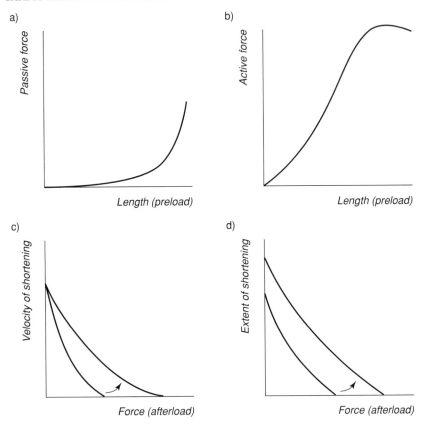

Fig 2.1 Force–length–velocity relationships of an isolated strip of myocardium. (a) Passive force builds up with increasing resting length; (b) active developed force increases with increasing resting length; (c) shortening velocity decreases with increasing load; (d) extent of shortening decreases with increasing load. Arrows indicate alterations caused by an increase in myocardial contractility.

characteristics on resting muscle length (preload) is a fundamental property of the myocardium and is known as the force–length relationship.[1][2] The ability of the myocardium to develop progressively more force with increasing sarcomere length has also been termed "length dependent activation" and appears to be related to an increase in the number of active actin–myosin cross bridges, increased sensitivity to intracellular calcium, and increased calcium release from sarcoplasmic reticulum.[3]

A second weight can be attached to the moving end of the isotonically contracting muscle strip. This additional weight is engaged only during contraction when it is lifted by the shortening muscle, and hence ensures a constant tension in the muscle during its shortening. This second weight

28

represents the afterload of the muscle. Similar to preload, afterload also has an important influence on muscle contraction. Both the extent of muscle shortening and that of shortening velocity are inversely related to afterload. Thus, an increase in afterload decreases, whereas a reduction in afterload increases, the extent and velocity of shortening.[1] The dependence of contractile performance on the shortening load is the second fundamental property of the myocardium.[4-6] The reduced shortening resulting from increased afterload can be reversed up to a given limit by an appropriate augmentation of the preload.[7]

When the preload and afterload are held constant, the developed tension (in isometric contraction) or extent and velocity of shortening (in isotonic contraction) can be increased by increasing the inotropic state of the muscle, for example, by adding calcium and consequently increasing myocardial contractility.[1] Thus, the contractile behaviour of the isolated heart muscle can be exhaustively described within the framework of a force–length relationship. It is determined by the interplay of preload, afterload, and contractility. This physiological concept is also most useful for the understanding of the function of the intact ventricle. Its too simplistic application to the human cardiovascular system may, however, be misleading.

Isolated ventricle

The principles determining contractile behaviour of an isolated strip of myocardium can also be applied to the intact isolated and perfused ventricle. The ventricle can contract either isometrically against an infinite outflow resistance (aortic clamp) or isotonically against a variable resistance. The first situation is called isovolumic contraction. The resting muscle fibre length can be increased or decreased by changing the diastolic filling, and consequently the volume of blood present in the ventricle at the end of diastole. In isovolumic preparations, the volume of a balloon positioned in the ventricular cavity can easily be changed. The passive distension of the ventricle induced by the increased filling volume leads to a progressive increase in passive tension in the ventricular wall opposing distension. Depending on the elastic properties of the myocardium and the ventricular chamber the pressure within the cavity will increase with the increasing volume. The relationship between resting pressure (P) and volume (V) is known as a diastolic P/V relationship, and describes the elasticity of the relaxed ventricle. During contraction, force is generated in the ventricular wall and transferred to the blood contained in the cavity, causing intraventricular pressure to rise (Fig 2.2). If the ventricle were severed in two equal parts along an imaginary plane, the intracavitary pressure would immediately tear both halves apart. Consequently, a force

29

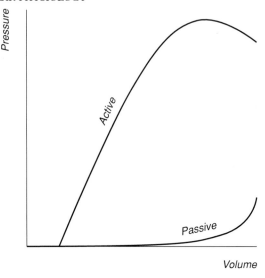

Fig 2.2 Passive (diastolic) and active (systolic) pressure–volume relationships of the ventricle. Curves illustrate filling and contractile behaviour of the ventricle for a given inotropic state.

of equal dimension but opposite direction must be operational in the virtual dividing plane of the ventricle that holds both parts together. On the basis of this assumption, mathematical models were developed that allow net wall forces to be calculated.[45] Depending on the orientation of the imaginary plane, circumferential, meridional, and radial forces can be estimated. When compared with the strip of myocardium in the isolated ventricle, the resting volume corresponds to the resting fibre length, and the developed pressure (or calculated wall force) corresponds to the directly measured force of the isolated muscle.

During isovolumic contraction, the developed ventricular pressure and wall force are directly proportional to the filling volume of the ventricle.[148] At a given volume, the maximal developed pressure will increase with positive inotropic stimulation. The ventricle, which is allowed to eject, also contracts under isovolumic conditions until the aortic (or pulmonic) valve opens. During this isovolumic contraction, the pressure increases while the ventricular volume remains unchanged, although the fibre length may change because the ventricle changes its geometry and assumes a more spherical shape. After the opening of the semilunar valve, myocardial fibres begin to shorten and volume (stroke volume) is expelled from the ventricle into the aorta or pulmonary artery. The fibre shortening (and ejection) is terminated when the maximal wall force that can be sustained by the myocardial fibres at the given level of contractility has been generated. This force is defined by the systolic or active P/V relationship of the isovolumically contracting ventricle and is independent of preload. Thus, the ventricle operates within the boundaries determined by the passive diastolic and active systolic P/V relationship.[9][10] Similar to an isolated muscle and isovolumic preparation, the contractile behaviour of the ejecting ventricle is also controlled by resting fibre length (preload), instantaneous wall force (afterload), and contractile state.[1][5] The wall force during ejection is a function of ventricular size and geometry, and of developed pressure. As ventricular size decreases in the course of ejection, the instantaneous wall force and hence the ventricular afterload decrease. Thus, a normally contracting ventricle unloads itself towards the end of ejection.[4]

Ventricle in situ

In clinical terms, the functions of the left and right ventricle are also described in terms of pressure and volume. Both variables are used for the construction of the pressure–volume diagram, which is an analogue of the force–length diagram of the strip of myocardium. In the P/V diagram, the volume plotted on the x axis is related to the myocardial fibre length, and the pressure plotted on the y axis corresponds to the generated force.[9] During one cardiac cycle of the ejecting heart, a P/V loop is inscribed (Fig 2.3). The cycle starts at end diastole, characterised by end diastolic volume and the corresponding end diastolic pressure (Fig 2.3, point 1). During isovolumic contraction, pressure increases whereas volume remains constant until the aortic valve opens (Fig 2.3, point 2) and ejection begins. Ejection continues until the end systolic P/V relationship line is reached (Fig 2.3, point 3). Ventricular relaxation causes the pressure to fall and the aortic valve to close. The intraventricular pressure falls further without changes in volume during the following isovolumic relaxation period. When the ventricular pressure falls below the atrial pressure, the mitral valve opens (Fig 2.3, point 4) and ventricular filling starts.[9-11] In the context of the P/V diagram, the effects of the three major determinants of the ventricular function (preload, afterload, and contractile state) can be illustrated.

Preload
An increase in end diastolic volume shifts the starting point 4 of the loop to the right along the passive P/V relationship, whereas the end systolic point remains unchanged. This results in an increase in ejected volume (stroke volume). A decrease in end diastolic volume shifts the loop leftwards and, because the end systolic P/V relationship line remains constant, this results in a decrease in stroke volume. This dependence of the

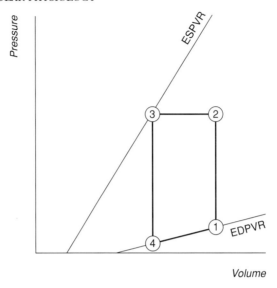

Fig 2.3 Left ventricular pressure–volume relationship. Points 1 to 4 demarcate the pressure–volume loop that is explained in the text. ESPVR (end systolic pressure–volume relationship) and EDPVR (end diastolic pressure–volume relationship) are curvilinear, but on this diagram, for simplification, they are approximated by straight lines.

ventricular performance on preload is an expression of the Frank–Starling law of the heart (see page 53).

Afterload

An increase in ejected stroke volume can also be achieved by a reduction of the afterload. A reduction in the force opposing ejection and, consequently, in the force developed by the contractile fibres (wall force) will result in a downward shift of the end systolic point of the loop along the active and systolic *P*/*V* relationship, and in an increase in stroke volume.[12] This phenomenon is the basis of the afterload reduction, a therapeutic principle applied to a failing ventricle. In contrast, an increase in afterload causes an upward shift of the end systolic point. As a consequence, the ventricle will not be able to empty completely and the stroke volume will decrease. A normal left ventricle responds to an acute increase in afterload by an immediate increase in end diastolic volume, which allows restoration of the stroke volume. The so called homoeometric regulation or Anrep effect will subsequently restore the end diastolic volume, in spite of the persisting higher afterload, by adjusting the intrinsic myocardial contractility.[13] More recent studies have shown that, during acute elevations in afterload, the end systolic *P*/*V* relationship does not remain constant but shifts to the left, a change compatible with enhanced inotropic state.[14] A failing ventricle is deprived of these compensatory mechanisms and, consequently, becomes exquisitely sensitive to any increase in afterload.

Contractility

The third major determinant of ventricular function is the contractile state of the myocardium. A change in myocardial contractility will breech the confines of the diastolic and end systolic P/V relationship. With an increase in contractility, the end systolic points of the P/V loop will shift upwards and to the left of the original active end systolic P/V relationship; consequently, stroke volume will increase despite unchanged preload and afterload. The new end systolic P/V relationship, which now determines the extent of ejection, is shifted to the left and its slope is steeper. Thus, the increase in contractility by positive inotropic stimulation causes the ventricle to empty more completely to a smaller end systolic volume.[9–11] With limited ventricular filling (for example, during hypovolaemia and reduced venous return), the end diastolic point of the P/V loop will also shift to the left, neutralising the increase in stroke volume. Under such circumstances, the positive inotropic stimulation will become evident by an increase in pressure rather than by an increase in stroke volume. Some positive inotropic agents may also exert vasodilating and afterload reducing effects, which further enhance the ventricular performance provided that a decrease in preload can be prevented. In addition, inhibitors of the enzyme phosphodiesterase exhibit a positive lusitropic effect. This effect, by virtue of improving ventricular relaxation, shifts the diastolic P/V relationship downwards, which facilitates ventricular filling and further enhances ventricular ejection.

Thus, P/V diagrams help the anaesthetist to have a better understanding of the changes in ventricular function under rapidly changing conditions of ventricular loading and contractility, and to predict the effects of his or her therapeutic interventions.

The heart as a pump

Functioning as a pump, the ventricle generates pressure and displaces volume. The fundamental mechanical properties of the ventricular pump are elasticity, resistance, and inertance.[4 12] Elasticity reflects the rate independent relationship between pressure and volume in the ventricle and determines the volume displaced from the ventricle during systole (stroke volume). Ventricular resistance is related to viscous properties of the ventricular pump that is operational during ejection, and is rate dependent because it changes with flow velocity. Finally, inertance describes the force required to accelerate the mass of the ventricle and the blood contained

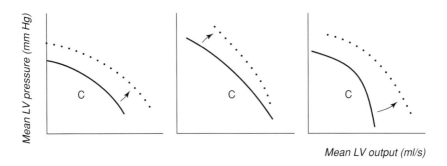

Fig 2.4 Pump function curve of the left ventricle. Ventricular pump output decreases with increasing developed pressure and eventually ceases when the pressure necessary to generate flow exceeds the capacity of the ventricular pump. Arrows indicate the effects of increased ventricular filling (left), contractility (middle), and heart rate (right).[14]

within its cavity at end diastole. These three properties of the ventricular pump determine the amount of pressure generated. In an isovolumically contracting ventricle, the maximum pressure is determined solely by the elasticity. In contrast, the ejecting ventricle develops less pressure because part of its contractile energy is used to overcome the resistive and inertial forces.[4]

The pump function of the ventricle can be described by means of a pump function graph plotting pressure against flow (Fig 2.4). The graph shows an inverse curvilinear parabolic relationship between mean left ventricular pressure and flow. Increased ventricular filling (preload) shifts the curve upwards and to the right; an increase in heart rate has the same effect. An increase in contractility causes the curve to rotate clockwise around the flow axis intercept.[15] Power output of the ventricular pump can be calculated as the product of mean ventricular pressure and flow. Knowing the myocardial oxygen consumption, which represents the power input, the efficiency of the ventricular pump can be calculated. On the basis of this pump model applied to a cat heart in situ, an efficiency of 20% was estimated.[16] It was also shown that the left ventricle tends to work at maximal power output, while minimising its volume. As maximal power is highly preload dependent, it must be normalised for end diastolic volume before it can be used as an index of myocardial contractility.[17]

Clinical evaluation of global ventricular pump function

In the perioperative period, the blood pressure resulting from the interaction between the left ventricle and the systemic vasculature often represents the only monitored index of ventricular performance. Nevertheless, when normal values of blood pressure are accompanied by normal heart rate and clinical signs of an adequate peripheral circulation (pulse quality, capillary refill time, skin temperature, urine output, pH), it can be assumed that ventricular performance is satisfactory. If more information on the cardiovascular function is required, intracardiac pressures and flows[18] as well as blood gases must be measured (Table 2.1).

Cardiac output can be measured invasively (contrast ventriculography, Fick's method, thermodilution) or non-invasively by rebreathing, ultrasonography, or impedance techniques. The output or work data obtained must be evaluated against the actual pulmonary capillary pressure (Frank–Starling relationship) and the adequacy of O_2 supply to the tissues as reflected by mixed venous O_2 tension or saturation. The most commonly used index of global left ventricular function is the ejection fraction (EF):[19]

$$EF(\%) = \frac{\text{Stroke volume}}{\text{End diastolic volume}} \times 100.$$

It can be measured non-invasively by radionuclide ventriculography or echocardiography. During anaesthesia, transoesophageal echocardiography allows continuous monitoring of the left ventricular cross sectional area and calculation of left ventricular fractional area change (FAC):

Table 2.1 Clinical assessment of left ventricular performance[18 113]

Assessment	Normal values
Symptoms	
Signs	
Haemodynamics	
Heart rate	50–90 beats/min
Systolic/diastolic arterial pressure	$\frac{140}{90} - \frac{100}{60}$ mm Hg
Mean arterial pressure	70–105 mm Hg
Left ventricular end diastolic pressure	4–15 mm Hg
Pulmonary capillary wedge pressure	5–15 mm Hg
Left ventricular end diastolic volume index	70 ml/m^2
Left ventricular end systolic volume index	25 ml/m^2
Cardiac index	2·6–4·2 l/min per m^2
Left ventricular stroke volume index	45–50 ml/m^2
Left ventricular ejection fraction	55–68%
Left ventricular mean systolic ejection rate	160 ml/s per m^2
Left ventricular stroke work index	40–60 g·m/m^2
Left ventricular stroke power index	170 g·m/m^2 per s
Oxygen transport parameters	
$\quad$ O_2 consumption	110–150 ml/min per m^2
$\quad$ Arteriovenous O_2 difference	40–55 ml/l
$\quad$ O_2 delivery	400–800 ml/min per m^2
$\quad$ Mixed venous O_2 saturation	65–75%
$\quad$ Mixed venous O_2 partial pressure	40–50 mm Hg

$$\text{FAC}(\%) = \frac{\text{End diastolic area} - \text{End systolic area}}{\text{End diastolic area}} \times 100.$$

This has been shown to correlate closely with simultaneously measured radionuclide ejection fraction.[20-22] The monitoring of FAC became easier after the introduction of automated border detection (Fig 2.5). The ejection fraction (or FAC) is the most useful and widely used index of global pump function. As an index of left ventricular contractility, however, it has the flaw of being load dependent. On the other hand, this dependency can guide the anaesthetist towards optimising the left ventricular function by primarily adjusting the left ventricular preload and afterload.

Determinants of ventricular function

What appears to be simple and easily understandable in an isolated papillary muscle preparation becomes a complex and sometimes controversial issue in the clinic. On the one hand, the indiscriminate use of the

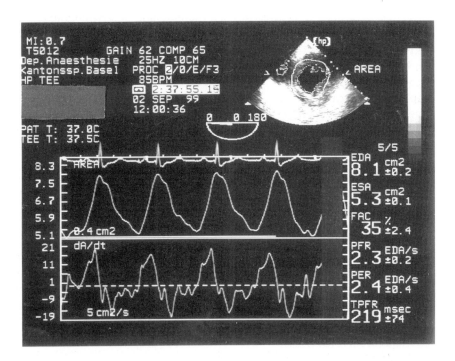

Fig 2.5 Automated border detection. Top: two dimensional, echocardiographic, short axis view of the left ventricle with left ventricular cavity area encircled by endocardial borders and the line drawn around the region of interest. Bottom: electrocardiogram and left ventricular area waveform—EDA (end diastolic area), ESA (end systolic area), and FAC (fractional area change).

physiologically well defined terms, such as preload, afterload, and contractility, by clinicians occasionally gives rise to ciriticism and confusion; on the other, many useful concepts of perioperative haemodynamic management are based on the interplay of these major determinants of ventricular function. Therefore, a detailed review of these determinants and the methods used for their assessment is warranted.

Preload

As already stated, preload is the force that stretches the resting myocardium and determines the resting length of its contractile fibres. In the intact ventricle, the fibre length cannot be measured. However, the end diastolic volume of the ventricle is proportional to the resting length of its contractile elements.[1 4 6 9] The measurement of end diastolic volume in patients undergoing surgery is difficult. Most data on left ventricular volume are based on contrast ventriculography, which requires radiography equipment, left heart catheterisation, and injection of contrast medium; it cannot be used for serial measurements. The calculated volumes depend on ventricular geometry, model and the mathematical formula used, and accurate identification of the endocardial borders. Inclusion of the volume of papillary muscles and trabeculae into the ventricular volume may lead to an overestimation of the volume. Furthermore, only a limited number of beats can be evaluated. Nevertheless, results obtained from ventriculography represent the standard to which the results from other less invasive and non-invasive methods have to be compared. Recently, ultrafast computed tomography (CT) and magnetic resonance imaging (MRI) have also been used for measurement of ventricular volumes.[23] Neither of these methods, although accurate, can be of use in the perioperative setting.

Equilibrium and first pass radionuclide ventriculography have been used in intensive care units. Although accurate with regard to determination of ejection fraction, radionuclide ventriculography can only approximate the absolute ventricular volume using either a geometric or a count based method. Moreover, the radionuclide methods are not suitable for intraoperative use. Echocardiography, in contrast, is much easier to use even in the operating room and allows measurements of ventricular volumes. A real breakthrough was the introduction of transoesophageal echocardiography, which permits continuous monitoring of ventricular size and function without interfering with the surgical field. Several studies have shown a good correlation between left ventricular volumes assessed by transoesophageal echocardiography and those obtained by contrast or radionuclide ventriculography or transthoracic echocardiography.[20 22 24 25] In spite of the good correlations found, transoesophageal echocardiography appears to underestimate absolute left ventricular volumes systematically. This results, in part, from foreshortening of the ventricular cavity in its long axis.

For perioperative online estimation of left ventricular filling volume, however, the calculation of end diastolic volume is not necessary. The area of the cross sectional view of the left ventricle in the transgastric short axis view has been shown to correlate reasonably well to left ventricular volume. The automated border detection method traces the changes of the left ventricular area throughout the cardiac cycle and displays, in real time, the end diastolic and end systolic area values together with the FAC (see Fig 2.5). The FAC represents the echocardiographic analogue of the radionuclide ejection fraction.[26][27] The most recent development, three dimensional echocardiography, has not yet been widely used in the perioperative setting.

Findings of a small ventricular size at end diastole, partial or complete obliteration of left ventricular cavity at end systole, and the "kissing papillary muscles" sign, all of which can be assessed usually by the naked eye, are most useful in the clinical online diagnosis of inadequate filling volume (preload). Furthermore, the dimensional data obtained by trans-oesophageal echocardiography (cavity radius and wall thickness), together with measured filling pressure (wedge pressure, pulmonary diastolic pressure, or mean left atrial pressure) allow calculation of the end diastolic wall stress, which may correlate even better to the end diastolic fibre length than the end diastolic volume.[28]

Without the possibility of monitoring left ventricular size, the filling pressure, usually measured as the mean pulmonary capillary wedge pressure by using a pulmonary artery catheter, remains the only means of estimating left ventricular filling volume during the perioperative period. The limitations of the wedge pressure as a measure of preload must, however, be kept in mind. The relationship between pressure and volume in diastole is curvilinear and changes when the ventricle moves along the P/V relationship.[9][10] Moreover, acute changes in ventricular stiffness may also substantially alter the relationship between filling pressure and volume (see section on "Diastolic performance"). Apart from monitoring ventricular size, echocardiography also provides additional information on left ventricular filling based on Doppler measurements of blood flow velocity across the mitral valve and in the pulmonary veins.

Afterload

It is difficult to apply the concept of ventricular afterload defined in an isolated heart muscle preparation to the patient's heart in situ. In heart muscle in vitro, the afterload remains constant during shortening and can be described by a single value of force. In the intact ventricle in situ, afterload represents the sum of forces opposing the shortening of myocardial fibres and the ejection of blood during systole. It is not constant during ejection and depends on the complex interplay of factors both internal and external to the myocardium. The internal factor (muscle load) refers to the instantaneous force or tension within the ventricular wall, which is related to the size and shape of the chamber, and the pressure within it according to the law of Laplace.[4 6 12] The external factor (arterial load) refers to the physical properties of the arterial system that the ventricle encounters during ejection.[29]

Another, although similar, concept of systolic load describes the total systolic load as comprising intrinsic and extrinsic components: the intrinsic component corresponds to intraventricular pressure gradients whereas the extrinsic component is related to the aortic root pressure waveform resulting from the interaction between ventricular ejection and aortic input impedance.[30] This total systolic ventricular load and the changing ventricular geometry determine the total muscle load that can be expressed in terms of systolic wall stresses. These stresses, in turn, determine the contractile behaviour of the ventricle within the framework of the force–velocity–length relationship. The novel aspect of this concept of the left ventricular systolic load is the incorporation of transient intraventricular pressure gradients related to both the blood inertia and impulsive flows in the early ejection and the convective flow acceleration in the left ventricular outflow tract at peak ejection. Instantaneous high fidelity measurements of pressure and flow did indeed demonstrate significant inhomogeneity of intraventricular pressure during ejection with local gradients up to 8 mm Hg at rest and 16 mm Hg at exercise.[30] These pressure gradients increase with diminishing chamber volume as a result of underfilling and/or concentric hypertrophy, as well as with positive inotropic stimulation. These findings are the basis for understanding the phenomenon of dynamic intraventricular obstruction associated with hypovolaemia and high adrenergic tone, which occasionally develops in the perioperative period. The intrinsic and extrinsic loads are complementary and competitive. Thus, a reduction in the extrinsic load by a vasodilator can be offset by a compensatory increase in the intrinsic component of the total load.

How can left ventricular afterload be assessed in the clinic? All of the following have been proposed as a measure of left ventricular afterload:

• arterial and ventricular systolic pressures
• peripheral vascular resistance
• aortic input impedance
• systolic wall stresses
• effective arterial elastance.

The meaning and the clinical use of each of these parameters are discussed below. Analogue parameters are valid for the right ventricle and the pulmonary vascular bed.

Arterial and ventricular systolic pressures The peripheral arterial pressure is an unreliable index of left ventricular afterload. The arterial pressure waveform results from a complex interaction between ventricular and vascular factors. Arterial pressure can remain unchanged in spite of relevant changes in the systolic load. Of all the ventricular pressures that can be measured (instantaneous, peak, end systolic, and mean), the mean left ventricular pressure reflects the afterload best.[31] The left ventricular pressure measurement is presently limited to the heart catheterisation laboratory.

Peripheral vascular resistance The peripheral resistance is calculated as the ratio of mean arterial pressure divided by flow (cardiac output) and is inversely related to the fourth power of the radius of the vascular bed. In a steady flow system, the peripheral resistance indeed represents the total load imposed on the ventricular pump. In the presence of intermittent ejection of blood into a distensible reservoir and of pulsatile blood flow, however, the total external load also includes elastic properties of the arterial system and wave reflections.[29 31]

Aortic input impedance The pulsatile characteristic of the cardiac pump flow is taken into account when aortic input impedance is calculated as a measure of the total ventricular load.[31 32] In general, impedance is a measure of opposition to flow present within a conducting system. In contrast to peripheral resistance, input impedance incorporates the oscillatory motion of blood. In the arterial system, oscillatory waveforms are superimposed on a mean non-pulsatile component, and the total opposition to flow is a sum of both. The aortic impedance relates the oscillatory or sinusoidal pressure in the aorta to the oscillatory flow and is affected by distensibility (compliance) of the arterial system and inertia of the blood. The impedance modulus is calculated as the ratio of oscillatory pressure and flow, and displayed graphically in the frequency domain by plotting the impedance moduli against their respective frequencies.(Fig 2.6). The frequencies are expressed as multiples of the frequency of the original pressure and flow waveform. In this input impedance spectrum, the modulus of zero frequency (obtained by dividing mean pressure by mean flow) represents the peripheral resistance. To calculate the other moduli, the original pressure and flow waveforms have to be reduced to a finite number of constituent sine waves (harmonics) by Fourier analysis. The oscillatory component of the load is expressed as characteristic impedance Z_0 (units dyn·s/cm^5) and is the arithmetic mean of the impedance moduli above the frequency of 2 Hz.[31 33] Aortic impedance moduli oscillate around the characteristic impedance line as a result of reflected waves (Fig 2.6). A decrease in resistance or an increase in aortic compliance will decrease the amplitude of reflected waves and moduli oscillation, whereas an increase in resistance or a decrease in aortic compliance will have the opoposite effect. The reflected waves exert a prominent influence on impedance moduli, particularly at low frequencies, and represent an additional component of ventricular afterload.[34] The overall contribution of the frequency dependent oscillatory impedance to flow in the normal systemic circulation is, however, only approximately 10% of the total external load. As a result of anatomical differences, it is significantly higher in the pulmonary vascular bed.

The oscillatory analysis can be completed by calculation of the phase of the harmonics that fluctuates between +1 and -1. A negative phase value indicates that the flow harmonic leads the pressure harmonic whereas a positive phase indicates that the flow harmonic lags behind the pressure harmonic. The phase is less than 0 at low frequencies and crosses 0 close to the frequency of the minimal impedance modulus.

In a study in normal subjects, the impedance modulus fell from the high level at zero (units dyn·s/cm^5) frequency (peripheral resistance) to a minimum at 4 Hz and slightly increased thereafter. The characteristic impedance was 90 (34) dyn·s/cm^5 where this represents the mean (SD), which corresponded to 8% of the total peripheral resistance.[33] In elegant

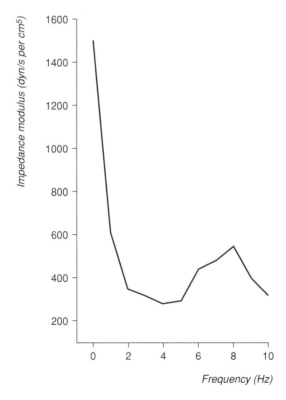

Fig 2.6 Aortic input impedance spectrum. The impedance moduli are plotted against their respective frequencies. The impedence modulus at zero frequency represents the peripheral vascular resistance. The impedance minimum for this example is 4 Hz.

studies, the aortic input impedance was shown to be a major determinant of left ventricular load and function. An increase in characteristic impedance with constant resistance clearly reduced the extent and velocity of shortening and decreased cardiac output.[32][35] However attractive from a physiological point of view, the need for continuous pressure and flow measurement, as well as its cumbersome calculation, renders aortic input impedance unsuitable for assessment of ventricular afterload under clinical conditions.

Systolic wall stresses The measurement of ventricular size and wall thickness by echocardiography allows assessment of the forces acting across the ventricular wall during systole as systolic wall stress.[28][36] Stress is defined as the force acting on a surface divided by the cross sectional area over which the force acts. The total stress can usually be reduced to component stresses acting perpendicular or parallel to the surface. The units of stress are dyn/cm^2 or g/cm^2. The theoretical calculation of ventricular wall stress relies on complex mathematical models based on Laplace's law. In practice, assumptions for simplifications are inevitable. The left ventricular geometry is usually approximated by a sphere or a prolate ellipsoid, and the ellipsoid has a stress distribution between that of a sphere and that of a cylinder. In the human ventricle, stress distribution at the equator more closely resembles that of a cylinder. Consequently, the models based on an ellipsoid or a sphere tend to underestimate the circumferential and overestimate the longitudinal (meridional) stress. According to Laplace's law, the force in the wall of a hollow, thin walled structure is proportional to the transmural pressure and the principal radii of curvature. In a thin walled structure, the bending and radial stresses can be neglected. The meridional and circumferential stresses in the wall of a prolate, thin walled ellipsoid can be calculated when systolic pressure, corresponding radii of curvature, and wall thickness are known.[36]

The basic assumption of the thin walled models is that the wall is thin relative to the cavity diameter. In an attempt to obtain a better approximation to the real stresses and to study the stress distribution across the wall, thick walled ventricular models were developed. The earlier models, which assumed isotropic (homogeneous) properties of the myocardium, showed that the stresses are apparently higher in the inner layers of the ventricular wall than in the outer layers. Newer models incorporating anisotropic properties of the myocardium, cylindrical geometry, and fibre direction revealed uniform distribution of stress across the ventricular wall.[37] The mechanism keeping the transmural distribution of the stress uniform is related to the interplay of the field of deformation and regional fibre orientation. When change in ventricular volume induces transmural gradients in fibre strain (relative elongation), an appropriate amount of torsion redistributes the fibre strain from the inner to the outer layers and equalises wall stresses. This uniformity of the mechanical load in the myocardium is not restricted to the left ventricular wall alone, but is found also in the papillary muscles and the free right ventricular wall.[37]

In animal experiments, systolic wall stress was compared with the aortic input impedance with regard to the determination of left ventricular afterload. It was found that alterations in ventricular stress more accurately predicted alterations in ventricular shortening than the aortic input impedance. Thus, systolic wall stress, which represents the internal load imposed on the contracting myocardium, also appears to reflect alterations in the external load reliably.[35]

In echocardiographic studies, the meridional end systolic wall stress is usually calculated according to the angiographically validated formula as follows:

$$\text{End systolic wall stress (dyn/cm}^2) = \frac{P \times D \times 1 \cdot 33}{4\text{WT}(1 + [\text{WT/D}])}$$

where P is end systolic pressure, D is the end systolic left ventricular diameter (dyn/cm^2), and WT the end systolic wall thickness.[24] Peak systolic and mean systolic wall stresses can also be calculated.

Although it is rather difficult to calculate the systolic wall stress in the perioperative setting, knowledge of at least directional changes of left ventricular afterload may help to evaluate the effects of therapeutic interventions and to optimise left ventricular function. For this purpose, the directional changes of the simple ratio [$P \times D$]/[WT] obtained by echocardiography can give us useful information on changes in left ventricular afterload. In the absence of major alterations in arterial pressure, even the end systolic size (diameter or cross sectional area) of the left ventricle alone will help to estimate online the directional changes in afterload.

Effective arterial elastance Another measure of left ventricular afterload has been introduced with the concept of the time varying elastance (see "Ventriculoarterial coupling"). The effective arterial elastance (E_a) relates end systolic arterial pressure to stroke volume. The concept of arterial elastance is a reflection of pressure that will be generated when the stroke volume is ejected into the arterial system. The greater the stroke volume ejected and the greater the opposition of the arterial system to the ejection, the greater the pressure increase in the arterial system. By plotting the developed pressures at end systole against varying stroke volumes, the arterial P/V relationship can be constructed. The term for the slope of this linear relationship is "effective arterial elastance" (E_a), and it is used in the end systolic P/V diagram as a measure of afterload to analyse the coupling of the left ventricle with the arterial system.[38]

Contractility

As previously mentioned, contractility is one of the fundamental properties of the heart muscle manifesting itself through the velocity and

43

extent of shortening. To ascribe an observed change in shortening to a change in contractility, the other determinants of pump function, that is, preload, afterload, and heart rate, must be held constant. This requirement disqualifies the ejection phase parameters such as stroke volume, ejection fraction, or the first derivative of the left ventricular pressure, dP/dt_{max}, as reliable measures of myocardial contractility.[39] The long search for a quantitative and reliable single index of contractility (see box) will probably be futile because it is most difficult to separate contractility from external factors and their feedback interactions with internal factors.[18] Future research will have to use a multivariate approach to this complex and salient issue.

Currently, the preferred way of assessing myocardial contractility in human studies is the determination of time varying elastance or of preload recruitable stroke work. Time varying elastance can be calculated from the instantaneous P/V relationship[38 40 41] (Fig 2.7). It represents the slope of the P/V relationship and increases towards the end of systole to a maximum: therefore, maximal elastance (E_{max}) or end systolic elastance (E_{es}) is an index of myocardial contractility. In isolated ejecting ventricles, E_{max} and E_{es} are almost identical over a wide range of varying preloads. When afterload is altered, they may differ considerably. This is frequently observed in vivo

---

Indices of ventricular contractility

Pre-ejection phase parameters
Maximum rate of change of ventricular pressure dP/dt_{max}
(dP/dt_{max})/IP (IP = developed pressure at dP/dt_{max} minus end diastolic pressure)
Left ventricular (dP/dt_{max})/end diastolic pressure
Pre-ejection period (PEP)

Ejection phase parameters
Ejection fraction (EF%)
Velocity of circumferential fibre shortening (V_{cf})
Ejection time (ET), PEP/ET
Peak systolic flow velocity, flow acceleration, time to peak flow (Doppler techniques)

Methods minimising load dependence
End systolic pressure/volume relationship (left ventricular elastance E_{max})
End systolic wall stress/volume relationship
Preload recruitable stroke work (SW/EDV relationship)
(dP/dt_{max})/end diastolic volume relationship
Maximal ventricular power
Velocity of circumferential fibre shortening/end systolic wall stress relationship
Ejection fraction/end systolic wall stress relationship

---

and is probably caused by resistive and inertial influences on the end systolic pressures and by the changes in time required to reach end systole as a function of load.[42] In such a case, E_{max} is steeper and does not fall on the end systolic (left upper corner) points of the P/V relationship. As E_{es} can be determined more easily, it represents the preferred index of myocardial contractility. To construct the P/V relationship of the left ventricle, several P/V loops must be recorded starting at different (usually decreasing) end diastolic volumes. To construct an end systolic P/V relationship in an isolated heart, the preload can be varied by changing the volume of saline in the balloon placed in the ventricle. During open chest conditions, preload can be changed by tightening a ligature around the inferior vena cava. During closed chest conditions, venous return and preload can be changed by briefly inflating a balloon at the tip of a catheter introduced into the inferior vena cava. Another possibility is to vary preload pharmacologically, for instance with glyceryl trinitrate (nitroglycerine).

It has been commonly assumed that the end systolic P/V relationship is linear and, therefore, can be described by two parameters: slope E_{es} and volume axis intercept V_0.[43] Recent studies, however, demonstrated significant non-linearity of the relationship under various conditions, for instance during myocardial ischaemia or a high contractile state.[42 44]

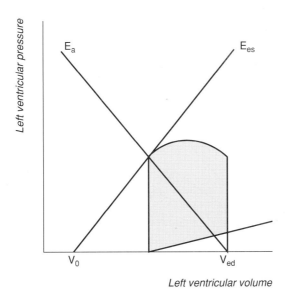

Fig 2.7 End systolic pressure–volume relationship and ventriculoarterial coupling. V_{ed} (left ventricular end diastolic volume), V_0 (volume intercept of the end systolic pressure–volume relationship), E_{es} (end systolic elastance), E_a (effective arterial elastance), grey area (area of the left ventricular pressure–volume loop). The intersection of the E_{es} and E_a lines defines the effective stroke volume.

Moreover, the end systolic P/V relationship is not completely load insensitive. Changes in afterload induce parallel shifts of the relationship and may even alter the slope. The changes in P/V relationships caused by load dependence have, however, been shown to be of minor importance compared with the substantial changes brought about by variation in the inotropic state.[42]

The development of the conductance catheter now allows determination of E_{es} in patients.[45] In the normal left ventricle, values of E_{es} of 3·5–4·5 mm Hg/ml were found, decreasing to 2·5 mm Hg/ml in patients with mildly depressed left ventricular function and to 1·5 mm Hg/ml in patients with severely depressed ventricles.[46] The E_{es} was used for evaluation of myocardial contractility in patients before and after open heart surgery. The E_{es} varied between 0·9 and 5·6 mm Hg/ml with a mean of 2·5 and standard deviation (SD) of 1·5, and showed individually variable changes after cardiopulmonary bypass.[47] E_{es} is very sensitive to positive inotropic stimulation, for example, to dobutamine, which clearly increases the slope without changes in V_0.[48] It has recently been shown that the use of a conductance catheter to measure ventricular volume can be replaced by the online measurement of cross sectional left ventricular area using trans-oesophageal echocardiography and automated border detection (Fig 2.8). In an open chest study in dogs using instantaneous echocardiographic left

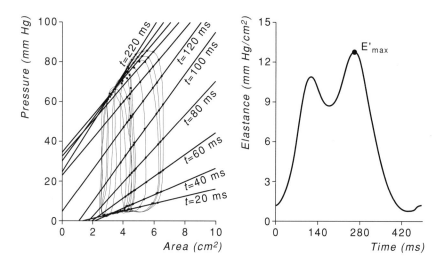

Fig 2.8 Left ventricular time varying elastance (E_{max}) obtained by instantaneous pressure–area relationship. Left: left ventricular pressure–area relationship demonstrating the increasing slope of the relationship (E) from the onset to the end of ejection. Right: the change in elastance (E) plotted against time with the maximal value of the elastance (E_{max}) occurring 250 ms after the onset of ejection. (Reproduced with permission from Gorcsan et al.[47]

ventricular area instead of volume, dobutamine markedly increased both E_{es} and E_{max}[49] (Fig 2.9). In a study in patients undergoing open heart surgery, significant decreases in E_{es} and E_{max} following cardiopulmonary bypass were observed. Such evidence of impaired left ventricular contractility was not reflected by any other haemodynamic parameter such as cardiac output, stroke work, or ejection fraction.[50]

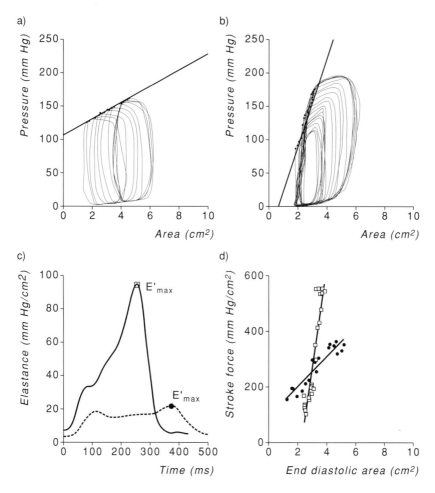

Fig 2.9 Effect of positive inotropic stimulation on the left ventricular pressure–area relationship (E_{max}). (a) Pressure–area loops and slope of the end systolic pressure–area relationship at control. (b) Increase in slope of the end systolic pressure–area relationship (E_{max}) after dobutamine administration. (c) Increase in E_{max} and shortening of the time to E_{max} after dobutamine administration (———) compared with control (——). (d) Increase in the slope of the stroke force–end diastolic area relationship after dobutamine administration (□) compared with control (●). (Reproduced with permission from Gorcsan *et al.*[46])

47

In patients with heart disease, the end systolic pressure may be an inaccurate index of ventricular afterload. In aortic stenosis or hypertensive cardiomyopathy, the end systolic pressure is high, although the afterload may be normal as a result of the development of ventricular hypertrophy, which is able to normalise the wall stress. Therefore, in these patients the systolic (peak or end systolic) wall stress is a more reliable reflection of ventricular afterload and should replace end systolic pressure in the P/V diagram. The end systolic wall stress/area relationship was used for estimating myocardial contractility in patients undergoing aortocoronary bypass surgery.[51] The relationship between end systolic pressure or wall stress and area or diameter of the left ventricle can be constructed from non-invasive data using cuff blood presssure and echocardiography. The use of systolic cuff blood pressure instead of end systolic pressure does not significantly alter the relationship. When the pressure in the radial artery is recorded perioperatively, the left ventricular end systolic pressure can be approximated with reasonable accuracy from the dicrotic notch pressure by adding 8 mm Hg.[52]

In the daily practice of anaesthesia, as well as in cardiology, it has not been possible to analyse the end systolic stress/volume relationship. However, it was suggested that the simple ratio of end systolic stress to end systolic volume, obtained by echocardiography, may be useful in evaluating left ventricular performance at the bedside. Although such a simple ratio must not be used as a substitute for the slope of the pressure, stress/volume, or area relationship, it can, however, provide simple but important information: a ventricle that can contract to a small end systolic volume at a normal or even high end systolic pressure or wall stress is in a better contractile state than one that remains large at end systole in spite of a similar or even lower pressure.[53 54] The maintenance of a low end systolic size (in the presence of adequate filling volume) should be the goal of perioperative haemodynamic management in patients with heart disease. Recently, a method for real time continuous monitoring of ventricular and arterial elastance, and their coupling ratio based on single-beat analysis, was developed.[55] The method, based on echocardiographic automated border detection and computation of isovolumic left ventricular pressure, obviates the need for preload manipulation and has a potential for use in the clinical setting.

The second index of myocardial contractility validated in patients is the preload recruitable stroke work. It is based on the linear relationship between left ventricular stroke work (product of mean systolic pressure and stroke volume) and left ventricular end diastolic volume.[56] The left ventricular stroke work is calculated as the area of the P/V loops, obtained in a similar fashion to elastance measurements by varying the end diastolic volumes. The slope of the stroke work/end diastolic volume relationship (denoted as M_w) is a measure of myocardial contractility. The relationship is highly linear and, in addition, the slopes and volume axis intercepts (M_o) are less variable than those of the end systolic P/V relationships.[57] In a study in patients, both preload recruitable stroke work and end systolic P/V relationships showed high and comparable linearity, and both responded to dobutamine by marked increases in E_{max} and M_w, respectively.[57] In contrast, following afterload reduction with captopril, the preload recruitable stroke work remained unchanged whereas the end systolic P/V relationship shifted to the right.[58] With increases in afterload, the preload recruitable stroke work relationship again does not change, but the end systolic P/V relationship shifts to the left. Thus, the independence of the afterload is the advantage of the preload recruitable stroke work relationship as a method of assessing myocardial contractility. Echocardiography using automated border detection allows the measurement of preload recruitable stroke force. End diastolic volume and stroke work are replaced by end diastolic area and stroke force, which is the integral of the pressure–area loop. In patients, there was a marked decrease in the slope of the preload recruitable stroke work relationship after cardiopulmonary bypass, not reflected by standard haemodynamic indices.[49 50]

Other validated methods for clinical assessment of myocardial contractility make use of the general principle of relating the parameter of left ventricular function to left ventricular afterload. One of these methods, which has been also applied in surgical patients, is the determination of the shortening velocity of circumferential fibres (V_{cf}) in relation to the actual systolic wall stress. V_{cf} is obtained by echocardiography applying the formula:

$$V_{cf} = \frac{\text{End diastolic} - \text{End systolic cavity circumference}}{\text{End diastolic circumference} \times \text{Ejection time}}.$$

When multiplied by the square root of the RR interval (where RR is the cardiac cycle), it becomes independent of heart rate. The relationship between end systolic stress and V_{cf} is inversely linear and reflects the force–velocity relationship. It shifts upwards with a positive inotropic intervention and downwards with impaired contractility.[59] A similar relationship exists between end systolic wall stress and ejection fraction.

More recently, left ventricular power was proposed as an index of myocardial contractility.[17] Power is work per unit time and the left ventricular power represents the rate of energy expenditure during the pressure–volume work of the ventricle. Maximal left ventricular power (PWR_{max}) is the peak instantaneous product of chamber pressure and rate of volume change obtained by simultaneous left ventricular pressure and volume measurements with a conductance catheter technique, and has been validated as an index of left ventricular contractility. It can be also measured non-invasively from the product of peak arterial pressure and flow.[60] The advantage of PWR_{max} is its afterload independence; on the other hand, it is highly sensitive to preload. This preload dependency can be eliminated by dividing PWR_{max} by EDV or EDV^2.[61]

Heart rate

An isolated strip of heart muscle responds to changes in frequency of electrical stimulation by changes in developed force. The ability of the heart muscle to develop force and/or to shorten clearly depends on the interval between preceding contractions. This dependence has been described as a force–interval, strength–interval, or a force–frequency relationship. The physiological phenomena reflecting this fundamental relationship are Bowditch's positive staircase response, Woodforth's negative staircase response, postextrasystolic potentiation, and the response to paired pacing. Basically, an increase in heart rate leads to an increase in myocardial contractility and vice versa. The short term effect is much more pronounced than the chronic steady state effects. The existence of these phenomena in intact, conscious animals and humans has been questioned.[62] Many earlier studies, however, were using unreliable, load dependent indices of contractility. When the less load sensitive, end systolic P/V relationship was used to look at the effects of heart rate on myocardial contractility in conscious dogs, a marked dependence of the contractility on the pacing rate was found.[63] The slope of the relationship, E_{max}, showed a positive correlation with heart rate. In addition, with increasing heart rate, the volume intercept (V_0) of the P/V relationship shifted to the right on the x axis. This may be partly responsible for the changes in stroke volume with changing heart rate. The increased slope of the relationship and the rightward shift of the V_0 point result in an increase in stroke volume at higher end systolic pressures, and in a decrease in stroke volume at low end systolic pressures.[63] The first effect may be beneficial during exercise by facilitating ejection despite an increase in afterload. Isotonic exercise has been shown to potentiate the effects of increasing heart rate on myocardial contractility.[64] As similar augmentation of the force–frequency relationship was observed during dobutamine infusion, these effects can be attributed to β-adrenergic stimulation.[65] Besides contractility, myocardial relaxation is also facilitated by increasing heart rate, and this effect is augmented by adrenergic stimulation.[66]

Except for patients with severe forms of bradycardia, it is not common practice to use cardiac pacing to improve systolic performance. Although short term increases in heart rate appear to have beneficial effects on ventricular performance, the opposite is true for chronic tachycardia. The development of myocardial stunning, dilated cardiomyopathy, and heart failure after prolonged fast pacing in animal experiments points to adverse effects of long term tachycardia.[67] A transient ventricular dysfunction also occurs in patients after successful conversion of a long lasting tachyarrhythmia.

It is interesting that heart muscle strips recovered from failing hearts do not respond to increases in stimulation rate; in contrast, a fall in developed force with increasing frequency was described, manifesting itself as a descending limb of the force–frequency relationship.[68]

Paired pacing that makes use of the phenomenon of postextrasystolic potentiation was, however, successfully applied in patients with severe heart failure to enhance ventricular performance. Postextrasystolic potentiation, as well as the positive staircase response, result from increased availability of intracellular calcium for binding to contractile proteins.

Ventriculoarterial coupling

The coupling of the left ventricle with the peripheral vascular system has been intensely studied in terms of the end systolic P/V relationship.[69] In this model, the left ventricle and the arterial system are regarded as two coupled elastic chambers. The distribution of blood between these chambers is determined by their relative elastances. The elastance E is a measure of respective chamber stiffness and is represented by the slope of the P/V relationship (see Fig 2.7). The instantaneous elastance increases from a low value during diastole to its maximum value (E_{max}) close to end systole. The pressure varies inversely and linearly with the stroke volume according the following equation:

$$P_{es} = E_{es} (V_{ed} - SV - V_0)$$

where E_{es} = end systolic elastance related to contractile properties of the ventricle, P_{es} = end systolic ventricular pressure, V_{ed} = end diastolic volume, SV = stroke volume and V_0 = volume–axis intercept of the P/V relationship.

The arterial system is characterised in this model by the relationship between end systolic pressure and stroke volume. The slope of this relationship, the effective arterial elastance ($E_a = P_{es}/SV$), serves as an index of total external load opposing ejection. E_a comprises resistance, compliance, and characteristic impedance of the arterial vascular bed. During the ejection phase, elastance varies with time; throughout ejection, ventricular elastance progressively increases from the onset to the end of ejection whereas arterial elastance progressively decreases (time varying elastance). The effective stroke volume resulting from the ventriculoarterial coupling is determined by the intersection of the ventricular end systolic P/V and arterial end systolic P/V relationships.[48 69] Graphic analysis of the ventriculoarterial coupling provides expeditious information on left ventricular function and its determinants during acute changes in loading conditions.[38 45] The left ventricle delivers maximal external work (stroke work) when the E_a/E_{es} ratio approximates 1. The mechanical efficiency of the ventricle, relating work to amount of energy consumed, is maximal when E_a is approximately half of E_{es}.[70] In normal subjects, E_{es} and E_a values of 3·5–7·0 and 1·6–4·0 mm Hg/ml, respectively, were found.[46 71] The E_a/E_{es} ratio was 0·4–0·6 and increased significantly with increasing afterload as a result of increased E_a. An afterload reduction caused E_a and the ratio E_a/E_{es} to decrease. Positive inotropic stimulation also decreased E_a/E_{es} as a result of an increase in E_{es}.[71]

The pressure/volume area (PVA) encompassed by the end systolic and diastolic P/V relationship and the systolic part of the P/V loop provides an interesting insight into myocardial energetics.[72–74] PVA is composed of the PE area (PE being the potential energy of an isovolumic contraction) and the EW area (EW being the external work of ejecting contraction) (Fig 2.10). PVA (= PE + EW) is a measure of the total mechanical energy of contraction and was shown to correlate linearly with left ventricular myocardial oxygen consumption ($M\dot{V}_{O_2}$). The slope of this relationship represents the oxygen cost of the PVA and its reciprocal represents the mechanical efficiency. This linear $M\dot{V}_{O_2}$/PVA relationship remains constant during changes in preload and afterload, but is shifted upwards in parallel manner by positive inotropic stimulation. In contrast, negative inotropic

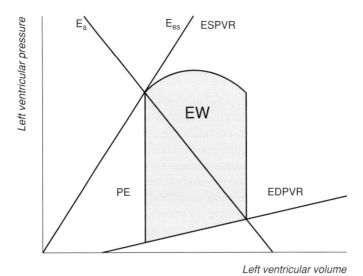

Fig 2.10 Left ventricular pressure–volume relationship and pressure–volume area (PVA): ESPVR (end systolic pressure–volume relationship), EDPVR (end diastolic pressure–volume relationship), E_{es} (end systolic elastance), E_a (effective arterial elastance), EW (left ventricular external work (stroke work)), PE (left ventricular potential energy). The PVA is the sum of EW and PE areas.

interventions shift the relationship downwards, again without changing its slope.[75] In patients with normal left ventricular function, a contractile efficiency of 40% was found.[76] A decrease in efficiency from 46% to 35% was demonstrated in healthy volunteers during positive inotropic stimulation with dobutamine.[77] The ratio of external work (EW or stroke work) to PVA can be used to express the mechanical efficiency of the whole left ventricle. In patients with normal left ventricular function, this ratio was 0·6. It decreased with an increase in afterload and increased when afterload was reduced.[71]

Ventricular function curves and the Frank–Starling law of the heart

Clinical evaluation of the overall pump function of the heart is usually based on the ventricular function curve, which relates a measure of ventricular performance (cardiac output, stroke volume, or stroke work) as a dependent variable to a measure of ventricular preload, such as ventricular filling pressure, end diastolic volume, end diastolic diameter, cross sectional area, or end diastolic wall stress.[9 10 78] The ventricular function curve describes the fundamental dependence of ventricular performance on ventricular preload and represents the expression of the Frank–Starling law of the heart: "the energy of contraction is a function of the length of the muscle fibre".[79] (Fig 2.11). This law is based on the length–tension relationship of myocardial sarcomeres, which at rest operate below the maximum length (L_{max}) on the ascending limb of their length–tension relationship. Increasing stretch on the sarcomeres towards L_{max} increases the number of activated cross bridges and the developed tension.

The dependence of ventricular performance on afterload and contractile state is reflected by displacement of the ventricular function curve with changing contractility and/or afterload. For example, with decreasing afterload and/or increasing contractility, the curve is shifted upwards and to the left; an opposite shift is observed with increasing afterload and/or deteriorating contractility.[78] Hence, the function of the ventricle cannot be described by one function curve; instead, a family of ventricular function curves, reflecting the changing load and inotropic states, gives a better characterisation of the ventricular function.[78 79] Incremental pacing also shifts the cardiac output curve upwards; the magnitude of the shift is, however, less than during exercise at a comparable heart rate, as a result of an additional positive inotropic effect of increased sympathetic tone during exercise.[80] At higher preloads the ventricular function curve tends to plateau and further augmentation in ventricular filling no longer enhances ventricular performance. The so called "descending limb of the Starling curve", which has given rise to considerable controversy in the past, is now

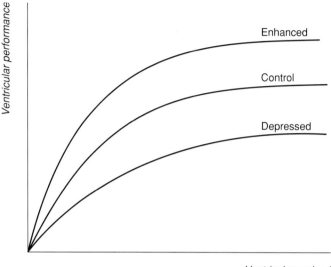

Ventricular preload

Fig 2.11 Ventricular function curves. The curves describe the relationship between resting length of contractile fibres (preload) and ventricular performance (cardiac output, stroke volume, stroke work), known as the Frank-Starling law. An enhanced inotropic state shifts the relationship leftward and upward; depressed inotropy has an opposite effect.

considered to be an artefact caused by non-physiological experimental conditions.[79]

Internal control mechanisms

Cardiac pump function or its output (cardiac output) is regulated by both internal and external factors. The Frank–Starling mechanism represents the internal control mechanism of the pump. It plays an eminent role in the maintenance of balance between right and left ventricular outputs, and the distribution of blood volume between the systemic and pulmonary circulation.[10 78 81] The Frank–Starling mechanism is also activated during early stages of exercise, possibly because of the delay in sympathetic activation, but it does not play a major role during later stages of vigorous exercise.[82] In normal supine subjects and in the presence of normal filling pressures (10–12 mm Hg), the left ventricle operates close to the maximum of its function curve. Attempts to increase the filling volume lead to an increase in filling pressure, but only to modest improvement in ventricular performance.[83 84] In contrast, in the upright position and in the presence of filling pressures that are lower than normal, the ventricle clearly operates on the ascending limb of its function curve and, consequently, fluid administration can markedly enhance pump function. In the presence of

54

myocardial depression, for example, resulting from anaesthesia and obtunded baroreflex function, the role played by the Frank–Starling mechanism becomes more important.[13]

External control mechanisms

In contrast to the internal control of the heart pump provided by the Frank–Starling mechanism, the external control factors interacting with ventricular performance reside within the systemic circulation.[78] During the steady state, the heart cannot pump more blood than it receives from the periphery. The flow of blood returning from the periphery is known as venous return and is equivalent to cardiac output except for very short periods of time, as during transient compression of the vena cava. Systemic venous return is described by the venous return curve, relating flow to right atrial pressure. In the negative filling pressure range, the venous return becomes maximal but soon levels out because of the limiting effect of venous collapse at the level of the thoracic inlet. In the positive pressure range, there is a linear decrease in venous return with increasing atrial pressure until a point is reached when the flow ceases. The pulmonary venous return curve, reflecting the relationship between left atrial pressure and cardiac output, is analogous to the systemic venous return curve.

When the heart pump stops and blood flow ceases, the pressures within the heart and circulation will equalise at the so called mean systemic pressure, which can be estimated by extrapolation during long diastoles. This mean systemic pressure depends on blood volume present in the circulation, vascular, notably venous tone, and external forces compressing the vessels. Venous return to the heart is directly proportional to this mean systemic pressure and to the difference between mean systemic pressure and right (or left) atrial pressure. The complex interplay of all major factors involved in cardiac output regulation, for instance during intraoperative changes in blood volume and intrathoracic pressure, can be studied on Guyton's graph where both ventricular function curves and venous return curves are combined. The points at which the curves cross represent respective equilibria and determine the actual value of cardiac output (Fig 2.12).

Afterload mismatch

As a result of the immediate upregulation in force generation in response to acute increases in afterload, the steady state relationship between stroke work and end diastolic volume remains insensitive to wide alterations in afterload.[85] This is true as long as there is a sufficient preload reserve; only then does the ventricular performance (generated stroke volume or stroke

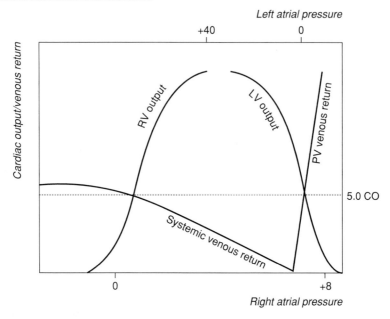

Fig 2.12 Guyton's diagram showing right and left ventricular function curves. At steady state, the output of both ventricles is identical and corresponds to cardiac output (CO). The outputs of the right and left ventricles are determined by the intersections of ventricular output curves with the corresponding systematic and pulmonary venous (PV) return curves.[68]

work) not decrease with increasing afterload, because the ventricle can maintain its stroke volume by mobilising its preload reserve and making use of the Frank–Starling mechanism. In contrast, when preload reserve is exhausted – for example, by overtransfusion or inadequate venous return – stroke volume becomes dependent on systolic pressure and linearly declines with any further increase in afterload. This can produce an apparent descending limb of the ventricular function curve.[84] The condition has been termed "afterload mismatch" and can be described as the inability of the ventricle at a given level of myocardial contractility to maintain a normal stroke volume against the prevailing systolic load.[86] A change in myocardial contractility will alter the afterload sensitivity of the ventricle, and the afterload mismatch will occur at different levels of systolic pressure and stroke volume. The concept of afterload mismatch is useful in the haemodynamic management of the perioperative phase even in patients with normal ventricular function. These patients may have a normal cardiac preload reserve, but peripheral factors may generate a venous return that is inadequate to maintain the end diastolic volume needed for adequate ventricular performance.[84]

Ventricular diastolic performance

During systole, the ventricle can pump only the amount of blood into the aorta that it has received during the preceding diastole. Furthermore, the ventricle, which fails to fill properly, is deprived of its intrinsic ability to increase the strength of its contraction by increasing the length of its contractile fibres. Therefore, the diastolic function of the ventricle is as important as the systolic one.[87 88] A normal diastolic function can be defined as the amount of filling of the ventricle that is necessary to produce a cardiac output commensurate with the body needs at normal pulmonary venous pressure.[89] Traditionally, diastole is defined as the part of the cardiac cycle between the closure of the aortic valve and the closure of the mitral valve. It comprises:

- isovolumic relaxation period
- rapid filling
- slow filling (diastasis)
- atrial systole.

An alternative concept assigns ventricular relaxation, which is an active, energy consuming process of myocardial inactivation, to the systole which, in turn, extends into the rapid filling phase.[90] The major determinants of diastolic function are:

- myocardial relaxation
- elastic recoil
- passive filling characteristics of the ventricle
- atrial function
- heart rate.

Isovolumic relaxation period

During relaxation, ventricular pressure is determined by two overlapping processes: the decay of the pressure actively developed during the preceding systole and the build up of the passive filling pressure. Together, these two components result in the effective pressure of the isovolumic relaxation period. The rapid fall in pressure can be approximated by a mono-exponential curve and described by its time constant τ.[88] Maximal negative dP/dt and the duration of the isovolumic relaxation period have been also used for the evaluation of ventricular relaxation. The rate of relaxation is modulated by sympathetic tone and circulating catecholamines. It increases with positive inotropic stimulation and increasing heart rate. Interventions causing an increase in the rate and extent of relaxation are called positive lusitropic effects.

A delay of ventricular relaxation can be caused by pressure or volume overload, which primarily prolongs the contraction. The *delayed relaxation*

57

can affect the early filling but does not cause diastolic failure. In contrast, the real impairment in the rate and extent of relaxation will compromise diastolic function. Such impairment becomes evident as an upward shift of the entire diastolic P/V relationship, reflecting increased resistance to ventricular filling.[91] Diastolic dysfunction and failure may result from disturbances of the mechanisms that control myocardial relaxation. They include intracellular calcium homoeostasis, function of sarcoplasmic reticulum and contractile proteins, loading conditions, and uniformity of relaxation.[92 93] The most common cause of impaired relaxation in the perioperative period is myocardial ischaemia.

Rapid filling

The driving force of early filling is the atrioventricular pressure gradient. The gradient is enhanced by the ventricular elastic recoil or suction. During contraction, potential energy is stored at end systole in the form of a longitudinal gradient of circumferential rotation (twist) and released during early diastole as elastic recoil.[94] Additional, so called restoring forces include myocardial compression and stretching of the mitral valve apparatus during contraction. The left ventricular twist is a special form of systolic deformation (torsion) and manifests itself as a counterclockwise rotation of the apex relative to the base of the left ventricle. At end systole the fast untwisting starts with a half of the twist already dissipated during the isovolumic relaxation period, followed by a slower untwisting during the early filling.[95] Consequently, 60–80% of the stroke volume enters the ventricle during the first third of diastole.[89] Restoring forces become more important when the end systolic volume is small, such as during exercise, tachycardia, and hypovolaemia.

Slow filling

The following phase of slow filling, diastasis, is characterised by only modest increases in pressure and volume in the ventricle (in accordance with the passive diastolic P/V relationship) and is caused by ongoing venous return.

Atrial contraction

At the end of diastole, atrial contraction raises the atrial pressure and hence the filling pressure gradient, and completes the filling. Atrial contraction represents a diastolic function reserve (atrial booster pump) that becomes increasingly important during shortening in filling time (such as during tachycardia) as well as in all situations of impaired ventricular filling, hence the importance of sinus rhythm for normal ventricular performance and the usually detrimental effect of its loss in patients with heart disease.

The contribution of the atrium to ventricular filling can be easily assessed by Doppler measurements of blood flow velocity across the mitral valve. The late diastolic flow velocity wave caused by atrial contraction (A wave) is normally lower than the early velocity (E wave).

The final amount of blood accommodated by the ventricle at end diastole depends on *passive characteristics* of the chamber, which are determined by the following:

- elastic properties of the myocardium
- geometry of the chamber
- thickness of the ventricular wall
- viscoelastic (flow velocity dependent) effects
- external constraints (pericardium, lungs).

These properties, taken together, can be expressed by *chamber stiffness*, which relates the instantaneous change in filling pressure to instantaneous change in filling volume ($\mathrm{d}P/\mathrm{d}V$) and reflects the pressure change induced by a unit change in volume (Fig 2.13). *Chamber compliance* ($\mathrm{d}V/\mathrm{d}P$) is the reciprocal of chamber stiffness.[96] The diastolic P/V relationship is exponential in shape and its slope increases as the end diastolic pressure increases more steeply at high filling volumes. The slope of the relationship at any part of the curve correlates linearly with the end diastolic pressure, allowing the calculation of the modulus of chamber stiffness as the slope of the ($\mathrm{d}P/\mathrm{d}V)/P$ relationship.[96] Changes in chamber stiffness may occur as a consequence of changes in operating end diastolic pressure (preload). With

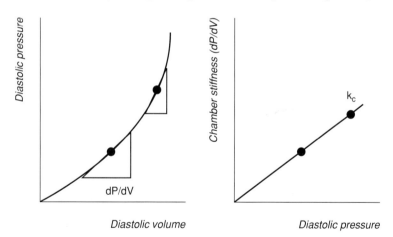

Fig 2.13 Diastolic (passive) pressure–volume relationship. Left: the slope of the pressure–volume relationship ($\mathrm{d}P/\mathrm{d}V$) represents the chamber stiffness and increases with increasing diastolic volume. Right: the relationship between chamber stiffness ($\mathrm{d}P/\mathrm{d}V$) and diastolic presure is linear and its slope represents the chamber stiffness constant k_c.[85]

progressive increase in end diastolic volume and a rightward and upward displacement of the ventricular P/V loop along the diastolic P/V line, the chamber becomes stiffer. In contrast, with a real alteration of chamber stiffness, the whole diastolic P/V relationship and its slope (modulus of chamber stiffness) are altered. A decrease in chamber stiffness is associated with a downward and rightward shift of the diastolic P/V relationship and vice versa.

Ventricular hypertrophy and myocardial infarction with ensuing remodelling represent the most common causes of increased chamber stiffness and diastolic dysfunction. In contrast to chamber stiffness, which is a measure of the ability of the ventricle to oppose distension, *myocardial stiffness* is a measure of the resistance to stretching of the myocardium itself.[88 97] The ventricular diastolic stress (σ), similar to systolic stress, is defined as force per unit of cross sectional area of the ventricular wall and is related to cavity pressure, radius, and wall thickness. Strain (ϵ) is the change in length with respect to a reference length and is expressed as a percentage. The stress/strain relationship (σ/ϵ) of the myocardium is non-linear and its shape resembles that of the diastolic P/V curve. The slope of any part of this exponential curve is termed the "elastic stiffness of the myocardium" ($d\sigma/d\epsilon$). When this elastic stiffness is plotted against the diastolic wall stress, the relationship becomes linear and its slope can be quantified by a single stiffness constant. An increase in the stiffness constant represents a true increase in myocardial stiffness, which is mostly caused by myocardial fibrosis.[28 88]

Heart rate

Heart rate is also a major determinant of diastolic performance. With progressively increasing heart rate and decreasing diastolic filling time, the diastolic reserve based on increased rate of relaxation and atrial booster becomes exhausted and cardiac output falls, even in patients with normal ventricular function. In patients with impaired diastolic function at rest, cardiac output may fall even with modest tachycardia.

Right ventricular performance

The right ventricle receives systemic and coronary venous return and pumps it into the left ventricle across the pulmonary vascular bed. The right and left ventricles can be described as two pumps in series coupled by the lungs and operating as one functional unit. Both parts of this unit have a common blood supply, a common muscular septum separating both cavities, and common intertwining myocardial bundles. Moreover, both ventricles are confined within the common pericardium and exposed to the same changes in intrathoracic pressure and lung volume. There are, however, important differences between both ventricles. Anatomically, the right ventricle consists of the free wall and septum arranged into the inflow tract (sinus) and the outflow tract (conus); the conus represents the phylogenic relic of the bulbus cordis.[98] The right ventricular outflow tract contracts after the inflow tract with a delay of up to 25–50 ms; this asynchrony causes the outflow tract to expand during the contraction of the inflow tract and to maintain right ventricular ejection by the time the inflow tract is beginning to relax. Under intense sympathetic stimulation, significant pressure gradients between inflow and outflow tracts can occur.[99–101]

Wall thickness and myocardial mass of the right ventricle are considerably less than those of the left ventricle, reflecting the lower external work of the former. Although the right ventricle pumps the same amount of blood (cardiac output) as the left ventricle, it does so into the low pressure pulmonary vascular bed with low resistance to flow. Pulmonary arteries are much more distensible than systemic arteries, and the pulse wave velocity in the pulmonary arteries is lower than in the systemic arterial tree. This causes the reflected pressure waves to return after the closure of the pulmonic valve. The pulmonary input impedance, representing the external load of the right ventricle, differs from the aortic impedance in that the oscillatory component (characteristic impedance) is relatively greater and makes up to 25–30% of the total pulmonary resistance.[102] The right ventricular ejection into the low impedance pulmonary vascular bed, together with the delayed return of the reflected waves, affect the right ventricular pressure waveform. There is a very short isovolumic contraction period, lower right ventricular dP/dt, and systolic peak pressure occurs early during the ejection. Furthermore, the ejection continues despite the rapid and marked decline in pressure.[103]

As a result of the low intraventricular and, consequently, low intramural pressure, the coronary blood flow in the right ventricle is continuous throughout the cardiac cycle. In spite of these differences, the mechanical behaviour of the right ventricle closely resembles that of its left companion. An increase in right ventricular filling (reflected by increases in end diastolic volume and pressure, and related to an increase in resting fibre length) leads to an augmentation of right ventricular stroke volume and stroke work according to the Frank–Starling law. Similar to the left ventricle, there is an inverse relationship between the impedance opposing ejection and the right ventricular function expressed as either ejection fraction or stroke volume.

An augmentation of right ventricular preload and positive inotropic stimulation will improve right ventricular performance.[99 101] The right ventricle is more sensitive to increases in afterload than the left one. With increasing resistance to ejection (for example, in pulmonary hypertension), the right ventricle readily uses up its preload reserve and dilates. As a result of the high chamber compliance of the thin walled right ventricle, the increase in end diastolic volume can be more pronounced than the increase in filling pressure. Thus, the right ventricle is able to maintain normal pulmonary blood flow and left ventricular filling without an undue increase in central venous pressure. The right ventricular ejection fraction will, however, exhibit a linear decrease with increasing afterload.[99 101] A prerequisite to the maintenance of flow is an adequate preload reserve. Yet, there is a limitation to right ventricular performance, as a normal, non-hypertrophied right ventricle will not sustain an acute increase in peak systolic pressure of more than 70–80 mm Hg without failing.[101]

Similar to the left ventricle and the systemic circulation, the coupling of the right ventricle and the pulmonary vasculature was studied by means of the time varying elastance model, which revealed an optimal matching between the right ventricle and its load under physiological conditions.[102] The right ventricular P/V loop reflects its ejection characteristics. Iso-volumic contraction is almost absent, and there is a continuous decrease in ventricular volume after the end systolic point. The slope of the end systolic P/V relationship (right ventricular E_{max}) is lower and the volume intercept (V_0) is higher in the right than in the left ventricle.[103]

The right ventricle appears to have better tolerance of acute decreases in pulmonary compliance (for example, occlusion of a central pulmonary artery branch) than of increases in resistance (for example, peripheral pulmonary embolisation or lung hyperinflation).[104 105]

Considering the close anatomical relationship between both ventricles, it is not surprising that changes in geometry, pressure, and volume of one ventricle directly affect the function of the other. This is known as ventricular cross talk or interdependence, and occurs in both diastole and systole.[106 107] An increase in filling volume of one ventricle causes an upward shift of the diastolic P/V relationship, a decrease in diastolic chamber compliance, and impaired filling of the other ventricle. For instance, an increase in right ventricular diastolic volume and pressure leads to an inversion of the diastolic trans-septal pressure gradient, flattening of the ventricular septum curvature, and a leftward shift of the septum during diastole; these effects increase the stiffness of the left ventricle and limit its filling. In patients with an overloaded and failing right ventricle, right ventricular filling pressure (right atrial pressure) exceeds left sided filling pressure (left atrial pressure or wedge pressure). Diastolic ventricular interdependence is more pronounced with the pericardium intact.[108 109]

The term "systolic interdependence" describes the observation that an increase in pressure in one ventricle leads to an immediate pressure increase in the other ventricle. The contribution of the left ventricle to pressure generation in the right ventricle exceeds the contribution of the right to the left ventricle and is estimated to be about one third of the right ventricular systolic pressure.[110] Although ventricular interdependence operates primarily through the interventricular septum, the free walls of both ventricles are also involved: in the case of the right ventricle, this is accomplished by pulling the right ventricular free wall against the septum during contraction of the intertwining muscle bundles shared by both ventricles.[108 111] This mechanism of "left ventricular assistance", combined with the force acting from behind ("vis a tergo") imparted by left ventricular contraction, explains why there is only a modest depression of haemodynamic function after total exclusion of the right ventricular free wall, provided that there is low pulmonary vascular resistance.[112]

The diastolic and systolic interdependence plays an important role in clinical conditions such as right ventricular volume or pressure overload and right ventricular ischaemia. In these conditions, both diastolic filling and systolic performance of the left ventricle are compromised and left ventricular support of the right ventricle reduced. Therapy aimed at improved left ventricular function and developed pressure will result in enhanced right ventricular function. That will result partly from the interdependence mechanism, and partly from the increase in right ventricular coronary perfusion pressure.

The right ventricle plays an important role in the perioperative period and critical care medicine where acute changes in loading conditions, gas exchange, ventilatory patterns, and coronary blood flow can often eventually lead to right ventricular failure. To assess the right ventricular function properly, to detect its dysfunction in time, and to treat it correctly, the measurement of pressures and flows in the right heart and lesser circulation is necessary (Table 2.2).[18 113]

The use of fast thermistor pulmonary catheters and the thermodilution method for assessment of right ventricular ejection fraction and volumes can provide additional useful information. The most valuable information on the structure and function of the right ventricle at the bedside is now obtained by transthoracic and transoesophageal echocardiography. With the help of echocardiography, and the end diastolic and end systolic size of the right ventricle, its ejection fraction, regional wall motion, septum shifts, and presence of tricuspid and pulmonic valve regurgitation can be evaluated. By means of Doppler measurements of forward and regurgitant

Table 2.2 Right ventricular pump function[18 113]

	Normal values
Right atrial pressure	5 mm Hg
Right ventricular pressure (systolic/diastolic)	25/5 mm Hg
Pulmonary artery pressure (systolic/diastolic)	25/9 mm Hg
Pulmonary artery pressure (mean)	15 (10–20) mm Hg
Right ventricular end diastolic volume index	65–100 ml/m^2
Right ventricular ejection fraction	48–66%
Right ventricular stroke work index	5–10 g·m/m^2

blood flow velocities across the tricuspid and pulmonic valve, estimates of right ventricular and pulmonary artery pressures can be made.

Ventricular performance during exercise

Exercise testing has proven useful as a method of preoperative assessment of cardiac reserve and cardiac risk stratification before anaesthesia and surgery. The ability of the heart to raise its output in response to the stress of trauma and surgery is a prerequisite to uneventful recovery and survival.

During exercise, the heart must increase its output in order to meet the increasing need of the body for oxygen and removal of metabolic end products. The metabolic demands of the exercising muscles are supported by the increased cardiac output and increased oxygen extraction in the tissues. During dynamic (isotonic) exercise, cardiac output increases linearly with increasing work performance and oxygen consumption ($\dot{V}o_2$). The relationship between $\dot{V}o_2$ and cardiac output as a dependent variable has an average y axis intercept of about 6 and a slope of 5–6.[113] For instance, a threefold increase in $\dot{V}o_2$ from 0·25 to 0·75 l/min is associated with an increase in cardiac output from 7·5 to 10·5 l/min. In healthy individuals, the change in cardiac output divided by the change in $\dot{V}o_2$ is more than 6. In this example, it is 3:0·5 = 6. Lower values indicate an inadequate augmentation of cardiac output in relation to oxygen demand.

Maximal oxygen consumption ($\dot{V}o_{2max}$) is reached when $\dot{V}o_2$ levels off despite a further increase in workload and represents the measure of the cardiac reserve (30–85 ml/min per kg depending on the level of physical fitness). Cardiac output increases three to four times to 20–25 l/min during peak exercise in young healthy subjects. In highly trained athletes, values up to 35 l/min were measured.[113] The increased oxygen extraction is reflected by the falling mixed venous oxygen saturation and a two- to threefold increase in the arteriovenous O_2 difference at peak exercise.[114 115]

The left ventricular and haemodynamic function during exercise is dependent on the position of the body.[116] In the supine position, the resting values of end diastolic, end systolic, and stroke volumes are higher than in the upright position, although the heart rate tends to be lower. During exercise in the supine position, there is only a modest initial increase (up to + 20%) in stroke volume, and the increased cardiac output results predominantly from tachycardia. In contrast, during upright exercise the Starling mechanism is more important. This is reflected by a marked increase in the initially lower end diastolic volume and a more pronounced increase (up to 50%) in stroke volume. There is a consistent reduction in end systolic volume and, consequently, an increase in ejection fraction.[117 118] The stroke volume levels off at about 40% of the maximum workload and, therefore, it is the progressive increase in heart rate to its maximum (180–200 beats/min) that is responsible for the attainment of the maximum cardiac output. The final maximal heart rate and cardiac output in both positions are the same, and ventricular volumes also become comparable.[116 117] Thus, the increase in preload (brought about by enhanced venous return from working muscles and mobilisation of blood volume, mostly from the splanchnic reservoir) and the increase in heart rate, together with sympathetically mediated enhancement of myocardial contractility, result in the required increase in cardiac output. Systemic vascular resistance progressively falls with an increasing level of isotonic exercise, reflecting vasodilation in the exercising muscles. Systolic blood pressure rises while diastolic pressure remains unchanged or falls.[113] Consequently, there is only a modest increase in left ventricular afterload during isotonic exercise. However, during isometric exercise (weight lifting, hand grip) systemic vascular resistance increases together with systolic and diastolic blood pressure, and this is associated with a marked augmentation of left ventricular afterload and myocardial oxygen consumption. There is also a difference between leg and arm exercise with the latter producing a more pronounced rate and pressure response despite a lower $\dot{V}o_{2max}$.

Endurance training based on isotonic exercise of adequate intensity and repetition frequency leads to increases in resting blood volume and oxygen carrying capacity, end diastolic and end systolic volumes, and ejection fraction. The heart rate is low at rest. The higher cardiac output achieved by trained individuals results primarily from a higher stroke volume, whereas the peak heart rates are similar in athletes and sedentary subjects.

Prolonged severe exercise produces alterations in ventricular function that can persist for up to 24 hours. In tests on athletes immediately after finishing a triathlon race, a decrease in left ventricular end diastolic dimension and shortening fraction associated with a depression of the wall stress/shortening velocity relationship was found, suggestive of decreased preload and impaired contractility.[119] In tests on runners after a high altitude mountain run, an isolated and marked right ventricular dilatation and depressed pump function associated with pulmonary hypertension were described in one third of them.[120] One can only speculate on the cardiac consequences of prolonged intensive therapy when accompanied by tachycardia comparable to that observed during strenuous exercise.

Changes in ventricular performance related to ageing

As age itself is rarely a contraindication to surgery, anaesthetists are increasingly encountering very old patients undergoing major surgery that puts formidable stress on the cardiovascular system. It is therefore important to understand the changes in cardiac function associated with ageing.[121]

On consideration of the high prevalence of clinically latent coronary artery disease and hypertension in elderly people, it is not easy to separate the effects of ageing from other pathological processes, and this may well explain some of the variations in the published data.[122] Ageing is associated with increasing stiffness of the great arteries, which in turn leads to increases in arterial pulse wave velocity and pulse wave amplitude. The ejection of stroke volume into a stiffer arterial tree and the accelerated reflected pulse waves returning before the aortic valve closure result in higher systolic pressures.[123] Thus, there is an increase in left ventricular systolic load manifesting itself as alterations in aortic input impedance. The characteristic impedance increases, there is increased fluctuation of the impedance moduli about the mean, and both the minimum modulus and the pressure–flow phase crossover shift to higher frequencies. The zero frequency impedance modulus, representing resistance to steady flow (systemic vascular resistance), was found to increase with age in some but not in all studies. The left ventricle responds to the augmented hydraulic load and wall stress by a modest increase in left ventricular wall thickness and mass, which, according to Laplace's law, will normalise the systolic wall stress. In experimental studies, changes in excitation–contraction coupling were found in senescent myocardium resulting in prolonged contraction.[122] At rest, ejection time, stroke volume, and ejection fraction are well preserved even in very old individuals. On the other hand, there are marked alterations in left ventricular filling.[124] Ageing prolongs the isovolumic relaxation time, reduces peak filling rate, and increases inhomogeneity in regional lengthening. Surprisingly, end diastolic volume remains well preserved despite these filling abnormalities and was even shown to increase with age. This may be related to the small increase in left atrial (wedge) pressure and increased atrioventricular pressure gradient and/or increased filling in the late diastole resulting from enhanced atrial contraction. The resting heart rate decreases with advancing age, accompanied by reduced heart rate variability and diminished intrinsic rate of the sinus node. Reports on changes in cardiac output with age vary, with both reductions and no change in cardiac output being described.[122] In elderly populations with maintained cardiac output, an increase in stroke volume associated with the reported increase in end diastolic volume presumably made up for the reduction in heart rate.

Ageing is associated with a progressive decline in both basal and maximal oxygen uptake ($\dot{V}o_{2max}$) and maximal heart rate, whereas the relationship between $\dot{V}o_2$ and heart rate during increasing workload remains linear and has the same slope in both old and young subjects. At peak exercise, increases in heart rate, cardiac output, and ejection fraction are lower in old compared with young subjects. Furthermore, the mechanism by which cardiac output rises during exercise is altered in old subjects: there is more reliance on the Frank–Starling mechanism manifesting itself as an increase in end diastolic volume. Furthermore, compared with younger subjects, end systolic volume increases at higher levels of exercise; together with the diminished heart rate response, these represent the principal age related alterations, resulting in blunted or even absent increase in ejection fraction and yet a well preserved stroke volume. In men at maximal workloads, end diastolic and end systolic volumes and systemic vascular resistance increased with increasing age, whereas inverse correlations between age and heart rate, cardiac index, ejection fraction, and contractility index were described.[125 126] There is also an inverse linear relationship between age and peak filling rate during exercise.[124] Thus, there is unequivocal evidence of a progressively diminished cardiac reserve in healthy ageing individuals.

1 Braunwald E, Ross J Jr, Sonnenblick EH. *Mechanisms of contraction of the normal and failing heart*. Boston: Little, Brown & Company, 1968:31–76.
2 Brady AJ. Mechanical properties of cardiac fibers. In: Berne RM, ed, *Handbook of physiology*, Section 2, *Cardiovascular system. The heart*, Vol 1. Bethesda, MD: American Physiological Society, 1979:461–74.
3 Lew WYW. Mechanisms of volume-induced increase in left ventricular contractility. *Am J Physiol* 1993;**265**:H1778–86.
4 Weber KT, Janicki JS, Hunter WC, Shroff S, Pearlman ES, Fishman AP. The contractile behavior of the heart and its functional coupling to the circulation. *Prog Cardiovasc Dis* 1982;**XXIV**:375–400.
5 Weber KT, Janicki JS. The dynamics of ventricular contraction: force, length, and shortening. *Fed Proc* 1980;**39**:188–95.
6 Weber KT, Hawthorne EW. Descriptors and determinants of cardiac shape: an overview. *Fed Proc* 1981;**40**:2005–10.
7 Strobeck JE, Krueger J, Sonnenblick EH. Load and time considerations in the force–length relation of cardiac muscle. *Fed Proc* 1980;**39**:175–82.
8 Weber KT, Janicki JS. The metabolic demand and oxygen supply of the heart: physiologic and clinical considerations. *Am J Cardiol* 1979;**44**:722–9.
9 Parmley WW, Talbot L. Heart as a pump. In: Berne RM, ed, *Handbook of physiology*, Section 2, *Cardiovascular system. The heart*, Vol 1. Bethesda, MD: American Physiological Society, 1979:429–60.
10 Braunwald E, Ross J Jr. Control of cardiac performance. In: Berne RM, ed, *Handbook of physiology*, Section 2, *Cardiovascular system. The heart*, Vol 1. Bethesda, MD: American Physiological Society, 1979:533–80.
11 Katz AM. Influence of altered inotropy and lusitropy on ventricular pressure–volume loops. *J Am Coll Cardiol* 1988;**11**:438–45.
12 Weber KT, Janicki JS. The heart as a muscle-pump system, and the concept of heart failure. *Am Heart J* 1979;**98**:371–84.
13 Vatner SFE, Braunwald E. Cardiovascular control mechanisms in the conscious state. *N Engl J Med* 1975;**293**:970–6.
14 Baan J, van der Velde EJ. Sensitivity of left ventricular end systolic pressure–volume relation to type of loading interventions in dogs. *Circ Res* 1988;**62**:1247–58.
15 Westerhof N, Elzinga G. Cardiac pump function. In: Strackee J, Westerhof N, eds, *The physics of heart and circulation*. Bristol: Institute of Physics, 1993:207–21.
16 Toorop GP, Van Den Horn GJ, Elzinga G, Westerhof N. Matching between feline left ventricle and arterial load: optimal power or efficiency? *Am J Physiol* 1988;**254**:H279–85.

17 Kass DA, Beyar R. Evaluation of contractile state by maximal ventricular power divided by the square of end-diastolic volume. *Circulation* 1991;**84**:1698–708.

18 Yang SS, Bentivoglio LB, Maranhao V, Goldberg H. *From cardiac catheterization data to hemodynamic parameters*, 2nd edn. Philadelphia: FA Davis Co., 1978:233–325.

19 Robotham JL, Takata M, Berman M, Harasawa Y. Ejection fraction revisited. *Anesthesiology* 1991;**74**:172–83.

20 Clements FM, Harpole DH, Quill T, Jones RH, McCann RL. Estimation of left ventricular volume and ejection fraction by two-dimensional transoesophageal echocardiography: comparison of short axis imaging and simultaneous radionuclide angiography. *Br J Anaesth* 1990;**64**:331–6.

21 Urbanowitz JH, Cahalan MK, Chatterjee KL, Schiller NB. Comparison of transoesophageal echocardiographic and scintigraphic estimates of left ventricular end-diastolic volume index and ejection fraction in patients following coronary artery bypass grafting. *Anesthesiology* 1990;**72**:607–12.

22 Smith MD, MacPhail B, Harrison MR, Lenhoff SJ, DeMaria AN. Value and limitations of transesophageal echocardiography in determination of left ventricular volumes and ejection fraction. *J Am Coll Cardiol* 1992;**19**:1213–22.

23 Pohost GM, O'Rourke RA. *Principles and practice of cardiovascular imaging*. Boston: Little, Brown & Co, 1991:383–503.

24 Leung JM, Schiller NB, Mangano D. Assessment of left ventricular function using two-dimensional transesophageal echocardiography. In: de Bruijn NP, Clements FM, eds, *Intraoperative use of echocardiography*. A Society of Cardiovascular Anesthesiologists Monograph. Philadelphia: JB Lippincott Co., 1991:59–75.

25 Nessly ML, Bashein G, Detmer PR, Graham, MM, Kao R, Martin RW. Left ventricular ejection fraction: single-plane and multiplanar transesophageal echocardiography versus equilibrium gated-pool scintigraphy. *J Cardiothorac Vasc Anesth* 1991;**5**:40–5.

26 Cahalan MK, Ionescu, P, Melton HE Jr, Adler S, Kee LL, Schiller NB. Automated real-time analysis of intraoperative transesophageal echocardiograms. *Anesthesiology* 1993;**78**:477–85.

27 Lindower PD, Rath L, Preslar J, Burns TL, Rezai K, Vandenberg BF. Quantification of left ventricular function with an automated border detection system and comparison with radionuclide ventriculography. *Am J Cardiol* 1994;**73**:195–9.

28 Mirsky I. Elastic properties of the myocardium: a quantitative approach with physiological and clinical applications. In: Berne RM, ed, *Handbook of physiology,* Section 2, *Cardiovascular system. The Heart,* Vol 1. Bethesda, MD: American Physiological Society, 1979:407–32.

29 Nichols WW, Pepine CJ. Left ventricular afterload and aortic input impedance: implications of pulsatile blood flow. *Prog Cardiovasc Dis* 1982;**XXIV**:293–305.

30 Pasipoularides A. Clinical assessment of ventricular ejection dynamics with and without outflow obstruction. *J Am Coll Cardiol* 1990;15:859–82.

31 Noble MIM. Left ventricular load, arterial impedance and their interrelationship. *Cardiovasc Res* 1979;**13**:183–98.

32 Covell JW, Pouleur H, Ross J Jr. Left ventricular wall stress and aortic input impedance. *Fed Proc* 1980;**39**:202–7.

33 Merillon JP, Fontenier GJ, Lerallut JF, et al. Aortic input impedance in normal man and arterial hypertension: its modification during changes in aortic pressure. *Cardiovasc Res* 1982;**16**:646–56.

34 O'Rourke MF, Kelly RP. Wave reflection in the systemic circulation and its implications in ventricular function. *J Hypertens* 1993;**11**:327–37.

35 Pouleur H, Covell JW, Ross J Jr. Effects of alterations in aortic input impedance on the force–velocity–length relationship in the intact canine heart. *Circ Res* 1979;**45**:126–36.

36 Yin FC-P. Ventricular wall stress. *Circ Res* 1981;**49**:829–42.

37 Arts T, Prinzen FW, Reneman RS. Mechanics of the wall of the left ventricle. In: Strackee J, Westerhof N, eds, *The physics of heart and circulation*. Bristol: Institute of Physics, 1993:153–74.

38 Sunagawa K, Sagawa K, Maughan ML. Ventricular interaction with the vascular system in terms of pressure–volume relationships. In: Yin FCP, ed, *Ventricular/Vascular coupling*. New York: Springer Verlag, 1987:210–39.

39 Kass DA, Maughan WL, Guo ZM, Kono A, Sunagawa K, Sagawa K. Comparative influence of load versus inotropic states on indexes of ventricular contractility: experimental and theoretical analysis based on pressure–volume relationships. *Circulation* 1987;**76**:1422–36.

40 Suga H, Sagawa K, Shoukas AA. Load independence of the instantaneous pressure–volume relation of the canine left ventricle and the effects of epinephrine and heart rate on the ratio. *Circ Res* 1973;**32**:314–22.

41 Grossman W, Braunwald E, Mann T, McLaurin LP, Green LH. Contractile state of the left ventricle in man as evaluated from end-systolic pressure–volume relations. *Circulation* 1977;**56**:845–52.

42 Kass DA, Maughan WL. From "Emax" to pressure–volume relations: a broader view. *Circulation* 1988;**77**:1203–12.

43 Mehmel HC, Stockins B, Ruffmann K, van Olshausen K, Schuler G, Kübler W. The linearity of the end-systolic pressure–volume relationship in man and its sensitivity for assessment of left ventricular function. *Circulation* 1981;**63**:1216–22.

44 Van Der Velde ET, Van Dijk AD, Steendijk P, et al. Nonlinearity and afterload sensitivity of the end-systolic pressure–volume relation of the canine left ventricle in vivo. *Circulation* 1991;**83**:315–27.

45 Kass DA. Clinical evaluation of left heart function by conductance catheter technique. *Eur Heart J* 1992;**13**(suppl E):57–64.

46 Asanoi H, Shigetake S, Kameyama T. Ventriculoarterial coupling in normal and failing heart in humans. *Circ Res* 1989;**65**:483–93.

47 Schreuder JJ, Biervliet JD, van der Velde ET, et al. Systolic and diastolic pressure–volume relationships during cardiac surgery. *J Cardiothorac Vasc Anesth* 1991;**5**:539–45.

48 Sasayama S. Matching of ventricular properties with arterial load under normal and variably depressed cardiac states. In: Lewis BS, Kimchi A, eds, *Heart failure mechanisms and management*. Berlin: Springer-Verlag, 1991:59–67.

49 Gorcsan J III, Romand JA, Mandarino WA, Deneault LG, Pinsky MR. Assessment of left ventricular performance by on-line pressure–area relations using echocardiographic automated border detection. *J Am Coll Cardiol* 1994;**23**:242–52.

50 Gorcsan J III, Gasior TA, Mandarino WA, Deneault LG, Hattler BG, Pinsky MR. Assessment of the immediate effects of cardiopulmonary bypass on left ventricular performance by on-line pressure–area relations. *Circulation* 1994;**89**:180–90.

51 O'Kelly BF, Tubau JF, Knight AA, et al. Measurement of left ventricular contractility using transesophageal echocardiography in patients undergoing coronary artery bypass grafting. *Am Heart J* 1991;**122**:1041–9.

52 Dahlgren G, Veintemilla F, Settergren G, Liska J. Left ventricular end-systolic pressure estimated from measurements in a peripheral artery. *J Cardiothorac Vasc Anesth* 1991;**5**:551–3.

53 Carabello BA, Spann JF. The uses and limitations of end-systolic indexes of left ventricular function. *Circulation* 1984;**69**:1058–64.

54 Carabello BA. Ratio of end-systolic stress to end-systolic volume: is it a useful clinical tool? *J Am Coll Cardiol* 1989;**14**:496–8.

55 Shih H, Hillel Z, Declerck C, Anagnostopoulos C, Kuroda M, Thys D. An algorithm for real time continuous evaluation of left ventricular mechanics by single-beat estimation of arterial and ventricular elastance. *J Clin Monit* 1997;**13**:157–70.

56 Glower DD, Spratt JA, Snow ND, et al. Linearity of the Frank–Starling relationship in the intact heart: the concept of preload recruitable stroke work. *Circulation* 1985;**71**:994–1009.

57 Feneley MP, Skelton TN, Kisslo KB, Davis JW, Bashore TM, Rankin JS. Comparison of preload recruitable stroke work, end-systolic pressure–volume and dP/dt_{max}–end-diastolic volume relations as indexes of left ventricular contractile performance in patients undergoing routine cardiac catheterization. *J Am Coll Cardiol* 1992;**19**:1522–30.

58 Takeuchi M, Odake M, Takaoka H, Hayashi Y, Yokoyama M. Comparison between preload recruitable stroke work and the end-systolic pressure–volume relationship in man. *Eur Heart J* 1992;**13**(suppl E):80–4.

69

59 Lang RM, Briller RA, Neumann A, Borow KM. Assessment of global and regional left ventricular mechanics: applications to myocardial ischemia. In: Kerber RE, ed, *Echocardiography in coronary artery disease*. Mount Kisco, NY: Futura, 1988:221–57.

60 Sharir T, Haber H, Feldman M, Marmor A, Kass DA. Ventricular systolic assessment in patients with dilated cardiomyopathy by preload-adjusted maximal power: validation and non-invasive application. *Circulation* 1994;**89**:2049–53.

61 Nakayama M, Chen C-H, Nevo E, Fetics B, Wong E, Kass DA. Optimal preload adjustment of maximal ventricular power index varies with cardiac chamber size. *Am Heart J* 1998;**136**:281–8.

62 Seed WA, Walker JM. Relation between beat interval and force of the heartbeat and its clinical implications. *Cardiovasc Res* 1988;**22**:303–14.

63 Freeman GL, Little WC, O'Rourke RA. Influence of heart rate on left ventricular performance in conscious dogs. *Circ Res* 1987;**61**:455–64.

64 Miura T, Miazaki S, Guth BD, Kambayashi M, Ross J Jr. Influence of the force–frequency relation on left ventricular function during exercise in conscious dogs. *Circulation* 1992;**86**:563–71.

65 Ross J Jr, Miura T, Kambayashi M, Eising GP, Ryu KH. Adrenergic control of the force–frequency relation. *Circulation* 1995;**92**:2327–32.

66 Kambayashi M, Miura T, Oh B-H, Rockman HA, Murata K, Ross J Jr. Enhancement of the force frequency effect on myocardial contractility by adrenergic stimulation in conscious dogs. *Circulation* 1992, **86**:572–80.

67 DePauw M, Bao SM, Heyndrikx GR. Reversible left ventricular dysfunction induced by short term (48 hrs) rapid pacing in conscious dogs: non-ischemic myocardial stunning (abstract). *Circulation* 1993;**88**(part 2):I29.

68 Erdmann E, Beuckelmann D, Boehm M, Schwinger HG. Klinische Gesichtspunkte der medikamentoesen Differentialtherapie der chronischen Herzinsuffizienz. *Z Kardiol* 1992;**81**(suppl 4):**97**–103.

69 Sunagawa K, Maughan WL, Burkhoff D, Sagawa K. Left ventricular interaction with arterial load studied in isolated canine ventricle. *Am J Physiol* 1983;**245**:H773–80.

70 Burkhoff D, Sagawa K. Ventricular efficiency predicted by an analytical model. *Am J Physiol* 1986;**250**:R1021–7.

71 Starling MR. Left ventricular–arterial coupling relations in the normal human heart. *Am Heart J* 1993;**125**:1659–66.

72 Suga H. Ventricular energetics. *Am J Physiol* 1990;**70**:247–77.

73 Nozawa T, Yasumura Y, Futaki S, et al. Relation between oxygen consumption and pressure–volume area of in situ dog heart. *Am J Physiol* 1987;**253**:H31–40.

74 Nozawa T, Cheng C-P, Noda T, Little WC. Relation between left ventricular oxygen consumption and pressure–volume area in conscious dogs. *Circulation* 1994;**89**:810–17.

75 Suga H. How we view systolic function of the heart: E max and PVA. 1994 CSDS Konrad Witzig Lecture. In: Ingels NB Jr, Daughters GT, Baan J, Covel JW, Reneman, RS, Yin FC-P, eds, *Systolic and diastolic function of the heart*. Amsterdam: IOS Press, 1995:215–25.

76 Takaoka H, Takeuchi M, Odake M, Yokoyama M. Assessment of myocardial oxygen consumption (Vo_2) and systolic pressure–volume area (PVA) in human hearts. *Eur Heart J* 1992;**13** (suppl E):85–90.

77 Vanoverschelde J-LJ, Wijns W, Essamri B, et al. Hemodynamic and mechanical determinants of myocardial O_2 consumption in normal heart: effects of dobutamine. *Am J Physiol* 1993;**265**:H1884–92.

78 Guyton AC, Jones CE, Coleman TG. *Circulatory physiology: cardiac output and its regulation*. Philadelphia: WB Saunders, 1973:137–252.

79 Elzinga G. "Starling's law of the heart" a historical misinterpretation. *Basic Res Cardiol* 1989;**84**:1–4.

80 Melbin J, Detweiler DK, Riffle RA, Noordergraaf A. Coherence of cardiac output with rate changes. *Am J Physiol* 1982;**243**:H499–504.

81 Jacob R, Dierberger B, Kissling G. Functional significance of the Frank–Starling mechanism under physiological and pathophysiological conditions. *Eur Heart J* 1992;**13** (suppl E):7–14.

82 Plotnick GD, Becker LC, Fisher ML, et al. Use of the Frank–Starling mechanism during submaximal versus maximal upright exercise. *Am J Physiol* 1986;251:H1101–5.

83 Parker JO, Case RB. Normal left ventricular function. *Circulation* 1979;60:4–11.

84 Lee J-D, Tajimi T, Patritti J, Ross J Jr. Preload reserve and mechanisms of afterload mismatch in normal conscious dog. *Am J Physiol* 1986;**250**:H464–73.

85 Feneley MP, Karunanithi M, Michniewicz J, Young J, Kalnins W. Rapid contractile upregulation rematches stroke work to increased afterload independent of ventricular geometry, afterload-related coronary perfusion pressure fluctuations and baseline contractile state. In: Ingels NB Jr, Daughters GT, Baan J, Covel JW, Reneman RS, Yin F C-P, eds, *Systolic and diastolic function of the heart*. Amsterdam: IOS Press, 1995:325–44.

86 Ross J Jr. Afterload mismatch and preload reserve: a conceptual framework for the analysis of ventricular function. *Prog Cardiovasc Dis* 1976;**28**:255–63.

87 Nishimura RA, Abel MD, Hatle LK, Tajik AJ. Assessment of diastolic function of the heart: background and current applications of Doppler echocardiography. Part II. Clinical studies. *Mayo Clin Proc* 1989;**64**:181–204.

88 Mirsky I, Pasipoularides A. Clinical assessment of diastolic function. *Prog Cardiovasc Dis* 1990;**XXXII**:291–318.

89 Little WC, Downes TR. Clinical evaluation of left ventricular diastolic performance. *Prog Cardiovasc Dis* 1990;**XXXII**:273–90.

90 Brutsaert DL, Sys SU. Relaxation and diastole of the heart. *Physiol Rev* 1989;**69**:1228–315.

91 Brutsaert DL, Sys SU, Gillebert TC. Diastolic dysfunction in post-cardiac surgical management. *J Cardiothorac Vasc Anesth* 1993;7(suppl 1):18–20.

92 Gillebert TC, Sys SU. Physiologic control of relaxation in isolated cardiac muscle and intact left ventricle. In: Gaasch WH, LeWinter MM, eds, *Left ventricular diastolic dysfunction and heart failure*. Philadelphia: Lea & Febiger, 1994:25–42.

93 Brutsaert DL, Sys SU, Gillebert TC. Diastolic failure: pathophysiology and therapeutic implications. *J Am Coll Cardiol* 1993;**22**:318–25.

94 Moon MR, Ingels NB Jr, Daughters GT, Stinson EB, Hansen DE, Miller DC. Alterations in left ventricular twist mechanics with inotropic stimulation and volume loading in human subjects. *Circulation* 1994;**89**:142–50.

95 Beyar R, Yin F C-P, Hausknecht M, Weisfeldt MC, Kass DA. Dependence of left ventricular twist–radial shortening relations on cardiac cycle phase. *Am J Physiol* 1989;**257**:H1119- 26.

96 Gaasch WH, Quinones MA, Waisser E, Thiel HG, Alexander JK. Diastolic compliance of the left ventricle in man. *Am J Cardiol* 1975;**36**:193–201.

97 Gaasch WH. Passive elastic properties of the left ventricle. In: Gaasch WH, LeWinter MM, eds, *Left ventricular diastolic dysfunction and heart failure*. Philadelphia: Lea & Febiger, 1994:143–9.

98 March HW, Ross JK, Lower RR. Observations on the behavior of the right ventricular outflow tract, with reference to its developmental origins. *Am J Med* 1962;**32**:835–45.

99 Morris JJ III, Wechsler AS. Right ventricular function: the assessment of contractile performance. In: Fisk RL, ed, *The right heart*. Philadelphia: FA Davis, 1987:3–18.

100 Furey SA III, Zieske HA, Levy MN. The essential function of the right ventricle. *Am Heart J* 1984;**107**:404–10.

101 Hurford WE, Zapol WM. The right ventricle and critical illness: a review of anatomy, physiology, and clinical evaluation of its function. *Intensive Care Med* 1988;**14**:448–57.

102 Piene H. Matching between right ventricle and pulmonary bed. In: Yin FC-P, ed, *Ventricular/Vascular coupling*. New York: Springer-Verlag, 1987:180–202.

103 Dell'Italia LJ, Santamore WP. Can indices of left ventricular function be applied to the right ventricle? *Prog Cardiovasc Dis*, 1998;**40**:309–24.

104 Pouleur H, Lefevre J, van Eyll C, Jaumin PM, Charlier AA. Significance of pulmonary input impedance in right ventricular performance. *Cardiovasc Res* 1978;**12**:617–29.

105 Ghignone M, Girling L, Prewitt RM. Effect of increased pulmonary vascular resistance on right ventricular systolic performance in dogs. *Am J Physiol* 1984;**246**:H339–43.

106 Bove A, Santamore WP. Ventricular interdependence. *Prog Cardiovasc Dis* 1981; **23**:365–88.

107 Olsen CO, Tyson GS, Maier GW, Spratt JA, Davis JW, Rankin JS. Dynamic ventricular interaction in the conscious dog. *Circ Res* 1983;**52**:85–104.

108 Weber KT, Janicki JS, Schroff S, Fishman AP. Contractile mechanics and interaction of the right and left ventricles. *Am J Cardiol* 1981;**47**:686–95.

109 Beyar R, Dong S-J, Smith ER, Belenkie I, Tyberg JV. Ventricular interaction and septal deformation: a model compared with experimental data. *Am J Physiol* 1993;**265**: H2044–56.

110 Santamore WP, Dell'Italia LJ. Ventricular interdependence: significant left ventricular contributions to right ventricular systolic function. *Prog Cardiovasc Dis* 1998; **40**:289–308.

111 Clyne CA, Alpert JS, Benotti JR. Interdependence of the left and right ventricles in health and disease. *Am Heart J* 1989;**117**:1366–73.

112 Jones DL, Guiraudon GM, Klein GJ. Total disconnection of the right ventricular free wall: physiological consequences in the dog. *Am Heart J* 1984;**107**:1169–77.

113 Lentner C. *Geigy scientific tables, the heart and circulation*, Vol 5. Basel: Ciba-Geigy Ltd, 1990:9–219.

114 Fleg JL, Schulman SP, O'Connor FC, et al. Cardiovascular responses to exhaustive upright cycle exercise in highly trained older men. *J Appl Physiol* 1994;**77**:1500–6.

115 Hammond K, Froelicher VF. Normal and abnormal heart rate responses to exercise. *Prog Cardiovasc Dis* 1985;**27**:271–96.

116 Poliner LR, Dehmer GJ, Lewis SE, Parkey RW, Blomquist CG, Willerson JT. Left ventricular performance in normal subjects: a comparison of the responses to exercise in the upright and supine positions. *Circulation* 1980;**62**:528–34.

117 Cotsamire DL, Sullivan MJ, Bashore TM, Leier CV. Position as a variable for cardiovascular responses during exercise. *Clin Cardiol* 1987;**10**:137–42.

118 Iskandrian AS, Hakki A-U, DePace NL, Manno B, Segal BL. Evaluation of left ventricular function by radionuclide angiography during exercise in normal subjects and in patients with chronic coronary heart disease. *J Am Coll Cardiol* 1983;**1**:1518–29.

119 ML Weisfeldt, ed, *The aging heart. Its function and response to stress.* Aging, vol 12, New York: Raven Press, 1980:1–6.

120 Douglas PS, O'Toole ML, Hiller WD, Hackney K, Reichek N. Cardiac fatigue after prolonged exercise. *Circulation* 1987;**76**:1206–13.

121 Davila-Roman VG, Guest TM, Tuteur PG, Rowe WJ, Ladenson JH, Jaffe AS. Transient right but not left ventricular dysfunction after strenuous exercise at high altitude. *J Am Coll Cardiol* 1997;**30**:468–73.

122 Lakatta EG. Cardiovascular regulatory mechanisms in advanced age. *Physiol Rev* 1993;**73**:413–53.

123 Fleg JL, Gerstenblith G, Lakatta EG. Pathophysiology of the aging heart and circulation. In: Messerli FH, ed, *Cardiovascular disease in the elderly*, 2nd edn, Boston: Martinus Nijhoff Publishing, 1988:9–35.

124 Schulman SP, Lakatta EG, Fleg JL, Lakatta L, Becker LC, Gerstenblith G. Age-related decline in left ventricular filling at rest and exercise. *Am J Physiol* 1992;**263**:H1932–8.

125 Rodeheffer RJ, Gerstenblith G, Becker LC, Fleg JL, Weisfeldt ML, Lakatta EG. Exercise cardiac output is maintained with advancing age in healthy human subjects: cardiac dilatation and increased stroke volume compensate for a diminished heart rate. *Circulation* 1984;**69**:203–12.

126 Fleg JL, O'Connor F, Gerstenblith G, et al. Impact of age on the cardiovascular response to dynamic upright exercise in healthy men and women. *J Appl Physiol* 1995;**78**:890–900.

3: Cardiac electrophysiology

JOHN L ATLEE

The heart's primary function is to generate contractile forces for the distribution of adequate amounts of blood to the lungs and systemic tissues. For contraction to occur, cells must first be excited – the function of the heart's specialised conducting system. Normally, excitation is initiated by spontaneous depolarisation (automaticity) of pacemaker cells located in the sinoatrial (SA) node. In turn, SA automaticity brings surrounding cells to the threshold for transient depolarisation – termed the "action potential" (AP). Action potentials propagate rapidly to excite atrial and ventricular muscle in preferential atrial pathways and the His–Purkinje conducting system, respectively. The atrioventricular (AV) node functions to slow AV impulse transmission, in order to provide sufficient time for ventricular filling.

The study of normal and abnormal mechanisms for generation and propagation of cardiac APs is termed "cardiac electrophysiology". It is the basis for understanding normal sinus rhythm and cardiac arrhythmias, and also antiarrhythmic drug or device actions. There are normal and abnormal cardiac electrophysiological processes; the latter can result from either an abnormal cardiac substrate (for example, accessory pathways or scar tissue) or a pathophysiological disease process (for example, ischaemia, adverse drug actions, or electrolyte imbalance).

Normal cardiac electrophysiology

Cardiac electrophysiology can be resolved at the macroscopic and cellular levels.[1][2] At the macroscopic level, the surface electrocardiogram (ECG) records electrical activity from an aggregate of myocardial cells. Slow depolarisation and delayed repolarisation are seen as QRS widening and prolongation of the QT interval, respectively. At the microscopic level, a single cardiac cell is impaled by a microelectrode, and an AP is recorded after a suitable excitatory stimulus. The rising AP upstroke reflects the rate of depolarisation, whereas final rapid AP repolarisation reflects the rate of repolarisation. Even higher resolution is provided by testing the effects of rapid changes in membrane voltage (voltage clamp) in single cardiac cells, and then recording the associated current – whole cell or macroscopic current.[3] Finally, most resolution is provided by the application of a highly polished microelectrode to a single cell to isolate electrically a small patch of the cell membrane (patch clamp).[4] Patch clamp permits resolution of the opening and closing transitions of individual ion channels.

Properties of cardiac ion channels

The basis for normal excitability (pacemaker potential) and conduction (AP) is the passage of Na^+, K^+, Ca^{2+}, and Cl^- ions across the cardiac plasma membrane (sarcolemma) through specialised voltage and ligand operated ion channels.[1 2 5-7] Ion channels are large membrane spanning proteins. They provide relatively low resistance pathways for the passive (not requiring energy) movement of ions across the lipid bilayer. In contrast, active ion transport mechanisms – such as the membrane Na^+/K^+ exchange pump – do require energy from the hydrolysis of adenosine triphosphate (ATP). Transmembrane ion fluxes probably occur through aqueous pores within the channel protein. It is hypothesised that ions move in single file through the channel pores in a discontinuous fashion, "hopping" between discrete selective binding sites. The variable size of hydrated ions and preferential binding possibly explain ion channel selectivity.[1]

Gating of cardiac ion channels

Based on the process that accounts for opening and closing (gating) of cardiac ion channels, the channels fall into three classes: (1) voltage gated ion channels; (2) ligand or receptor gated ion channels; and (3) stretch activated ion channels.[1 2] These mechanisms are not mutually exclusive. Neurotransmitters and hormones may modulate voltage gated channels, whereas ligand gated channels may show voltage dependence.

Voltage gated ion channels

Voltage gated channels are the largest group of cardiac ion channels. They have charges (dipoles) that sense changes in membrane potential, causing a conformational change in charged ion channel regions, generating small "gating" currents.[8] These precede voltage dependent changes in ion conductance through the ion specific channel. Voltage gated ion channels occupy open or closed conductance states; these are termed the resting state. Most resting channels open in response to depolarisation. The open channel permits ion movement across the cell membrane, with the direction determined by a particular ion's electrochemical gradient (Table 3.1).

The number of closed states preceding channel opening determines the activation kinetics. With a single closed state, the rate of ion conductance

Table 3.1 Ion concentration and equilibrium potentials in cardiac fibres

Ion	Extracellular (mmol/l)	Intracellular (mmol/l)	Ratio (E/I)	E_i (mV)
Na^+	145	15	9·7	+60
K^+	4	150	0·027	−94
Cl^-	120	5	24	−83
Ca^{2+}	2	0·0001	20000	+129

increase is maximal at the onset of depolarisation (Fig 3.1a). With multiple closed states, there is a delay in the rise in conductance (Fig 3.1b). Some ion channels maintain their high state of conductance for the duration of depolarisation. With others, conductance declines despite persistent depolarisation as a result of channel inactivation (Fig 3.1c).

The inactivated state is a second non-conducting state, different from the resting state, because inactivated channels do not usually open in response to membrane depolarisation.[1] Some resting channels bypass the open state, and pass directly into the inactivated state. To reverse inactivation, the membrane must be repolarised to highly negative values – termed "recovery from inactivation". This process is highly voltage dependent, and hastened by membrane hyperpolarisation (that is, repolarisation to a level of resting membrane potential that is more negative than normal). Further, the nature of the voltage dependence of inactivation is characteristic for each channel type. Factors such as temperature, pH, and the concentration of divalent cations may influence the voltage dependence of inactivation.

Hodgkin–Huxley model of Na⁺ channel gating

Nearly 50 years ago, Hodgkin and Huxley proposed a model for the Na^+ channel to account for the transient nature of Na^+ current in response to depolarisation.[9] Despite extensive studies using more complex methods, the basic tenets of their proposal still account for more than 95% of Na^+ channel behaviour.[1] Hodgkin and Huxley suggested that ion movement through the Na^+ channel is controlled by activation (m) and inactivation (h) gates. The behaviour of the channel in response to depolarisation is illustrated in Fig 3.2. A similar model may hold true for other ion channels.[1]

Ligand gated ion channels

Neurotransmitters, ATP or Ca^{2+} ions are ligands for membrane bound receptors and gate ion channels.[1,2] The K^+ selective ion channel opened by muscarinic (M_2) receptor activation is a well studied example.[10] Acetylcholine (ACh) interacts with the muscarinic receptor initiating a sequence of events that result in the dissociation of the α and β–γ subunits of a guanine nucleotide, regulatory G protein – Gi. The α and β–γ subunits of

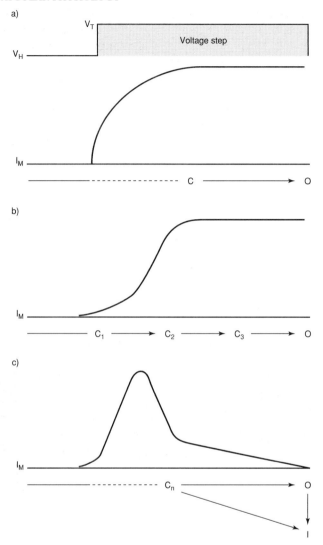

Fig 3.1 Depiction of membrane current (I_M) waveforms generated in response to a voltage step form the holding potential (V_H) to test potential (V_T) in voltage gated ion channels. (a) Non-inactivating channel with a single closed state (C) preceding opening (O). Ion conductance (g) is a function of a single activation variable (n) and maximal from the outset. (b) Non-inactivating channel with several closed states (C_1, C_2, C_3). Ion conductance remains a function of a single activation variable; however, there is a delay in the rise in ion conductance. (c) Inactivating channel with multiple closed states and a single inactivated state (I). Activation (m) and inactivation (h) variables are required for a full description of conductance changes. As in (b), there is a delay in the rise in ion conductance to a maximal value. Current then declines to zero at I, despite maintenance of voltage step depolarisation.

Gi open a K^+ channel.[10] This process is rapid, being limited by hydrolysis of ACh in the synaptic cleft and desensitisation – a sequence of intracellular processes that collectively result in a diminution of the effect of ACh receptor interaction, despite the continued presence of ACh.

Other ligands bind to receptors to *close* an ion channel. The K^+ ATP sensitive channel is closed by normal intracellular levels of ATP; however, a reduction in intracellular ATP concentration to below 0.5 mmol/l results in channel opening.[11] Intracellular pH and the ADP/ATP ratio modulate the sensitivity of the K^+ ATP channel to ATP. Activation of this channel by

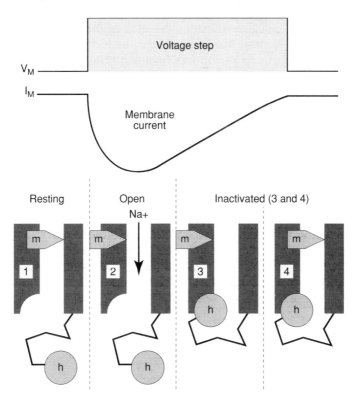

Fig 3.2 Hodgkin-Huxley model of Na^+ channel gating. Depiction of membrane current (I_M) and single channel gating behaviour in response to a step in cell membrane potential (V_M). The Na^+ channel is shown as a pore spanning the sarcolemma bilayer in resting, open, and two inactivated states. (1) Resting state: the activation or m gate is closed, and the inactivation or h gate open. (2) Open state: upon depolarisation, the h gate remains open and the m gate opens to allow movement of Na^+ into the cell. (3) First inactivated state: the h gate then closes to block further Na^+ movement into the cell. (4) Second inactivated state: when the membrane potential has returned to its resting level, the m gate also closes. After a variable time interval, the h gate moves into the open position – a process termed "recovery from inactivation" – returning the Na^+ channel to the resting state.

77

low ATP during myocardial ischaemia shortens the duration of the action potential (APD) of ischaemic fibres, thereby increasing disparity of APD among myocardial fibres. Finally, physical factors such as stretch can activate ion channels,[1] and second messenger systems are involved in signal transduction.

Structure–function relationships of ion channels

The simplest ion channel carries the slow component of the delayed rectifier current (I_K) in cardiac muscle.[12] It consists of a single chain of 130 amino acids spanning the sarcolemmal membrane. The larger family of voltage gated K^+ channels provides the next higher order of structural complexity.[1] Each channel has four subunits, each consisting of 500–1000 amino acids that form six membrane spanning helices. The four subunits may be the same – a homotetramer – or different – a heterotetramer.[13]

The voltage gated Na^+ and Ca^{2+} channels have the highest order of complexity.[1 6 14–16] They consist of the α, β_1, and β_2 subunits. The α subunit is, however, sufficient to form a functional channel. It consists of four homologous domains (I–IV). Each domain has six sarcolemma spanning segments (S1–S6). The structure of each segment is highly conserved between domains; however, peptide chains connecting the segments show more variability. The β subunit of the Na^+ channel modulates the level of expression and kinetics of inactivation of the α subunit,[17] the structure of which is shown in Fig 3.3. The fourth sarcolemma spanning segment has a positively charged amino acid in every fourth position (Fig 3.3), and acts as the voltage sensor ("m" gate) for the activation process.[5 15] The loop between S5 and S6 extends for some distance in the membrane, and is believed to form the channel pore. The loop between the third and fourth homologous domains plays a central role in normal inactivation.[5 15]

Terminology

Three types of cardiac transmembrane potentials (TMPs) can be recorded by inserting a microelectrode (tip diameter = 0.5 μm) into a single cell:

Resting membrane potential (RMP) – The membrane potential during electrical quiescence (diastole) in most fast response fibres.

Action potential (AP) – The changes in transmembrane potential (TMP) that occur when the cell has been brought to threshold for regenerative excitation.

Automatic TMP – Spontaneous, diastolic depolarisation brings some specialised conducting system cells to threshold for an AP. Instead of an RMP, these fibres have a maximum diastolic potential (MDP).

APs for quiescent and automatic cardiac fibre types are shown in Fig 3.4, and a comparison of TMP characteristics for these fibre types in Table 3.2.

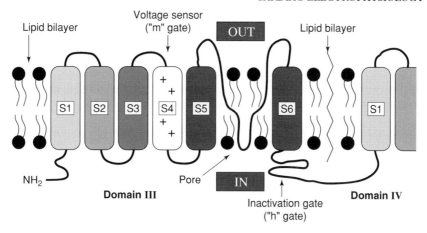

Fig 3.3 Structure of portion of the α subunit of a Na$^+$ channel. Voltage gated ion channels (Na$^+$, K$^+$, and Ca^{2+}) are glycosylated proteins. Each subunit of these contains four covalently linked domains (except for K$^+$ channels) designated I – IV – shown are domain III and a portion of domain IV. Each domain contains six α-helical trans-sarcolemmal segments (S1–S6). S4 is thought to represent the voltage sensor ("m" gate) for the activation process, and the cytoplasmic peptide chain between domains III–S6 and IV–S1 the inactivation or "h" gate.

TMPs may be depolarised, repolarised, or hyperpolarised with respect to a reference or immediately preceding level of TMP (Fig 3.5).

Cardiac action potential

The action potential of a quiescent Purkinje fibre has five phases:

1 *Phase* 0: upstroke or rapid depolarisation phase.
2 *Phase* 1: early rapid repolarisation.
3 *Phase* 2: plateau phase.
4 *Phase* 3: final rapid repolarisation.
5 *Phase* 4: resting or diastolic membrane potential.

That portion of phase 0 when the membrane potential is positive to 0 mV is termed the AP overshoot. Cardiac AP phases, major ionic currents

Cellular cardiac electrophysiology

AP	action potential	LMP	loss of membrane potential
AV	atrioventricular	MDP	maximum diastolic potential
DAD	delayed after depolarisation	RMP	resting membrane potential
DFR	depressed fat response	SA	sinoatrial
EAD	early after depolarisation	TMP	transmembrane potential

Terms

Action potential:	change in TMP after excitation of cell
Automaticity:	spontaneous diastolic depolarisation
Fast response fibre:	atrial, ventricular, or Purkinje fibres with AP upstroke dependent on fast Na$^+$ current
Maximum diastolic potential:	most negative diastolic TMP (automatic fibres)
Resting membrane potential:	stable TMP during diastole (most fast response fibres)
Slow response fibre:	SA and AV node cells with AP upstroke mostly dependent on slow Ca^{2+} current
Transmembrane potential:	electrical potential across cell membrane

---

responsible for generation of the APs, and ion exchange pumps that help to restore ion gradients during phase 4 are depicted in Fig 3.6.[1 19 20]

Resting membrane potential (phase 4)

K$^+$ is the major ion determining RMP, because the cell membrane is quite permeable to K$^+$ during phase 4, but relatively impermeable to other ions. A membrane bound, Na$^+$/K$^+$ exchange pump (Fig 3.6), fuelled by the hydrolysis of ATP, transports three Na$^+$ out of the cell for two K$^+$ into the cell during phase 4. As this pump generates a net outward movement of positive charges, it is "electrogenic". As a result, [Na$^+$]$_i$ and [K$^+$]$_i$ are kept low and high, respectively, with the inside of the cell being negative with respect to the outside. Indeed, in most cardiac cell types, were it not for a small leak of Na$^+$ ions (Fig 3.6), RMP would approach the equilibrium potential for a K$^+$ electrode ($-$ 96 mV). Also, depending on TMP, and Na$^+$ and Ca^{2+} concentrations inside and outside the cell, a passive Na$^+$/Ca^{2+} exchanger can run in the forward or reverse modes to move Na$^+$ or Ca^{2+} into or out of cells (Fig 3.6). This exchanger depends partly on maintenance of the Na$^+$ concentration gradient by the Na$^+$/K$^+$ exchange pump. Under normal conditions, one intracellular Ca^{2+} is exchanged for three or more external Na$^+$ ions. If [Na$^+$]$_i$ is abnormally high – for example, with digitalis toxicity – external Ca^{2+} may be exchanged for internal Na$^+$.

Action potential

The cardiac AP is a propagating wave of transient depolarisation, which begins when an excitatory stimulus (propagating AP, an external stimulus) depolarises the cell membrane beyond threshold potential. The AP is inscribed by the movement of Na$^+$, K$^+$, Ca^{2+}, and Cl$^-$ ions through at least nine distinct voltage or ligand operated ion channels.[1] The Na^+/K^+ pump and Na^+/Ca^{2+} exchanger also contribute to the genesis of the AP by: (1) maintaining membrane ion gradients essential for excitability; (2) generating small currents as the result of net ion movements; and

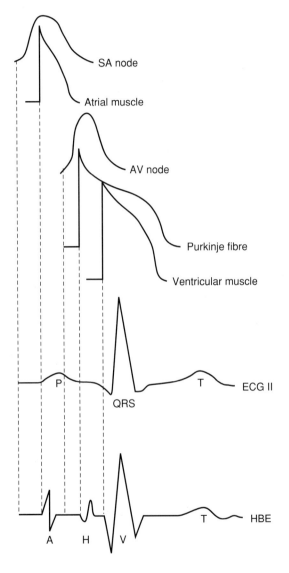

Fig 3.4 Schematic representation of action potentials (APs) from various cardiac fibre types. Approximate timing of APs in relationship to events of surface ECG lead II and His bundle ECG (HBE) for one cardiac cycle is shown. Note that SA and AV nodal activation is electrically silent in both ECG II and HBE.

Table 3.2 Comparison of transmembrane potentials and other action potential characteristics from various cardiac fibre types[a]

	SA node	Atrial	AV node	Purkinje	Ventricular
RMP or MDP (mV)	-50 to -60	-80 to -90	-60 to -70	-90 to -95	-80 to -90
Amplitude (mV)	60–70	110–120	70–80	120	110–120
Overshoot (mV)	0–10	100–200	5–15	30	30
Duration (ms)	100–300	100–300	100–300	300–500	200–300
Upstroke (V/s)	1–10	100–200	5–15	500–700	100–200
Conduction (m/s)	<0·05	0·3–0·4	0·1	2–3	0·3–0·4

[a] Data from Sperelakis.[18] SA, sinoatrial; AV, atrioventricular; RMP or MDP, resting membrane potential (quiescent fibres) or maximum diastolic potential (automatic fibres). Upstroke, maximum upstroke velocity.

(3) restoring normal intracellular ion concentration once the AP is inscribed.

By convention, *inward* (depolarising) currents during the AP reflect movement of positive charges into the myocyte. I_{Na} and I_{Ca} (below) are the major physiological inward currents. *Outward* currents reflect movement of positive charges out of the cell, and repolarise the cell during AP phase 3. K^+ ions are the major charge carrier for outward current in heart.

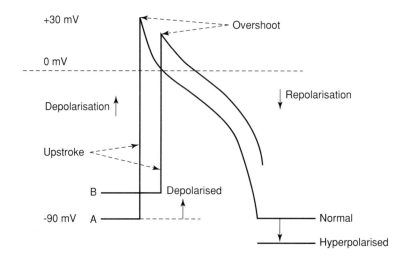

Fig 3.5 Terminology used to describe changes in transmembrane potential (TMP) during cardiac action potential (AP). Depolarisation is towards a more positive (low) level of TMP, and repolarisation towards a more negative (high) level of TMP. Note that action potential "B" arises from a depolarised membrane potential compared with action potential "A". As a result, some Na^+ channels are inactivated, less Na^+ current can flow, and action potential "B" has a slower rate of rise and less overshoot compared with action potential "A". See text for further discussion.

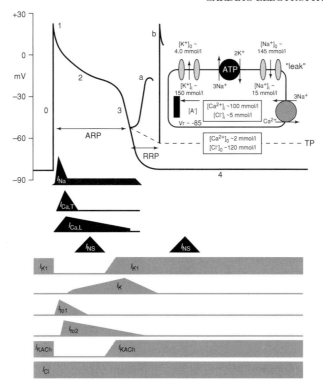

Fig 3.6 Transmembrane currents, ion exchange pumps, and refractory periods in a typical fast response fibre. Inward currents (black) include the fast Na^+ current (I_{Na}); transient or tiny Ca^{2+} current ($I_{Ca,T}$); long-lasting or large Ca^{2+} current ($I_{Ca,L}$); and a non-selective cation current (I_{NS}) carried by a channel activated by intracellular Ca^{2+} loading. Outward currents (grey) include the inward rectifier current (I_{K1}); delayed rectifier current (I_K – shown as the sum of its two components); a rapidly activated, time dependent, non-Ca^{2+} dependent K^+ current (I_{to1}); a transient current that is dependent on $[Ca^{2+}]_i$, and carried by Cl^- in some species (I_{to2}); and a hyperpolarising K^+ current activated by acetylcholine (I_{ACh}). A chloride conductance (I_{Cl}) dependent protein kinase A can be activated in some species. Typical intra- and extracellular ion concentrations during phase 4 are shown (top right). The predominant intracellular anions (A^-) are large, impermeable proteins. The ATP dependent Na^+/K^+ pump maintains the steep outwardly and inwardly directed gradients for K^+ and Na^+, respectively, and also generates a small net outward current. The passive Na^+/Ca^{2+} exchanger generates a small net inward current. The resting membrane potential (V_r) results from high membrane permeability to K^+ relative to other ions and the transmembrane concentration gradient for K^+. A small inward "leak" of Na^+ ions keeps V_r slightly positive to the K^+ equilibrium potential. Finally, the fibre cannot be excited during the absolute refractory period (ARP). During the relative refractory period (RRP), excitation produces action potentials with reduced amplitude, slower upstrokes, and no overshoot (AP "a"). These either fail to propagate or do so slowly. Following the RRP, the threshold potential (TP) returns to normal, so that a fully regenerative AP (AP "b") occurs with excitation. See the text for further discussion.

Finally, we must define the term "rectification" before describing ionic mechanisms for the AP. Rectification describes the voltage dependence of resistance to ion flow through some ion channels. For example, the delayed rectifier K$^+$ current (I$_K$) and transient outward currents (I$_{to1}$ and I$_{to2}$) (Fig 3.6) exhibit outward going rectification, that is, more current flows with increasing depolarisation. In contrast, current flow progressively decreases with increasing depolarisation for the inward rectifier K$^+$ current (I$_{K1}$).

Phase 0: AP upstroke (rapid depolarisation)

There are two types of fibres, depending on the primary mechanism for generation of the AP upstroke – "fast" (Na$^+$) and slow (Ca^{2+}) response fibres. The first includes atrial, Purkinje, and ventricular muscle fibres, and the second SA and AV nodal cells.

In fast response fibres, depolarisation increases the probability of Na$^+$ channel activation. It must be sufficient to bring the membrane to threshold potential (TP), where enough inward Na$^+$ current is activated to overcome the repolarising influence of the outward K$^+$ conductances. TP ranges from −70 to −65 mV in normal Purkinje fibres. Once reached, the escalating influx of Na$^+$ ions causes regenerative depolarisation – whereby movement of a little Na$^+$ into the cell further depolarises the cell membrane, allowing more and more Na$^+$ to enter the cell. Depolarisation approaches, but never actually reaches, the Na$^+$ equilibrium potential (+70 mV). Purkinje fibres, with the highest AP upstroke velocities (see Table 3.2), have a significantly higher density of Na$^+$ channels than atrial or ventricular muscle fibres. AP upstroke velocity and amplitude are major determinants of myocardial conduction velocity. Finally, smaller depolarising stimuli that do not bring fast response fibres to threshold for regenerative excitation can result in non-propagated APs (local or "electrotonic effects"). Non-propagated APs, however, may impair conduction of subsequent propagating APs.

Slow response fibres have a lower RMP, slower upstrokes, and little or no overshoot (see Table 3.2 and Fig 3.4). Depolarisation during phase 0 is dependent primarily on the slow inward current (I$_{si}$) carried predominantly by Ca^{2+} (I$_{Ca}$). Its threshold for activation is about −30 to −40 mV. In fast response fibres, this current is activated during phase 0 by regenerative depolarisation caused by I$_{Na}$. Although current flows through both the fast (I$_{Na}$) and slow channels (I$_{si}$) during the second half of phase 0, I$_{si}$ is much smaller than peak I$_{Na}$, and therefore contributes little to the AP until after inactivation of I$_{Na}$ (following completion of phase 0). In addition, I$_{si}$ can be activated and may play a prominent role in incompletely depolarised fast response fibres ("depressed fast response" – see below) in which I$_{Na}$ has been inactivated, provided that conditions are appropriate for I$_{si}$ activation. I$_{si}$ passes through protein membrane channels that are selective for Ca^{2+}. Two types of Ca^{2+} inward current exist in cardiac fibres:

84

1 A slowly inactivating, high threshold, dihydropyridine sensitive current (long lasting, large or "L type" Ca^{2+} current – $I_{Ca,L}$). $I_{Ca,L}$ contributes to depolarisation and impulse propagation in slow response fibres. In fast response fibres, $I_{Ca,L}$ contributes to the AP plateau and triggering the release of Ca^{2+} from the sarcoplasmic reticulum.[2] Ca^{2+} channel blockers block $I_{Ca,L}$, but it is stimulated by drugs that increase cyclic AMP levels (β-adrenergic agonists and phosphodiesterase inhibitors).

2 A fast inactivating, low threshold, dihydropyridine insensitive current (transient, tiny, or "T type" – $I_{Ca,T}$). $I_{Ca,T}$ is activated at thresholds intermediate between those for I_{Na} and $I_{Ca,L}$. It probably contributes inward current to the later stages of phase 4 depolarisation in SA node cells and Purkinje fibres.[2]

Phase 1: early rapid repolarisation

In fast response fibres, the AP upstroke peak is followed by rapid, early repolarisation (phase 1). This brings the membrane potential back to $+10 \pm 10$ mV.[1 2] Phase 1 results from inactivation of I_{Na} along with activation of I_{to}. I_{to} consists of at least two components:[21]

1 I_{to1} is a voltage dependent, rapidly activating K^+ current with outward going rectification. It undergoes voltage and time dependent inactivation, and its channels are notably slow to recover from inactivation – diminishing its importance to phase 1 at fast heart rates.

2 I_{to2} is believed to be a Ca^{2+} dependent Cl^- current.[22] I_{to2} activation correlates with Ca^{2+} release from the sarcoplasmic reticulum, triggered by Ca^{2+} influx from L type Ca^{2+} channels.

There is marked regional variation in the prominence of I_{to2}. For example, AP of ventricular epicardial cells have prominent I_{to2} and phase 1 repolarisation. In contrast, I_{to2} is small and phase 1 negligible in endocardial cells.[23] Cl^- ions, along with I_{to2}, may contribute to early rapid repolarisation during adrenergic stimulation via rapidly activating–non-inactivating Cl^- current.[24]

Phase 2: AP plateau

The AP plateau phase (phase 2) may last several hundred milliseconds. Membrane conductance for all ions falls to rather low levels.[1 2] Decreased Na^+ conductance (caused by inactivation of I_{Na}) along with decreased outward K^+ conductance (consequent to I_{K1} inward going rectification – so that little K^+ leaves the cell) are primarily responsible. Minor currents during phase 2 include:

1 Ca^{2+} current ($I_{Ca,T}$, $I_{Ca,L}$): current through T type channels, activated at cell membrane potentials positive to -70 mV, is negligible, but may contribute to the pacemaker potential (see below). Current through the

L type channels, activated at cell membrane potentials positive to -40 mV, inactivates slowly. Its primary role is to trigger the release of Ca^{2+} from the sarcoplasmic reticulum to initiate contraction.

2 ATP dependent Na^+/K^+ pump: this does not turn on and off with each AP, but instead restores the ionic gradient over a cumulative time period. It pumps 3 Na^+ ions out for 2 K^+ ions into the cell.

3 Cl^- current: Ca^{2+} dependent Cl^- current (I_{to2}) also contributes to phase 2.[22]

4 Slowly inactivating or "late" Na^+ current: a small, persistent inward Na^+ current that continues to flow during phase 2 in ventricular muscle and Purkinje fibres.[25] It is unknown whether it results from delayed or failed inactivation of some Na^+ channels (I_{Na}), or is carried by a distinct subpopulation of Na^+ channels that open with long latencies.[1] Inhibition of this "late" Na^+ current is thought to be responsible for the shortening of the ventricular AP duration by lidocaine (lignocaine) and other class IB antiarrhythmic drugs.[26]

5 Passive Na^+/Ca^{2+} exchanger: this exchanger generates a small membrane current by virtue of its 3:1 Na^+:Ca^{2+} transport ratio.[27] The direction of the current flow is determined by the relationship of the membrane potential to the Na^+/Ca^{2+} equilibrium potential. Inward current (Na^+ influx/Ca^{2+} efflux) flows at rest because RMP is negative to E_{Na-Ca} (-30 to -40 mV). Outward current flows (Na^+ efflux/Ca^{2+} influx) towards the end of phase 0 and during phase 1 because RMP is positive to E_{Na-Ca}. As $[Ca^{2+}]_i$ increases (phase 2), E_{Na-Ca} becomes more positive and the exchanger reverts to its Na^+ influx/Ca^{2+} efflux mode.

Phase 3: final rapid repolarisation

Progressive decay of $I_{Ca,L}$ with increased outward K^+ current terminates phase 2 and initiates phase 3.[1][2] Outward current is generated by I_K (early phase 3) and I_{K1}, along with a small contribution from the ATP dependent Na^+/K^+ pump. I_{K1} channels, closed during phase 2, progressively reactivate during phase 3 to cause regenerative repolarisation back to the RMP.

Automaticity: phase 4 (diastolic) depolarisation

Pacemaker fibres in the SA node and latent (also subsidiary or secondary) pacemakers spontaneously depolarise during phase 4 towards threshold for regenerative excitation – termed "automaticity".

Sinus node automaticity

The SA nodal action potential with underlying currents is shown in Fig 3.7.[20] From a maximum diastolic potential of -50 to -60 mV, the cell undergoes slow diastolic (phase 4) depolarisation. This phase merges smoothly with the AP upstroke (phase 0), and there is no distinct AP overshoot, phase 1, or phase 2 (Fig 3.7).

SA node automaticity must be the result of a net gain in intracellular positive charges during diastole.[1][2] Contributing to this change is a voltage dependent channel activated at membrane potentials negative to −50 to −60 mV, with a reversal potential of around −20 mV. This pacemaker current (I_f) is carried mostly by monovalent cations (Na^+, K^+). Hyperpolarisation increases the I_f rate of activation, so that it carries only about 20% of phase 4 depolarising current in SA nodal cells. Therefore, automaticity is primarily dependent on I_K, $I_{Ca,L}$, $I_{Ca,T}$, and an unidentified background current (I_b). Repolarisation results in the closure or deactivation of the K^+ channels (I_K) opened during the preceding AP. This causes K^+

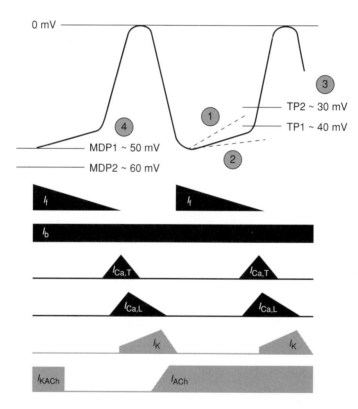

Fig 3.7 Membrane currents underlying SA node automaticity and the modulation of automaticity. Inward currents (black) include the pacemaker current (I_f), background current (I_b), transient Ca^{2+} current ($I_{Ca,T}$), and long lasting Ca^{2+} current ($I_{Ca,L}$). Outward currents include two inward rectifying K^+ currents – the delayed rectifier (I_K) and a hyperpolarising K^+ current that is activated by vagal stimulation (I_{ACh}). (1) The rate of SA node discharge can be increased by increasing the slope of phase 4 depolarisation. (2) The rate can be slowed by reducing the slope of phase 4 depolarisation, (3) reducing threshold potential (TP), or (4) by increasing maximum diastolic potential (MDP).

conductance to decline during phase 4, contributing to net depolarising current. The proposed Na^+ background current (I_b) is carried by a voltage independent channel in SA nodal cells – one that is different from the one responsible for I_{Na}. Finally, $I_{Ca,L}$ and $I_{Ca,T}$ contribute to the SA node AP upstroke.

Purkinje fibre automaticity

The MDP of automatic Purkinje fibres is hyperpolarised (-70 to -90 mV) compared with that of SA nodal cells.[1][2] Consequently, I_f is the major pacemaker current in automatic Purkinje fibres, and I_{Na} is also the primary carrier for the AP upstroke.

Modulation of automaticity

The intrinsic rate of SA nodal pacemaker discharge is determined by: (1) maximum diastolic potential (MDP); (2) threshold potential (TP); and (3) the slope of phase 4 depolarisation (Fig 3.7). Vagal stimulation slows SA node automaticity by: (1) activation of inward rectifying, hyperpolarising K^+ current (I_{KACh}), (2) reduction of $I_{Ca,L}$, and (3) reduction of I_f.[28] I_{KACh} hyperpolarises MDP and shortens AP duration. This, together with the reduction in I_f, slows the rate of phase 4 depolarisation, causing it to take longer to reach TP for a regenerative AP (Fig 3.7). Reduced $I_{Ca,L}$ slows the rate of phase 0 depolarisation. Catecholamines accelerate automaticity by moving the potential for I_f activation to a more positive value, and by increasing I_K and I_{Ca} – both increase the slope of phase 4 depolarisation.

Subsidiary (latent) pacemakers

In addition to Purkinje fibres, cells in certain portions of the atria (sulcus terminalis, Bachman's bundle, coronary sinus ostia), muscle of the tricuspid and mitral annuli, and distal AV node cells may undergo gradual phase 4 depolarisation, The SA node discharge normally exceeds that of these pacemakers, so that they are kept from reaching threshold potential. This is termed "overdrive suppression" of automaticity. The mechanisms for automaticity in latent pacemakers are probably similar to those for SA node cells and Purkinje fibres, with the actual mechanism most dependent on fibre MDP. Compared with the SA node, latent pacemakers are not as subject to the influence of neurotransmitters and the autonomic nervous system.

Impulse propagation

The SA node impulse must be propagated to excite the rest of the heart. AP propagation is dependent on excitability, conduction, and refractoriness.

Excitability

The term excitability describes the ease with which a regenerative AP capable of propagation to the rest of the heart is initiated in response to a depolarising stimulus.[29] Excitability depends upon the complex interplay of membrane active ("generator") and passive ("resistive") properties.[30] The former include: (1) the kinetics and amplitude of ionic currents responsible for the AP; (2) threshold potential for activation of I_{Na} (fast response fibres) or I_{Ca} (slow response fibres); and (3) the difference between RMP (or MDP) and TP, which determines the amount of current needed to evoke an AP. Passive properties refer to the impedance elements or cable properties of the myocyte: (1) membrane resistance, (2) intra- and extracellular resistance, and (3) membrane capacitance.[31][32] The last comprises the myoplasmic and gap junctional channel resistances. Gap junctions connect adjacent myocytes, and provide low resistance electrical coupling between cells by establishing aqueous pores that directly link their respective cytoplasms.[2] Gap junctions permit the multicellular heart to function electrically like an orderly, synchronised, interconnected unit. Electrolyte abnormalities (especially K^+ and Mg^{2+} imbalance), antiarrhythmic drugs, general and local anaesthetics, and ischaemia may influence excitability by affecting one or more of its determinants.[1][2][29][30][33][34]

Conduction

AP propagation by local circuit currents is best understood by assuming that electrical behaviour of a small segment of cell membrane – the unit membrane – is equivalent to resistance (R_m) and capacitance (C_m) arranged in parallel.[35] Resistive properties arise from the presence of ion channels, and capacitance properties from the lipid bilayer – as a result of its hydrophobic core and polar cytoplasmic and extracellular surfaces. The entire cell is then considered as a cable, consisting of many unit membranes – each coupled to adjacent units by the resistances of cytoplasm (R_i) and the extracellular fluid (R_o).

Local circuit current is initiated by I_{Na} or I_{Ca}, depending on cell type. The resulting influx of positive charges moves longitudinally through the cytoplasmic resistance R_i and discharges the capacitance C_m of the adjacent non-excited membrane segment This brings it to threshold for activation of Na^+ or Ca^{2+} inward current. The local circuit is completed when positive charges (released to the extracellular space by discharge of C_m) and flow through gap junctions (see above) return to the initiating active membrane segment through R_o. Local currents within the cell are carried by K^+ ions, which are by far the most predominant intracellular cation.

Propagation between adjacent cells occurs by specialised, low resistance, gap junctional channels (see above), which are located most densely at the ends of ventricular muscle and Purkinje fibres.[1][2] Gap junctions are probably partly responsible for the fact that conduction in the heart is anisotropic – namely, its anatomical and biophysical properties vary according to the direction in which they are measured. Usually, conduction is two to three times faster longitudinally than transversely (perpendicular to long axis). However, the safety factor for conduction is greater transversely, and conduction delay or block occurs more commonly in the longitudinal direction. As a result of anisotropy, propagation is discontinuous and can be a cause of re-entry.

The velocity of impulse propagation is determined by several factors.[1][2] Active membrane properties include: (1) the amplitude and kinetics of I_{Na} and I_{Ca}; and (2) the difference between RMP and TP. Passive properties include: (1) the excitability threshold; (2) R_i and gap junctional resistance; and (3) cross-sectional area of the cell. Conduction velocity may be increased by factors that enhance the magnitude of inward current during phase 0: (1) hyperpolarisation of RMP or MDP; (2) increase in R_m – for example, with hypokalemia; or (3) decrease in R_i – for example, with catecholamines. Finally, direction of impulse propagation is crucial to the influence of anisotropy – as mentioned earlier.

Refractoriness

Refractoriness describes the ability to re-excite a cell (or tissue) after previous excitation. A cell may be absolutely (no response to stimulation), relatively (partial response), or no longer refractory (normal response). The state of refractoriness depends on Na^+ or Ca^{2+} channel availability in fast or slow response fibres, respectively, as well as the ability of the depolarising stimulus to bring the membrane potential to threshold for activation of the available Na^+ or Ca^{2+} channels. In fast response fibres, almost all Na^+ channels are inactivated beginning with the AP upstroke and continuing through AP phase 2 to phase 3. Consequently, a regenerative AP cannot be initiated regardless of stimulus strength. Once the cell has repolarised during phase 3 to about –50 mV, however, an increasing proportion of Na^+ channels recovers from inactivation as a function of time and voltage. This defines the end of the absolute refractory period (ARP), and the beginning of the relative refractory period (RRP) (see Fig 3.6). During the RRP, a regenerative AP may occur, but this requires a suprathreshold stimulus. Also, APs initiated during the RRP have a reduced AP upstroke velocity, amplitude, and overshoot, and are conducted more slowly (see Fig 3.6).

In fast response fibres, the time course for recovery of excitability closely follows that for membrane repolarisation – usually full recovery within approximately 50 ms of achievement of the normal RMP. This reflects the rapid time course for Na^+ channel recovery from inactivation. Deactivation of K^+ repolarisation currents may also, however, affect Na^+ channel recovery from inactivation and excitability. Delmar[36] has shown that dynamic changes in I_K and I_{K1}, by altering R_m, exert an important role in determining the ease with which the membrane depolarises to threshold.

Further, I_K inactivates slowly during the AP, so that complete deactivation can extend beyond restoration of the normal RMP. If so, current through still open I_K channels may oppose inward stimulating current, despite full recovery of the Na^+ channels from inactivation.[36]

The time course for recovery from inactivation is much slower for Ca^{2+} channels of slow response fibres (SA and AV nodes), so that relative refractoriness outlasts the return to MDP by more than 100 ms. Fast response fibres that have been partially depolarised by ischaemia or other factors that slow recovery of Na^+ channels (for example, long acting local anaesthetics and class 1C antiarrhythmic drugs) may also exhibit prolonged post-repolarisation refractoriness.

Abnormal cardiac electrophysiology

Abnormal cardiac electrophysiological phenomena include impaired conduction and uneven refractoriness associated with the depressed fast response, and repetitive impulse formation arising *de novo* in fibres that do not normally exhibit automaticity (that is, abnormal automaticity) or *triggered* by early or delayed after depolarisations, and re-entry of excitation. Such abnormal phenomena result from the disruption of normal cardiac electrophysiological processes, as a result of either altered physiological states or myocardial disease. The first is considered to be "imbalance", implying that the cause is at least potentially reversible (see box). The second is considered a "substrate" – a more or less fixed defect that is conducive to arrhythmogenesis (see box).

Loss of membrane potential and depressed fast response

Loss of membrane potential (LMP) is the partial depolarisation of fast response fibres resulting from a metabolic abnormality (for example, ischaemia, hyperkalaemia). LMP reduces Na^+ channel availability.[2] LMP reduces AP upstroke velocity, amplitude, and overshoot, and prolongs conduction time of propagating AP – even to the point of block. APs with their upstrokes dependent on I_{Na} flowing through partially inactivated Na^+ channels are called depressed fast responses (DFR). DFR AP contours resemble those of slow response fibres (see Fig 3.4). AP changes with LMP are likely to be heterogeneous, as a result of variable inactivation of the I_{Na}. As a result, there is uneven conduction and refractoriness – conditions especially favourable for re-entry arrhythmias. LMP may also contribute to the genesis of abnormal automaticity and triggered activity (see below).

Cellular mechanisms for arrhythmias

Arrhythmias are disorders of impulse initiation (automaticity, triggered activity – from early or delayed after depolarisations), propagation, or both

91

Myocardial imbalance

Autonomic imbalance
Electrolyte imbalance
Metabolic imbalance
Acid–base imbalance
Temperature extremes
Adverse drug effects
Adverse PCD effects
Drug interactions
Myocardial ischaemia
Too light anaesthesia
Too deep anaesthesia
Hypo- or hypercapnia
Cerebral hypoxia
Microshock

Myocardial substrates

Healed myocardial infarction
Hypertrophic cardiomyopathy
Dilated cardiomyopathy
Restrictive cardiomyopathy
Sick sinus syndrome
Ventricular pre-excitation (WPW)
Pericarditis, myocarditis
Congenital long QT syndrome

PCD, pacemakers and cardioverter defibrillators; WPW, Wolff–Parkinson–White syndrome.

(for example, a focus of abnormal automaticity protected by entrance block – parasystole). Automaticity may be normal (SA node, latent pacemakers), altered normal, or abnormal. "Altered normal" simply means that the ionic mechanisms for automaticity are normal; only the rate of automaticity has changed as a result of an increase or decrease in current magnitude. Re-entry is the only disorder of impulse propagation, although some authorities also include deceleration dependent block (block at slow heart rates – possibly caused by reduced AP amplitude or excitability), tachycardia dependent block (resulting from refractoriness caused by incomplete recovery of excitability), and decremental conduction (whereby properties of a fibre change along its length so that the propagating AP loses its efficacy as a stimulus to excite the fibre ahead of it).[2]

Abnormal automaticity

Abnormal automaticity is different from normal automaticity because: (1) it occurs in fibres that do not normally exhibit automaticity; or (2) ionic mechanisms for abnormal automaticity are dissimilar to those for normal automaticity in the same fibre type (for example, Purkinje fibres). It occurs in fibres with reduced MDPs – often at potentials positive to –50 mV, when $I_{Ca,L}$ and I_K may be operative.[2] Electrotonic effects from surrounding, more depolarised or normally polarised myocardium will influence the development of automaticity. Application of constant depolarising current can produce abnormal automaticity in atrial and ventricular muscle, and Purkinje fibres. If so, loss of membrane potential, along with a background inward current provided by declining I_K and activating I_{Ca}, possibly explain abnormal spontaneous phase 4 depolarisation.[1 2] This mechanism has been observed in experimental canine infarction, rat myocardium damaged by epinephrine (adrenaline), diseased human atrium, and ventricular myocardium from patients undergoing ventricular aneurysectomy or endocardial resection for tachyarrhythmias.[2]

Triggered activity

Triggered activity is repetitive impulse formation that is initiated by depolarising oscillations in membrane potential induced by one or more APs. These oscillatory potentials are also referred to as after potentials or after depolarisations. After depolarisations can occur before or after full repolarisation of the fibre (Fig 3.8). Those arising during phase 2 or 3 of the AP are termed "early after depolarisations" (EADs), whereas those that arise after full repolarisation (phase 4) are termed "delayed after depolarisations" (DADs).[37] Not all after depolarisations reach the threshold for

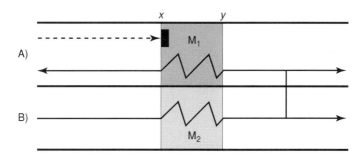

Fig 3.8 Depiction of linear re-entry in a fibre bundle with a local region of depressed excitability (M_1), similar to that first proposed by Schmitt and Erlanger.[61] Region M_1 is also the zone of unidirectional conduction block. The impulse propagates in fibre A from left to right, and blocks at x – the proximal border of M_1. In adjacent fibre B, however, excitability is less depressed (M_2); therefore, the impulse conducts slowly beyond the more depressed region (M_1) in fibre A. It continues to propagate in fibre B, and also crosses back to distal fibre A via lateral connections. In fibre A it propagates distally as well as slowly back through the former site of block – with excitability restored (that is, y to x in M_1) to re-excite proximal fibre A, before it is excited by another impulse arriving from above.

regenerative depolarisation, but, if they do, they may trigger another AP and repetitive impulse formation. Such repetitive impulse formation is termed "triggered activity" because, in contrast to automaticity, it is critically dependent on prior impulses (EAD, DAD) or stimulation.[2]

Early after depolarisations

EADs arise from incompletely repolarised membrane during phase 2 (type 1 EAD) and 3 of the AP (type 2 EAD).[1 2 38] EADs and triggered activity are associated with bradycardia and drugs that prolong the QT interval – acquired long QT syndrome (A-LQTS) – particularly when associated with hypokalaemia and hypomagnesaemia.[38] Quinidine, the prototype class 1A antiarrhythmic, is well-known to cause QT prolongation and *torsade de pointes* ventricular tachycardia attributed to EADs and triggered activity.[2 38 39] Other drugs that have caused *torsade de pointes* in association with a long QT interval and *torsade* include other type 1A and some class III antiarrhythmics, non-sedating antihistamines (terfenadine, astemizole), and erythromycin.[38 40]

Not all drugs that prolong the QT interval[38] are associated with *torsade de pointes* ventricular tachycardia caused by EADs.[39] Class 1C antiarrhythmics also cause QT interval prolongation and may be associated with ventricular proarrhythmia (the term used to describe paradoxical ventricular arrhythmia formation with antiarrhythmic drugs[38 39 41–43]). However, with 1C drugs, the polymorphic ventricular tachycardia *resembling torsade de pointes* is more likely as a result of re-entry – attributed to depression and delayed recovery from inactivation of I_{Na}, as well as prolonged refractoriness.[39] Either facilitates re-entry (see below), especially in patients with poor left ventricular function, acute myocardial ischaemia, or pre-existing ventricular arrhythmias,[39 41–43]

The mechanism for EADs and triggered activity is uncertain, especially given that EADs may arise from two ranges of membrane potential (type 1 EAD, potentials < -40 mV; type 2 EAD, potentials between -50 and -70 mV). At least type 1 EAD must involve activation (or reactivation) of $I_{Ca,L}$ in conjunction with delayed repolarisation as a result of block of I_K.[2 39] At least with quinidine, however, EADs and triggered activity are enhanced at slower heart rates.[40 44] Quinidine blocks both I_{Na} and I_K at sites within the channel pores; only receptor occupancy within the K^+ channel is greater at slow rates[44] – possibly as a result of reduced extracellular K^+ accumulation.[40 45] This phenomenon – greater block at slower heart rates – is termed "reverse use dependence", because this denotes greater block at faster heart rates.

Finally, EADs (also delayed after depolarisations – see below) and triggered activity, and *torsade de pointes* ventricular tachycardia, are associated with QT interval prolongation in the congenital (idiopathic) long QT syndrome (C-LQTS). QT prolongation is attributed to defects in the genes encoding K^+ and Na^+ channels, left sided sympathetic predominance, or both.[46-50] β-Adrenergic stimulation facilitates EADs and triggered activity, and *torsade de pointes* with C-LQTS, hence the use of β-blockers for the management of patients with this syndrome. β-Adrenergic stimulation is expected to increase $I_{Ca,L}$ (and amplitude of EAD), and possibly also inhomogeneity of repolarisation.[47]

Delayed after depolarisations

In contrast to EADs, DADs are secondary depolarisations that arise from a fully repolarised membrane.[1 2] Triggered activity resulting from DADs has been observed in atrial and ventricular muscle and Purkinje fibres under a wide variety of experimental conditions (for example, digitalis intoxication, one day after experimental myocardial infarction, exposure to catecholamines). It has also been observed in vitro in diseased human atrial and ventricular fibres. DADs and triggered activity are believed to be responsible for at least some tachyarrhythmias precipitated by digitalis toxicity, and possibly accelerated junctional or idioventricular rhythms with acute myocardial infarction.

The mechanism believed to be responsible for DADs involves an increase in $[Ca^{2+}]_i$, which activates a transient inward current (I_{ti}) mediated either by the Na^+/Ca^{2+} exchanger or a Ca^{2+} dependent non-specific ion channel.[51 52] This current (I_{ti}) is small or absent normally, but activated by an increase in intracellular Ca^{2+} ("Ca^{2+} overload"),[53 54] such as might occur with myocardial ischaemia or injury, catecholamines, or digitalis excess. Na^+ is the primary carrier for I_{ti}. Drugs that (1) reduce diastolic Ca^{2+} transient, by reducing Ca^{2+} overload (Ca^{2+} channel blockers, β-blockers), (2) inhibit Ca^{2+} release from the sarcoplasmic reticulum (caffeine, ryanodine), or (3) reduce I_{Na}, and consequently $[Na^+]_i$, inhibit DADs.[2]

In contrast to the behaviour of EAD triggered activity, pacing at a rate faster than the rate of triggered activity or premature stimulation increases the amplitude and prematurity of subsequent DADs.[2] This is in contrast to normal automaticity, which is temporarily suppressed (for example – sinus pause or bradycardia after termination of paroxysmal supraventricular tachycardia). Further, because a single premature stimulus can both initiate and terminate DAD triggered activity, the differentiation of this mechanism from re-entry may be difficult.

Re-entry of excitation

The excitatory wavefront emanating from the SA node continues until all of the heart has been activated and become completely refractory. If for some reason a group of fibres is not activated by the propagating impulse, and it returns by another pathway to excite them, this process is termed "re-entry of excitation". It is also termed "circus movement or reciprocation", and extrasystoles caused by re-entry reciprocal or echo beats. Three basic criteria for ascribing abnormal beats or rhythm to re-entry were first formulated by Mines:[55][56]

1 There must be an area of unidirectional conduction block.
2 The re-entrant pathway must be defined – namely, the movement of the excitatory wavefront should be observed to progress through the pathway, return to its point of origin, and then return to re-excite the same pathway.
3 It must be possible to terminate re-entry by interrupting the circuit at some point to rule out a focal origin (that is, automatic, triggered).

These criteria have been satisfied for many clinical tachyarrhythmias, because it is now possible to map tachycardia circuits (electrophysiological studies) and interrupt the circuits by surgical or radiofrequency catheter ablation techniques. Discussed here are the basic requirements for re-entry (slow conduction, unidirectional block), anatomical and functional re-entry, re-entry involving the SA and AV nodes, and atrioventricular re-entry with accessory pathways.

Slow conduction

It has long been known that a basic requirement for re-entry is sufficient delay of the propagating impulse in an alternative pathway to permit proximal tissue a site of unidirectional block to recover from refractoriness. If so, re-entry would be facilitated by conduction that was slower than normal. In fast response fibres, the speed of conduction is dependent on the magnitude of I_{Na} during phase 0, and the rapidity with which I_{Na} reaches its maximum. This will depend on the number of available Na^+ channels, which in turn is dependent on the level of TMP. For example, membrane depolarisation in a fast response fibre to levels of –60 to –70 mV may inactivate half the Na^+ channels, whereas depolarisation to –50 mV or less may inactivate all the Na^+ channels.[2] Further, time is required for Na^+ channels to regain excitability after inactivation. If so, conduction of a premature AP can be slowed in distal tissue as a result of decreased Na^+ channel availability and/or incomplete recovery from inactivation.

The amplitude and upstroke velocities of premature AP initiated before full repolarisation are reduced (see Fig 3.6), as is their speed of propagation. Re-entry may occur during propagation of premature AP in regions with different AP durations, as a result of slowed conduction and unidirectional block (see below). Re-entry may also occur in fibres with persistent low levels of membrane potential (namely slow response or depressed fast response fibres), caused by slow conduction (reduced Na^+ channel availability) and refractoriness that extends beyond full repolarisation. Finally, coupling resistance between adjacent cells is another factor that may influence the speed of conduction. As coupling resistance is increased, the speed of conduction decreases. Increased $[Ca^{2+}]_i$ and acidosis are two factors that may increase coupling resistance.[57]

Unidirectional conduction block

Unidirectional block of conduction may occur as the result of non-uniform recovery of excitability, geometric factors, or asymmetrical depression of conduction and excitability.[57]

Non-uniform recovery of excitability – When an impulse propagates through tissue with regional differences in refractoriness, conduction may fail in the regions with the longest refractory periods. These regions will, however, be available for re-excitation, provided the propagating impulse can somehow return to the site of former block. This is unlikely in normal working myocardium, even at fast heart rates, because there is still enough time during diastole when tissue is non-refractory. Re-entry induced by premature extrasystoles may, however, be facilitated because refractory periods shorten with short cycle lengths resulting from prematurity or fast heart rates. It follows that the pathways over which the impulse propagates are also shortened. The amount of refractory period non-uniformity needed for unidirectional conduction block after a premature impulse may be quite small – with minimal differences of 10–40 ms reported for atrial and ventricular fibres, respectively.[57]

Geometric factors – When a thin bundle of fibres inserts into a larger muscle mass – for example, the Purkinje fibre–ventricular muscle junction ("junction") – the insertion point can be the site for unidirectional block of conduction.[57] Such block has not been observed in normal fibres, even though the anterograde junctional conduction delay may be longer than in the retrograde direction. With reduced Na^+ channel availability, however, anterograde block may occur at the junction whereas retrograde conduction remains possible.[58] More recent studies indicate that the Purkinje fibre–muscle junction is better represented by a three dimensional model of overlying two dimensional sheets of fibres, rather than terminal Purkinje fibres inserting into a three dimensional ventricular muscle mass.[59] If so, activation of the ventricular muscle layer occurs only at specific junctional sites; otherwise, a considerable resistive barrier exists between the two cell layers.[57] It follows that reasons for unidirectional block between Purkinje and ventricular fibres include differences in excitability and fibre thickness between the two layers, as well as increased coupling resistance at sites of unidirectional conduction block.[60] Sites where the cross sectional area of interconnected cells suddenly increases may also be sites for unidirectional conduction block (for example, ventricular insertion points for accessory pathways in patients with the Wolff–Parkinson–White syndrome, as well as sites of fibre branching and junctions of separate muscle bundles).[57] Finally, the way in which myocardial cells are connected to one another influences the speed of conduction, with longitudinal conduction velocity being about three times transverse conduction velocity.[57]

Asymmetrical depression of excitability and conduction – There may be an asymmetrical region of depressed excitability and conduction, which can also result in unidirectional conduction block (see Fig 3.8), first suggested by Schmitt and Erlanger.[61]

Anatomical re-entry

The simplest model of re-entry involving a fixed anatomical obstacle (Fig 3.9a) was proposed by Mines in 1913.[55] He suggested that re-entry could occur in an anatomically defined circuit, provided that conduction was sufficiently slowed along with shortened refractoriness. An important

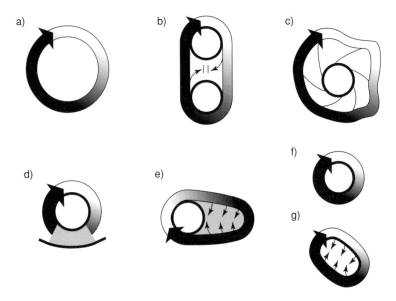

Fig 3.9 Schematic depiction of variations on anatomical and functional re-entry. The arrows represent the crest of the circulating wavefront, and in its wake are areas of absolute (black) or relative refractoriness (stippled). White areas represent excitable tissue, that is, the "excitable gap" (see also fig 3.10). (a) Circus movement around a gross anatomical obstacle, as envisioned by Mines.[55] (b) Circus movement around the caval orifices, separated by a zone of functional block. (c) Circus movement in a loop composed of bundles of fibres having a greater conduction velocity than surrounding tissue. (d, e) Circus movement based on a combination of an anatomical obstacle (circle) and an adjacent area of diseased tissue (hatched area) with depressed conduction. (f) Circus movement around a relatively small anatomical obstacle becomes possible as a result of a shortened refractoriness and reduced conduction velocity – thereby shortening the wavelength of the circulating impulse. (g) Leading circle concept of re-entry, with no need for an anatomical obstacle. See the text for further discussion. (Reproduced from Allessie et al,[62] with permission.)

feature of Mines' model was the presence of an *excitable gap* (Figs 3.9 and 3.10). The excitable gap implies that an impulse originating outside the re-entry circuit can penetrate it and influence the rhythm.[57] But, normal pacemakers of the heart are suppressed (that is, overdriven) during re-entrant tachycardia. Consequently, the impulse that can penetrate the circuit must come from another source (extrastimulation, burst pacing, etc).

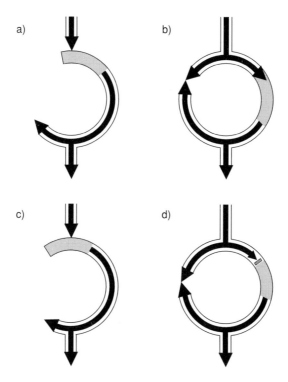

Fig 3.10 The excitable gap, and how a single premature stimulus can reset or terminate re-entry tachycardia. The arrows represent the crest of the circulating wavefront, and the black tails the zones of absolute refractoriness. Relative refractoriness within the excitable gap (stippling) decreases with increasing distance from the tail of absolute refractoriness. (a) A premature stimulus reaching the circuit relatively late, when tissue within the excitable gap has almost regained full excitability. (b) A moment later, the stimulus wavefront has penetrated the circuit in both directions, and blocks in the retrograde (left) limb as it encounters the advancing tachycardia wavefront, but advances in the anterograde (right) limb to change the phase or *reset* the tachycardia. (c) The premature stimulus reaches the re-entry circuit earlier, when tissue behind the tail of absolute refractoriness is only partially excitable (relatively refractory). (d) This stimulus blocks in both the retrograde and anterograde limbs as a result, respectively, of the advancing tachycardia wavefront and relative refractoriness – terminating the tachycardia. (Reproduced from Janse et al,[63] with permission.)

There are several variations on re-entry involving a fixed anatomical obstacle.[57 62] Lewis and co-workers used rapid atrial pacing or alternating current to initiate re-entrant tachycardia (that is, atrial flutter) around the caval orifices in dogs (Fig 3.9b), but the question remained whether such natural obstacles were large enough for sustained re-entry to occur. Moe's group suggested that *anisotropic atrial conduction* would remove the need for a large anatomical obstacle (Fig 3.9c).[64] For example, anatomically distinct, interatrial or intranodal, preferential conducting pathways, with faster conduction velocities than surrounding atrial myocardium, could form the loops required for re-entry. It is now believed that such anatomically distinct pathways do not exist; rather, preferential conduction is the result of different electrophysiological properties or geometrical arrangements among the fibres. Allessie and co-workers[62] proposed that re-entry would be facilitated by an anatomical obstacle with an adjacent area of depressed conduction (Fig 3.9d,e). Finally, it has been suggested that altered electrophysiological properties of fast response fibres (namely, loss of membrane potential – see above) might reduce the size of an anatomical obstacle needed for re-entry.[57]

Anatomically defined re-entry circuits might occur in fibrotic regions of the atria or ventricles, or in surviving muscle fibres of healed infarctions.[65] Critical slowing of conduction and unidirectional block for re-entry may be caused by loss of membrane potential (above) with atrial cardio-myopathies,[66] or by increased effective axial resistivity with healed infarcts.[67] Defined anatomical circuits are also involved in ventricular tachycardia as a result of bundle branch re-entry,[68] supraventricular tachycardia caused by atrioventricular re-entry involving accessory path-ways,[69] and atrial flutter resulting from re-entry confined to the right atrium.[70]

Functional re-entry

Functional re-entry lacks restrictive anatomical boundaries, and occurs in contiguous fibres with heterogeneous electrophysiological properties caused by local differences in APs.[2 65] Dispersed excitability and/or refractoriness, and anisotropic distribution of intercellular resistances, allow the initiation and maintenance of re-entry.[71–73]

Leading circle re-entry – Leading circle re-entry (Fig 3.9g) was first described by Allessie and co-workers in experiments on atrial muscle,[74–76] and is an important mechanism in clinical atrial fibrillation.[2 64] Re-entry is initiated by a precisely timed premature beat in regions that are activated normally at regular spontaneous or paced rates. Sustained re-entry is made possible by different refractory periods of atrial fibres in close proximity to one another.[75] The premature beat initiating re-entry blocks in fibres with long refractory periods, although propagating in those with shorter ones. It eventually returns to the former site of block after excitability has recovered there. The impulse may continue to circulate around a central core that is kept refractory because it is constantly bombarded by impulses propagating towards it from all sides of the circuit (Fig 3.9g). The circumference of the smallest leading circle is as small as 6–8 mm, and is a pathway in which the circulating wavefront is just able to excite relatively refractory tissue ahead of it.[2 64] No, or only a very short, excitable gap exists, which distinguishes this from other mechanisms for re-entry.[2] Therefore, impulses propagating outside the circuit cannot easily enter the circuit to terminate or reset the tachycardia.[77] Theoretically, drugs that prolong refractoriness but do not delay conduction (for example, dofetilide, ibutilide, bretylium, and sotolol) would slow tachycardia as a result of the leading circle mechanism, although not affecting re-entry tachycardia with an excitable gap.[2] Conversely, an antiarrhythmic drug that primarily slows conduction with little effect on refractoriness (for example, class 1 drugs – Na^+ channel blockers) would have major effects on tachycardia with an excitable gap, but little effect on leading circle re-entry.[2] These examples illustrate how an antiarrhythmic drug may be targeted against specific mechanisms for clinical arrhythmias (see below) – the approach advanced by the Sicilian Gambit.[20 78]

Random re-entry – Random re-entry is also an important mechanism in atrial fibrillation.[2 64] It occurs when the impulse propagates randomly and continuously, re-exciting areas that were excited shortly before by another wavelet. Examples of random re-entry include anisotropic and spiral wave re-entry. *Anisotropic re-entry* is the result of the structural features responsible for variations in conduction velocity and the time course of repolarisation – such as concentration of gap junctions at the ends rather than sides of cells – which can result in slowed conduction, unidirectional conduction block, and re-entry. Therefore, in contrast to leading circle re-entry, the functional characteristic that leads to re-entry is not spatial differences in refractory period but rather spatial differences in effective axial resistivity caused by non-uniform anisotropy.[64] Anisotropic re-entry has been shown in atrial and ventricular muscle, and an excitable gap may be present.[2 64] In contrast to anisotropic re-entry, *spiral wave re-entry* (*scroll wave* re-entry in three dimensions) does not require any permanent heterogeneities for its initiation or maintenance.[79–82] Instead, transient heterogeneities can be created in normally uniform tissue. Similar to anisotropic or leading circle re-entry, however, electrical activity with spiral waves is organised around a central fulcrum (the core). But, in contrast to leading circle re-entry, in which the central core is inexcitable, the central core during spiral wave re-entry is excitable but not excited. The mechanism of the core of the spiral is the pronounced curvature of the wavefront at the tip of the spiral, which is higher than the critical curvature for successful propagation. As a result, the rotating wave cannot invade the core because of its inability to stimulate it, not because the core is

101

refractory. Another important difference between leading circle re-entry and spiral waves is the presence of a fully excitable gap with the spiral waves. In the heart these have three distinct dynamics: (1) stationary, whereby the core remains in the same position, giving rise to a rhythmic pattern of activation; (2) drifting, whereby the core drifts away from the site of origin, giving rise to complex and irregular patterns of activation; and (3) anchored, whereby a drifting core becomes stationary by anchoring to small areas of discontinuity in cardiac muscle (for example, blood vessel, connective tissue). Finally, "anchoring" of a drifting spiral possibly explains the transition between polymorphic and monomorphic ventricular tachycardia.[80]

SA and AV node re-entry

As the result of slow conduction and prolonged refractoriness, the SA node has the potential for dissociation of conduction – whereby an impulse can propagate in some but not other fibres, permitting re-entry to occur.[2 57 83] The re-entrant circuit may be located entirely within the SA node or involve both the SA node and the atrium. Supraventricular tachycardia (SVT) caused by SA node re-entry is generally tolerated better than other types of SVT resulting from slower tachycardia rates. SVT caused by SA node re-entry accounts for 3–16% of paroxysmal SVT referred for electrophysiological study.[83]

Although longitudinal electrophysiological dissociation of the AV node into two or more pathways has been demonstrated in animal investigations,[84] whether such dissociation accounts for paroxysmal SVT resulting from AV nodal re-entry in humans is more dubious.[2] The presence of dual AV nodal pathways is not disputed,[85 86] but whether they are intranodal and undergo functional longitudinal dissociation, or are extranodal – involving separate inputs to the AV node – has been the question.[2] Results of clinical electrophysiological investigation, and radiofrequency catheter and surgical ablation, are now conclusive – the slow and fast AV nodal pathways have their origins well outside the limits of the compact AV node, and consist of ordinary atrial muscle fibres.[2 87–89] Thus, these pathways are atrial to nodal approaches or connections, not distinct intranodal pathways. Target sites for ablation of the fast pathway in AV nodal re-entry tachycardia (AVNRT) are located along the anterosuperior portion of the interatrial septum near the tricuspid annulus, just proximal to the compact AV node (that is, the anterosuperior atrial approach – Fig 3.10a).[88 89] Target sites for ablation of the slow pathway in AVNRT are found more posteriorly along the tricuspid annulus, close to the ostium of the coronary sinus (that is, the posteroinferior atrial approach – Fig. 3.10a). During the *common form* of AVNRT, atrial to AV nodal (anterograde) conduction occurs via the posteroinferior (slow) atrial approach, with AV nodal to atrial (retrograde) conduction over the anterosuperior (fast) atrial approach. With the *uncommon form* of

AVNRT, the reverse occurs. (The distinction between common and uncommon forms of AVNRT is moot as far as recognition – P waves are usually non-apparent with either, and both are narrow QRS tachycardias, or treatment – which is the same for both forms). Either or both atrial approaches can be selectively ablated by catheter or surgical methods to cure AVNRT.[88 89] In patients with dual AV nodal physiology, anterograde conduction probably occurs over the anterosuperior atrial approaches during sinus rhythm, and the premature impulse that initiates AVNRT blocks in this pathway (with longer refractoriness) as well.[2] Finally, paroxysmal SVT caused by AV nodal re-entry accounts for 28% to 50% of paraoxysmal SVT referred for electrophysiological study.[90]

Atrioventricular re-entry with accessory pathways (see Fig 3.11)

Accessory atrioventricular connections (accessory pathways – AP) are the anatomical substrate for ventricular pre-excitation and AV reciprocating tachycardia (AVRT) in the Wolff–Parkinson–White (WPW) syndrome – that is, short PR interval, slurred QRS complex upstroke (δ wave), prolonged QRS duration, and associated paroxysmal tachyarrhythmias.[2 91–96] APs consist of small fibres that resemble ordinary atrial tissue, and can bridge the AV groove at any location along the mitral or the tricuspid annulus, except for the region where the mitral annulus is contiguous with the aorta. Thus, APs provide abnormal electrical continuity between the atrium and ventricle. AP conduction is normally rate independent – a contributing factor to the extremely rapid ventricular rates sometimes seen during atrial flutter and fibrillation. Such rates can be the cause for sudden death, and the ECG may be difficult to differentiate from polymorphic ventricular tachycardia or coarse fibrillation. In this regard, however, it should be noted that primary ventricular arrhythmias are unusual in WPW patients, unless they have other heart disease – often coronary artery disease.[94]

In patients who present to the emergency room with paroxysmal SVT, but with no evidence of ventricular pre-excitation in sinus rhythm, about 30% have AVRT, 60% have AVNRT, and the remainder have SVT caused by SA or intra-atrial re-entry.[92] APs may be capable of anterograde and retrograde conduction. Alternatively, they may be incapable of anterograde conduction, and only participate in antidromic AVRT or not at all (see below), or they may conduct only in the retrograde direction during orthodromic AVRT (see below). If so, there could be no ventricular pre-excitation, and the AP re-entry would be "concealed". As already noted, paroxysmal SVT resulting from concealed AV re-entry is about half as common as that caused by AV node re-entry.

Finally, AV reciprocating tachycardia can be orthodromic or antidromic, depending on the direction of impulse propagation in the AP. With the former (Fig 3.11b), activation of the ventricles during tachycardia is by the

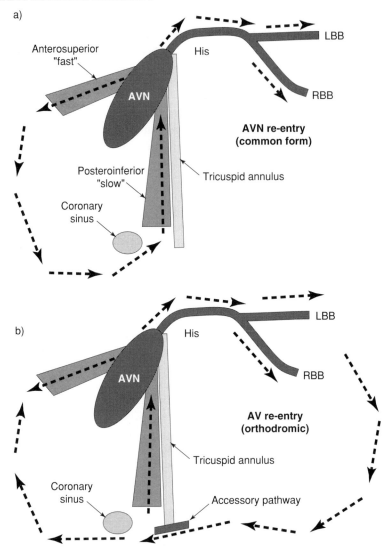

Fig 3.11 Depiction of the usual mechanisms for AV node re-entry tachycardia: (a) AVNRT and (b) AV reciprocating tachycardia AVRT. With the common form of AVNRT, the re-entry loop involves the AV node, possibly the atria (still debated[2]), and the anterosuperior and posteroinferior atrial approaches. The latter are the fast and slow pathways in AVNRT, respectively. With orthodromic AVRT, the anterosuperior and posteroinferior atrial approaches may or may not participate in tachycardia. Anterograde conduction is from the atrium (and/or AV nodal approaches) to the AV node, His bundle, left and right bundle branches (LBB, RBB), and the ventricles – resulting in a narrow QRS tachycardia. See the text for further discussion.

104

normal pathway (AV node to His bundle, etc). The circulating impulse returns to the atria via the AP. This gives rise to a narrow QRS tachycardia. With antidromic tachycardia ($\leq$ 10% of AVRT[91]), the ventricle is activated by anterograde impulses in the AP, giving rise to a wide QRS (pre-excited) tachycardia, which can be difficult to distinguish from ventricular tachycardia. This, however, is quite unusual in the WPW patient without other heart disease,[94] which is worth remembering when confronted with a *regular* wide QRS tachycardia in a patient known to have the WPW syndrome.

Conduction block

There can be block of conduction anywhere within the specialised AV conducting system. SA, atrial, AV nodal, bundle branch, fascicular, and intraventricular block can be diagnosed or inferred – primary or secondary SA block only – by inspection of the surface ECG. Diagnosis of tertiary SA block, intra-atrial block, or block within the His bundle requires catheter electrode recording techniques. SA and AV heart block is classified as: primary, delayed conduction; secondary, some but not all beats are conducted with (type 1) or without delay (type 2); tertiary, no beats are conducted to the atria (SA block) or ventricles (AV block). Advanced secondary SA or AV block is two or more successive non-conducted beats to the atria or ventricles, respectively. Bundle branch block is block in the right or left bundle branches. Block in the left anterior or posterior fascicle of the left bundle branch is fascicular block. Bifascicular block is a block in either both fascicular branches (that is, left bundle branch block) or one branch and the right bundle branch.

The site of conduction block has clinical and prognostic significance. The ratio of conducted beats with SA or AV nodal block may be increased with antimuscarinic drugs or β_1-agonists. Intra-atrial and infranodal (AV node) block is not as likely to respond favourably. Block within or below the His bundle carries a worse long term prognosis than block within the AV node or higher. Further discussion of conduction block and literature citations can be found elsewhere.[40]

Mechanisms for clinical arrhythmias

Clinical arrhythmias most certainly result from the abnormal cellular electrophysiological phenomena discussed above. Involvement of a particular mechanism in specific arrhythmias – with some exceptions – can, however, never be certain because in vitro cardiac electrophysiological studies cannot model circumstances of the intact heart. Nowhere is this more true than in perioperative and critical or emergent care situations, where drugs and imbalance – metabolic, electrolyte, autonomic – combine to affect the genesis of arrhythmias.[33 34 38] Thus, a patient with hypertension and healed myocardial infarction from coronary artery disease, who develops monomorphic ventricular tachycardia (VT) after a difficult tracheal intubation, could have several mechanisms involved in the genesis and maintenance of VT:

1 *Re-entry of excitation*: islands of normal myocardium interspersed with regions of fibrosis provide an anatomical substrate for re-entry, likely to be the mechanism which sustains monomorphic VT in this setting.

2 *Loss of membrane potential and depressed fast response*: increased heart rate and blood pressure act in concert to increase myocardial O_2 demand and reduce supply (reduced diastolic time). This and occlusive coronary disease cause acute myocardial ischaemia and, in turn, loss of membrane potential and the depressed fast response.

3 *Abnormal automaticity*: depolarisation induced (abnormal) automaticity in ischaemic Purkinje or ventricular muscle fibres could be the cause for slow monomorphic VT. Catecholamines released in response to endotracheal intubation can increase the rate of abnormal automaticity.

4 *Triggered activity*: increased $[Ca^{2+}]_i$ with ischaemia and catecholamines might underlie DAD or EAD triggered activity.

5 *Re-entry initiated by automatic or triggered beats*: finally, automatic or triggered premature beats might initiate re-entry of excitation involving anatomical (fibrous scar tissue) or functional re-entry loops (caused by varying depression of the fast response and inhomogeneous conduction and refractoriness). Ideal drug treatment for VT in this example is not at all obvious – although treatment may be successful, it can just as easily produce proarrhythmia (see below).

In contrast to this complexity, the genesis and treatment of paroxysmal SVT caused by AV node or AV re-entry are far more clear. Re-entry pathways are defined by electrophysiological mapping, and subsequently ablated by catheter or surgical means to "cure" SVT. Acute paroxysms of SVT can be readily terminated by drugs that increase AV node conduction time and refractoriness. So, mindful that cellular mechanisms may vary for the same disturbance, depending on the setting, postulated mechanisms for specific clinical arrhythmias are given in the box.

Antiarrhythmic drug action

There is no question that the emphasis on therapy for arrhythmias, especially ventricular tachyarrhythmias with coronary artery disease, has moved from drugs to "electricity" (implanted pacemakers, cardioverter defibrillators), or catheter–surgical ablation. When the heart is structurally normal, antiarrhythmic drugs have proved safe and effective. However, in the structurally abnormal heart (for example, myocardial infarction and

Postulated mechanisms for specific clinical arrhythmias

Mechanism	Arrhythmias
Altered normal automaticity	Sinus bradycardia/tachycardia; sinus arrhythmia; AV junctional/idioventricular escape rhythms; wandering atrial pacemaker
Abnormal automaticity	Slow monomorphic VT; accelerated AV junctional or idioventricular rhythm with acute myocardial infarction; some ectopic atrial tachycardia
Triggered activity (DAD)	Some VT in first 24 hours after infarction; atrial/ventricular tachycardias with digitalis toxicity; catecholamine mediated VT
Triggered activity (EAD)	Polymorphic VT insetting of QT interval prolongation (*torsade de pointes*)
Re-entry (anatomical)	SVT to SA, AV node, or AV re-entry; VT with healed infarction; atrial flutter (possibly anatomical and functional)
Re-entry (functional)	Atrial fibrillation; monomorphic and polymorphic VT with acute myocardial infarction; ventricular fibrillation

congestive heart failure), drug efficacy has been modest. Indeed, their use has been associated with increased mortality.[98–100] Nevertheless, drugs are an important adjuvant to electrical therapy for management of ventricular tachyarrhythmias, and the mainstay of treatment for atrial fibrillation.[101] In this brief overview of antiarrhythmic drugs, the decided emphasis is on ion channels as targets for antiarrhythmic drug action.

Antiarrhythmic treatment: role of structure of the myocardium

Antiarrhythmic drug therapy is least effective in structurally abnormal heart.[39 41–43 101] The myocardium is terminally differentiated. Replacement microfibrosis and a reduction in the number of gap junctions follow cell loss between surviving fibres ("myocardial remodelling"). The implications of changes in the normal distribution of gap junctions for the genesis of arrhythmias – namely, emergence of discontinuous conduction phenomena resulting from increased cellular electrical loading – are discussed by Spach and Boineau.[102] So, if structural heart disease is a primary culprit in the genesis of arrhythmias, perhaps one goal of pharmacological treatment should be the prevention of myocardial remodelling secondary to ischaemia and infarction, hypertrophy, and probably heart failure.[101] At least atrial remodelling seems to be a part of ageing, and may be important in the increased prevalence of atrial fibrillation in elderly people.[103] Although development of means to reduce myocardial remodelling with disease (for example, drugs that influence gap junction expression[101]) has been neglected as part of the antiarrhythmic strategy, and this is a promising new area for investigation.

Antiarrhythmic treatment: desirable drug properties

Ion channels and neurohormonal receptors that modulate their function, and not electrophysiological phenomena themselves,[98 99] have now become the primary targets for antiarrhythmic drug action.[20 42 78 100 101 104] The goal of drug therapy is, as far as possible, to restore normal impulse initiation and propagation – or to slow the effective ventricular rate (chronic atrial fibrillation). The following are desirable properties of an antiarrhythmic drug:

- specificity: the drug should interact with the specific ion channel(s) involved in the genesis of the arrhythmia
- pharmacodynamics: the kinetics of association and dissociation should be such that effects (slowing of conduction, prolongation of refractoriness) are maximal during tachycardia
- pharmacokinetics: brief onset and duration of action (parenteral administration); high bioavailability, rapid onset of action, and infrequent dosing (oral administration). [101]

Specific ion channels as targets for antiarrhythmic drug action

Pacemaker currents

The pacemaker current (I_f) helps initiate automaticity in SA node cells and subsidiary pacemaker fibres. Although specific blockers of this current have been identified,[105] their use is quite limited because sinus tachycardia is usually a compensatory rhythm disturbance. Both T type and L type Ca^{2+} current also contribute to the pacemaker potential and conduction in SA node and subsidiary pacemakers, but clinically effective antagonists (verapamil, diltiazem) block only L type current. Verapamil and diltiazem have low lipid solubility, and access their intracellular Ca^{2+} channel binding site predominantly via the open channel.[104] Either is effective for slowing AV conduction with atrial fibrillation–flutter, and terminating SA and AV node re-entry. Dihydropyridine Ca^{2+} antagonists (nifedipine, nicardipine) are neutral compounds that are highly lipid soluble, and ineffective blockers of L type current in the heart. They occupy receptors on the extracellular surface of the Ca^{2+} channel, and bind preferentially to the channel in depolarised tissue (that is, in its inactivated state).[104] As they are neutral and lipid soluble, they also dissociate rapidly, especially from more polarised tissue. Hence, dihydropyridine Ca^{2+} blockers are primarily effective for blocking Ca^{2+} channels in more depolarised vascular smooth muscle.

Na$^+$ channel: fast inward current

Block of the fast Na$^+$ inward current (I_{Na}) is useful against re-entrant arrhythmias involving atrial, ventricular, and Purkinje fibres – with AP upstrokes largely dependent on I_{Na}. There is, however, recognised potential for proarrhythmia with Na$^+$ channel blockers, which appears to be greatest with class 1A (quinidine-like) and 1C (flecanide-like) drugs. These drugs have intermediate or slow dissociation kinetics – consequently, lesser block at relatively slow heart rates may be substantially enhanced at faster rates (that is, use-dependent block). This might promote re-entrant tachycardia, and in part explain increased mortality with 1C drugs in the Cardiac Arrhythmia Suppression Trial (CAST) studies.[98 99]

The antiarrhythmic efficacy of Na$^+$ channel blockers is determined mainly by how they interact with the multiple states of the Na$^+$ channel (see Fig 3.2). This has a number of clinical ramifications. For one, high affinity binding states may be accessible only phasically, so that drug binding occurs primarily during depolarisation. If so, a fast binding drug may compete with and displace one with slower kinetics – as shown in a patient with propoxyphene overdose in whom marked QRS widening was reversed by lidocaine.[106] Also, ischaemia or stretch with consequent partial depolarisation may incompletely inactivate Na$^+$ channels. Compared with primarily open state blockers (disopyramide and quinidine), drugs that block both open and inactivated Na$^+$ channels (lidocaine and mexiletine) depress AP phase 0 and conduction more in partially depolarised fibres.[105] Consequently, inactivated state blockers may be more effective against re-entrant ventricular tachyarrhythmias with acute myocardial infarction and ischaemia.[107] Open channel Na$^+$ blockers penetrate the Na$^+$ channel pore a significant distance to produce block, and Na$^+$ ions bind to specific sites as they transit the pore.[104] Competition between the open channel blocker and the permeating Na$^+$ ions may result. If so, administration of Na$^+$ lactate or bicarbonate solutions may decrease the rate of association of open but not inactivated state Na$^+$ channel blockers with the Na$^+$ channel.

In addition to producing open state Na$^+$ channel blockade, class 1A drugs (quinidine and disopyramide) prolong AP duration. This increases the period of inactivation of Na$^+$ channels. If so, open state blockers may enhance the blocking action of inactivated state blockers (lidocaine and mexiletine),[104] which is the rationale behind combining class 1A and 1B drugs.[108 109]

Action potential plateau currents

Both the Na$^+$ and Ca^{2+} channels contribute inward current during the AP plateau. Increasing either current component will prolong AP duration, and directly (Ca^{2+}) or indirectly (Na$^+$) cause positive inotropy.[101] This might occur in a patient receiving a positive inotrope for ventricular dysfunction and lidocaine for arrhythmia suppression after cardiopulmon-

109

ary bypass. There is, however a downside to this. If Na^+ or Ca^{2+} activators bind during the AP plateau, AP prolongation could become regenerative and EAD with triggered activity result.[101]

K+ channel blockers

The emphasis of antiarrhythmic drug research and development has shifted away from drugs that are primarily Na^+ channel blockers to those that prolong AP duration and refractoriness by blocking voltage gated K^+ channels (class 3 effect). The basis of this shift is multifactorial:[104]

Class 1 proarrhythmia – There is accumulating evidence of relative inefficacy and increased proarrhythmia with class 1 agents.[98 99]

Class 3 efficacy – Prolongation of AP duration and refractoriness is particularly efficacious for arrhythmias with an excitable gap (atrial flutter, monomorphic VT).[104 110] Class 3 drugs appear to be more effective than class 1 drugs in preventing death and arrhythmia recurrence in patients with ventricular tachyarrhythmias,[111] and in experimental models of atrial flutter and lethal ventricular arrhythmias.[104]

Contractility – In contrast to class 1A and 1C drugs, which depress myocardial contractility, class 3 drugs either do not affect contractility or slightly increase it.[104] This effect is attributed to AP prolongation, which increases Ca^{2+} current during the AP plateau, thereby enhancing Ca^{2+} release from the sarcoplasmic reticulum.

Defibrillation threshold (DFT) – Class 3 drugs have been reported to decrease DFT in canine models, thereby facilitating defibrillation.[104]

The K^+ channel blockers are a diverse group of compounds that share the property of prolonging AP duration and refractoriness in fast response fibres. They include drugs traditionally grouped as class 1A, 1C, and 3 agents in the modified Vaughan Williams classification.[112 113] The degree of AP duration prolongation is quite variable among class 1A and 1C drugs, despite the fact that all block the delayed rectifier (I_K), and some (quinidine and disopyramide) block the inward rectifier (I_{K1}) and transient outward currents (I_{to1}) as well.[104] This is attributed to the concomitant influence of these drugs on I_{Na}, particularly the slowly inactivating or late component.[104] Potent block of this component by flecainide shortens AP duration, which counters AP duration prolongation by block of I_K.[104] Increased Ca^{2+} or Na^+ current during the AP plateau can also prolong AP duration. Indeed, part of the effect of the class 3 drug ibutilide – a drug recently approved for chemical conversion of atrial flutter and fibrillation – is mediated by block of the late component of I_{Na}.[104 114] Ibutilide may also prolong AP duration by blocking I_K.

Quinidine and disopyramide (class 1A) are non-specific blockers of K^+ current, blocking all three components (I_K, I_{K1}, and I_{to1}).[104] Procainamide (class 1A) and flecainide (class 1C) are selective blockers of I_K. The class 3 drugs, sotolol, amiodarone and bretylium are relatively non-selective K^+ blockers. Sotolol is also a non-selective β-blocker (β_1, β_2), and bretylium causes initial release of norepinephrine (noradrenaline). Amiodarone exhibits all four class actions. In addition to blocking I_K and I_{K1}, amiodarone also blocks Na^+ and Ca^{2+} channels, and has non-competitive α- and β- adrenergic blocking effects. This non-specificity may in part explain the lower proarrhythmic potential of amiodarone compared with other antiarrhythmic agents.[104 110]

Most Na^+ channel blockers, especially in higher concentrations, cause use-dependent block, that is, depression of Na^+ current and AP upstroke velocity (hence, AP propagation or conduction) is greater at faster heart rates. The "ideal" K^+ channel blocker should also display use-dependent block. Most available ones (except, amiodarone and flecainide) do just the opposite, however, produce maximal prolongation of AP duration and refractoriness at slow heart rates, with progressively diminishing effects at faster heart rates.[104] This has been termed "reverse use dependence".[115] In fact, it really isn't "reverse use dependence".[104] Most K^+ channel blocking drugs (including amiodarone and flecainide) block I_K in a use-dependent fashion. Furthermore, block is increased at depolarised potentials, when channels are in the open state. Accordingly, drug *block* (what occurs at the K^+ channel level, the conventional meaning for "use dependence"[116]) shows normal use dependence.[104] If so, the term "reverse rate dependence"[117] may be the more appropriate way to describe K^+ channel blocker behaviour.[104]

Reverse rate dependence is expected to limit the efficacy of most K^+ blockers for terminating sustained tachyarrhythmias. It may also help predispose to development of bradycardia dependent prolongation of the QT interval and *torsade de pointes*.[104 107 110 115] Nevertheless, as a group the K^+ channel blockers are moderately effective antiarrhythmics, possibly because prolongation of refractoriness decreases the diastolic window of excitability for initiation of tachycardia.[115] Finally, the fact that amiodarone does not exhibit reverse rate dependence over a wide range of heart rates may explain its greater efficacy and lower proarrhythmic potential compared with other antiarrhythmic drugs.[104]

Finally, and of possible relevance to further development of cardiac K^+ channel blockers, several mechanisms have been proposed to explain the disparity between use dependent block of I_K and reverse rate dependent prolongation of AP duration and refractoriness.[104] First, at faster heart rates, the relative contribution of other ionic processes (for example, the inactivation of $I_{Ca,L}$) may exceed that of I_K. Second, at fast heart rates, as a result of incomplete activation, the slowly activating component of I_K (I_{Ks}) assumes more importance than its faster component (I_{Kr}) in mediating AP repolarisation.[104] As most selective I_K blockers target I_{Kr} and have little affinity for I_{Ks}, they should be less effective at fast heart rates.[104 118 119] In this regard, it is noteworthy that amiodarone primarily blocks I_{Ks}. This may partly explain why the drug prolongs AP duration over a range of heart rates.[104] Third, preferential block of open K^+ channels does not necessarily result in prominent use dependent block, especially if recovery from block is slow (dofetilide) or onset of block is very rapid (quinidine).[104] This results because, as for the Na^+ channel blockers, the kinetics of onset and offset of K^+ channel block are key determinants of use dependent block. Thus, if the onset of block is rapid, steady state block could be achieved during a single AP, and there would be little increase in block at faster rates. Similarly, with slow offset of block, there would be little dissipation of the block between beats, and steady state block would be achieved at relatively slow heart rates. It has been suggested that the "ideal" K^+ channel blocker should block the open channel with depolarisation, thereby permitting rapid recovery from inactivation with repolarisation.[119] Kinetic properties such as these are expected to result in a normal use dependent (not reverse rate dependent) pattern of APD prolongation. This has the potential for greater antiarrhythmic efficacy with less proarrhythmia.[120]

Anaesthetic arrhythmic potential

Anaesthetic drugs can have both pro- and antiarrhythmic actions.[33 34 38] Proarrhythmic actions include the facilitation of catecholamine mediated ventricular arrhythmias, suppression of normal automaticity in primary and secondary pacemaker fibres, and depression of AV conduction. Examples of antiarrhythmic actions include suppression of abnormal automaticity and DAD triggered activity, and ventricular tachyarrhythmias in canine models of myocardial ischaemia and infarction. Discussion of these in more detail is beyond the scope of this chapter. Suffice it to say, no anaesthetic drug, inhalational or otherwise, could be introduced into clinical practice today were it discovered in preclinical trials to cause *de novo* arrhythmias in normal heart. Nor would it enjoy a very long clinical life if it were proarrhythmic in subsets of patients with cardiovascular disease, especially with myocardial remodelling. In this vein, it is disheartening that very little is really known about anaesthetic drug effects in patients with arrhythmias or susceptibility to arrhythmias. Finally, one cannot presume that an anaesthetic drug will be proarrhythmic in a patient with heart disease, especially the patient with coronary disease and a history of ventricular arrhythmias, just because it is sensitising (for example, halothane).[121]

1 Whalley DW, Wendt DJ, Grant AO. Basic concepts in cellular cardiac electrophysiology: Part I: Ion channels, membrane currents, and the action potential. *Pace* 1995;**18**:1556–74.

2 Zipes DP. Genesis of cardiac arrhythmias: Electrophysiological considerations. In: Braunwald E, ed, *Heart disease*, 5th edn. Philadelphia, WB Saunders, 1997:548–92.

3 Brown AM, Lee KS, Powell T. Voltage clamp and internal perfusion of single rat heart muscle cells. *J Physiol (Lond)* 1981;**318**:455–77.

4 Hamill OP, Marty A, Neher E, Sachmann B, Sigworth FJ. Improved patch-clamp techniques for high-resolution current recording from cells and cell-free membrane patches. *Pflügers Arch* 1981;**39**:85–100.

5 Katz AM. Cardiac ion channels. *N Engl J Med* 1993; **328**:1244–51.

6 Catterall WA. Cellular and molecular biology of voltage-gated sodium channels. *Physiol Rev* 1992;**72**:515–48.

7 Hille B. *Ionic channels of excitable membranes.* Sunderland Sinauer Association, Inc., 1984:1–19.

8 Armstrong CM. Sodium channels and gating currents. *Physiol Rev* 1981;**61**:544–683.

9 Hodgkin AL, Huxley AF. A quantitative description of membrane current and its application to conduction and excitation in nerve. *J Physiol (Lond)* 1952;**117**:500–44.

10 Brown AM. Ion channels as g protein effectors. *News Physiol Sci* 1991;**6**:158–61.

11 Nichols CG, Lederer WJ. Adenosine triphosphate-sensitive potassium channels in the cardiovascular system. *Am J Physiol* 1991;**261**: H1675–86.

12 Freeman LC, Kass RC. Expression of a minimal K^+ channel protein in mammalian cells and immuno-localization in guinea pig heart. *Circ Res* 1993;**73**:968–73.

13 Po S, Roberds S, Snyders DJ, et al. Heteromultimetric assembly of human potassium channels. Molecular basis of a transient outward current? *Circ Res* 1993;**72**:1326–36.

14 Cohen SA, Barchi RL. Voltage-dependent sodium channels. *Int Rev Cytol* 1993;**137C**:55–103.

15 Stuhemer W, Conti F, Suzuki H, et al. Structural parts involved in activation and inactivation of the sodium channel. *Nature* 1993;**339**:597–603.

16 Backx PH, Yue DT, Lawrence JH, et al. Molecular localization of an ion-binding site within the pore of mammalian sodium channels. *Science* 1992;**257**:258–51.

17 Isom LL, De Jongh KS, Patton DE, et al. Primary structure and functional expression of the β1 subunit of the rat brain sodium channel. *Science* 1992;**256**:839–42.

18 Sperelakis N. Origin of the cardiac resting potential. In: Berne RM, ed, *Handbook of physiology*, Section 2, *The cardiovascular system. The heart*, Vol 1. Bethesda, MD: American Physiological Society, 1979:187–267.

19 Boyden PA. Cellular electrophysiologic basis of cardiac arrhythmias. *Am J Cardiol* 1996;**78**(suppl 4A):4–11.

20 Task Force of the Working Group on Arrhythmias of the European Society of Cardiology. The Sicilian Gambit. A new approach to the classification of antiarrhythmic drugs based on their actions on arrhythmogenic mechanisms. *Circulation* 1991;**84**:1831–51.

21 Coraboeuf E, Carmeleit E. Existence of two transient outward currents in sheep cardiac Purkinje fibres. *Pflügers Arch* 1982;**352**:9.

22 Zygmunt AC, Gibbons WR. Calcium-activated chloride current in rabbit ventricular myocytes. *Circ Res* 1991;**68**:424–37.

23 Litovsky SH, Antzelvitch C. Transient outward current prominent in canine ventricular epicardium but not endocardium. *Circ Res* 1988;**62**:116–26.

24 Harvey RD, Clark CO, Hume JR. A chloride current in mammalian cardiac myocytes: Novel mechanisms for autonomic regulation of action potential duration and resting membrane potential. *J Gen Physiol* 1990;**95**:1077–102.

25 Patlak JB, Ortiz M, . Slow current through single Na^+ channels of adult rat heart. *J Gen Physiol* 1988;**86**:89–104.

26 Wasserstrom JA, Salata JJ. Basis for tetrodotoxin and lidocaine effects on action potentials in dog and ventricular myocytes. *Am J Physiol* 1988;**254**:H1157-66.

27 Eisner DA, Lederer WT. Na-Ca exchange: stoichiometry and electrogenecity. *Am J Physiol* 1985,**248**:C189-202.

28 Irisawa H, Brown HF, Giles W. Cardiac pacemaking in the sinoatrial node. *Physiol Rev* 1993;**73**:197–227.

29 Arnsdorf MF. Arnsdorf's paradox. *J Cardiovasc Electrophysiol* 1990;**1**:42–52.

30 Arnsdorf MF. Basic understanding of electrophysiological actions of antiarrhythmic drugs: Sources, sinks and matrices of information. *Med Clin North Am* 1988;**68**:1247–80.

31 Kleber AG, Riegger CB. Electrical constants of arterially perfused rabbit papillary muscle. *J Physiol (Lond)* 1987;**385**:307–24.

32 Weidmann S. Passive properties of cardiac fibres. In: Rosen MR, Janse MJ, Wit AL, eds, *Cardiac electrophysiology: A textbook*. Mount Kisco, NY: Futura Publishing Co., 1990:415–25.

33 Atlee JL III, Bosnjak ZJ. Mechanisms for cardiac dysrhythmias during anesthesia. *Anesthesiology* 1990;**72**:347–94.

34 Turner LA, Bosnjak ZJ. Autonomic and anesthetic modulation of cardiac conduction and arrhythmias. In: Lynch C III ed, *Clinical cardiac electrophysiology. Perioperative considerations*. Philadelphia: JB Lippincott Co., 1994:53–84.

35 Fozzard HA, Arnsdorf MF. Cardiac electrophysiology. In: Fozzard HA, Jennings RB, Haber E, Katz AM, Morgan HE, eds, *The heart and cardiovascular system*, 2nd edn. New York: Raven Press, 1992:63–98.

36 Delmar M. Role of potassium currents on cell excitability in cardiac ventricular myocytes. *J Cardiovasc Electrophysiol* 1992;**3**:474–86.

37 Cranefield PF. Action potentials, afterpotentials, and arrhythmias. *Circ Res* 1977;**41**:415–23.

38 Patterson E, Szabo B, Scherlag BJ, Lazzara R. Arrhythmogenic effects of antiarrhythmic drugs. In: Zipes DP, Jalife J, eds, *Cardiac electrophysiology: from cell to bedside*. 2nd edn. Philadelphia: WB Saunders, 1995: 496–511.

39 Grace AA, Camm AJ. Quinidine. *N Engl J Med* 1998;**338**:35–44.

40 Atlee JL. Perioperative cardiac dysrhythmias. *Anesthesiology* 1997;**86**:1397–424

41 Morganroth J. Proarrhythmic effects of antiarrhythmic drugs: evolving concepts. *Am Heart J* 1992;**123**:1137–9.

42 Kerin N, Somberg J. Proarrhythmia: Definition, risk factors, causes, treatment, and controversies. *Am Heart J* 1994;**128**:575–86.

43 De Luna A, Guindo J, Vinolas X, et al. Proarrhythmic effects of anti-arrhythmic agents. *Postgrad Med J* 1994;**70**:S84-8.

44 Colatsky TJ, Follmer CH, Starmer CF. Channel specificity in antiarrhythmic drug action: mechanism of potassium channel block and its role in suppressing and aggravating cardiac arrhythmias. *Circulation* 1990;**82**:2235–42.

45 Yang T, Roden DM. Extracellular K^+ modulation of drug block by I_{Kr}: implications for *torsade de pointes* and reverse use-dependence. *Circulation* 1996;**93**:407–11.

46 Schwartz PJ, Stramba-Badiale M, Segantini A, et al. Prolongation of the QT interval and the sudden infant death syndrome. *N Engl J Med* 1998;**338**:1709–14.

47 Schwartz PJ, Locati EH, Napolitano C, Priori SG. The long QT syndrome. In: Zipes DP, Jalife J, eds, *Cardiac electrophysiology: from cell to bedside*, 2nd edn. Philadelphia: WB Saunders, 1995:788–811.

48 Schwartz P, Priori S, Locati, EH, et al. Long QT syndrome patients with mutations of the SCN5A and HERG genes have differential responses to Na^+ channel blockade and to increases in heart rate. *Circulation* 1995;**92**:3381–6.

49 Rosen M. Long QT syndrome patients with gene mutations. *Circulation* 1995;**92**:3373–5.

50 Moss A, Zareba W, Benhorin J, et al. ECG T-wave patterns in genetically distinct forms of the hereditary long QT syndrome. *Circulation* 1995;**92**:2929–34.

51 Kass RL, Lederer WJ, Tsien RW, Weingurt R. Role of calcium ions in transient inward currents and aftercontractions induced by acetylstrophanthidin in cardiac Purkinje fibres. *J Physiol* 1978;**281**:187–208.

52 Kass RL, Tsien RW, Weingurt R. Ionic basis of transient inward current induced by strophanthidin in cardiac Purkinje fibres. *J Physiol* 1978;**281**:209–26.

53 Luo CH, Rudy Y. A dynamic model of the cardiac ventricular action potential: I. Simulations of ionic currents and concentration changes. *Circ Res* 1994;**74**:1071–96

54 Luo CH, Rudy Y. A dynamic model of the cardiac ventricular action potential: II. Afterdepolarizations, triggered activity and potentiations. *Circ Res* 1994;**74**:1097–113

55 Mines GR. On dynamic equilibrium in the heart. *J Physiol (Lond)* 1913;**46**:349–82.

56 Mines GR. On circulating excitations in heart muscles and their possible relation to tachycardia and fibrillation. *Trans R Soc Canada, Section IV,* 1914:43–52.

57 Fozzard HA, Haber E, Jennings RB, et al, eds. *The heart and cardiovascular system: Scientific foundations,* 2nd edn. New York: Raven Press, 1991:63–98, 863–1169, 2021–193.

58 Mendez C, Mueller WJ, Urguiaga X. Propagation of impulses across the Purkinje fibre–muscle junctions in the dog heart. *Circ Res* 1970;**36**:135–50.

59 Veenstra RD, Joyner RW, Rawling DA. Purkinje and ventricular activation sequences of canine papillary muscle: Effects of quinidine and calcium on Purkinje–ventricular conduction delay. *Circ Res* 1984;**54**:500–15.

60 Joyner RW, Overhold VD, Ramza B, Veenstra RD. Propagation through electrically coupled cells: Two inhomgeneously coupled cardiac tissue layers. *Am J Physiol* 1984;**247**:H596–609.

61 Schmidt FO, Erlanger J. Directional differences in the conduction of the impulse through heart muscle and their possible relation to extrasystoles and fibrillary contractions. *Am J Physiol* 1929;**87**:326–47.

62 Allessie MA, Lammers WJ, Bonke IM, Hollen J. Intra-atrial reentry as a mechanism for atrial flutter induced by acetylcholine and rapid atrial pacing in the dog. *Circulation* 1984;**70**:123–35.

63 Janse MJ, Van Cappele FJ, Freud GE, Durrer D. Circus movement within the AV node as a basis for supraventricular tachycardia as shown by multiple microelectrode recording in the isolated rabbit heart. *Circ Res* 1971;**28**:403–14.

64 Pastelin G, Mendez R, Moe GK. Participation of atrial specialized conduction pathways in atrial flutter. *Circ Res* 1978;**42**:386–93.

65 Cabo C, Wit AL. Cellular electrophysiologic mechanisms of cardiac arrhythmias. *Cardiol Clin* 1997;**15**:517–38

66 Boyden PA, Tilley LP, Albala A, Liu SK, Fenoglio JJ Jr, Wit AL. Mechanisms for atrial arrhythmias associated with cardiomyopathy: A study of feline hearts with primary myocardial disease. *Circulation* 1984;**69**:1036–47.

67 Ursell PC, Gardner PI, Albala A, Fenoglio JJ Jr, Wit AL. Structural and electrophysiological changes in the epicardial border zone of canine myocardial infarcts during infarct healing. *Circ Res* 1985;**56**:436–51.

68 Blanck Z, Sra J, Dhala A, Deshpande S, Jazayeri MR, Akhtar M. Bundle branch reentry: Mechanisms, diagnosis, treatment. In: Zipes DP, Jalife J, eds, *Cardiac electrophysiology: from cell to bedside,* 2nd edn. Philadelphia: WB Saunders, 1995:878–85.

69 Miles WM, Klein LS, Rardon DP, Mitrani RD, Zipes DP. Atrioventricular reentry and variants: Mechanisms, clinical features, and management. In: Zipes DP, Jalife J, eds, *Cardiac electrophysiology: from cell to bedside,* 2nd edn. Philadelphia: WB Saunders, 1995: 638–41, 642–55.

70 Waldo AL. Atrial flutter: Mechanisms, clinical features, and management. In: Zipes DP, Jalife J, eds, *Cardiac electrophysiology: from cell to bedside,* 2nd edn. Philadelphia: WB Saunders, 1995:666–81.

71 El-Sherif N. Reentrant mechanisms in ventricular arrhythmias. In: Zipes DP, Jalife J, eds, *Cardiac electrophysiology: from cell to bedside.* 2nd edn. Philadelphia: WB Saunders, 1995: 567–82.

72 Janse MJ, Opthof T. Mechanisms of ischemia induced arrhythmias. In: Zipes DP, Jalife J, eds, *Cardiac electrophysiology: from cell to bedside* 2nd edn. Philadelphia: WB Saunders, 1995:489–96.

73 Wit AL, Dillon SM, Coromilas J. Anisotropic reentry as a cause of ventricular tachyarrhythmias in myocardial infarction. In: Zipes DP, Jalife J, eds, *Cardiac electrophysiology: from cell to bedside,* 2nd edn. Philadelphia: WB Saunders, 1995:511–26.

74 Allessie MA, Bonke FIM, Schopman FJG. Circus movement in rabbit atrial muscle as a mechanism of tachycardia. *Circ Res* 1973;**33**:54–62.

75 Allessie MA, Bonke FIM, Schopman FJG. Circus movement in rabbit atrial muscle as a mechanism of tachycardia: II. The role of nonuniform recovery of excitability in the occurrence of unidirectional block, as studied with multiple microelectrodes. *Circ Res* 1976;**39**:168–77.

76 Allessie MA, Bonke FIM, Schopman FJG. Circus movement in rabbit atrial muscle as a mechanism of tachycardia: III The leading circle concept: A new model of circus movement in cardiac tissue without the involvement of an anatomical obstacle. *Circ Res* 1977;**41**:9–18.

77 Allessie MA. Re-entrant mechanism underlying atrial fibrillation. In: Zipes DP, Jalife J, eds, *Cardiac electrophysiology: from cell to bedside*, 2nd edn. Philadelphia: WB Saunders, 1995: 562–6.

78 The Sicilian Gambit. *Antiarrhythmic therapy: a pathophysiologic approach.* Armonk, NY: Futura Publishing, 1994:3–337

79 Davidenko JM, Pertsov AM, Salomonsz R, Baxter W, Jalife J. Stationary and drifting spiral waves of excitation in isolated cardiac muscle. *Nature* 1992;**335**:349–51.

80 Davidenko JM. Spiral waves in the heart: Experimental demonstration of a theory. In: Zipes DP, Jalife J, eds, *Cardiac electrophysiology: from cell to bedside* 2nd edn. Philadelphia: WB Saunders, 1995:478–88.

81 Davidenko JM. Spiral wave activity: A possible common mechanism for polymorphic and monomorphic ventricular tachycardias. *J Cardiovasc Electrophysiol* 1993;**4**:730–46.

82 Chen P-S, Garfinkel A, Weiss JN, Karagueuzian HS. Spirals, chaos, and new mechanisms of wave propagation. *PACE* 1997;**20**:414–21.

83 Naccarelli GV, Shih HT, Jalal S. Sinus node reentry and atrial tachycardias. In: Zipes DP, Jalife J, eds, *Cardiac electrophysiology: from cell to bedside*, 2nd edn. Philadelphia: WB Saunders, 1995:607–19.

84 Watanabe Y, Watanabe M. Impulse formation and conduction of excitation in the atrioventricular node. *J Cardiovasc Electrophysiol* 1994;**5**:517–31.

85 Janse MJ, Anderson RH, McGuire MA, Ho SV. "AV nodal" reentry: 1. "AV nodal" reentry revisited. *J Cardiovasc Electrophysiol* 1993;**4**:561–72.

86 McGuire MA, Janse MJ, Ross DL. "AV nodal" reentry: 2. AV nodal, AV junctional or atrial nodal reentry? *J Cardiovasc Electrophysiol* 1993;**4**:573–86.

87 Jackman WM, Nakagawa H, Heidbuuchel H, et al. Three forms of atrioventricular nodal (junctional) reentrant tachycardia: Differential diagnosis, electrophysiological characteristics, and implications for anatomy of the reentrant circuit. In: Zipes DP, Jalife J, eds, *Cardiac electrophysiology: from cell to bedside*, 2nd edn. Philadelphia: WB Saunders, 1995: 620–37.

88 Kalbfleisch SJ, Morady F. Catheter ablation of atrioventricular nodal reentrant tachycardia. In: Zipes DP, Jalife J, eds, *Cardiac electrophysiology: from cell to bedside*, 2nd edn. Philadelphia: WB Saunders, 1995:1477–99.

89 Mahomed Y. Surgery for atrioventricular nodal reentrant tachycardia. In: Zipes DP, Jalife J, eds, *Cardiac electrophysiology: from cell to bedside*, 2nd edn. Philadelphia: WB Saunders, 1995:1577–83.

90 Wellens HJJ. Supraventricular tachycardia with reentry in the AV node. In: Kastor JA, ed, *Arrhythmias*. Philadelphia: WB Saunders, 1994:250–61.

91 Gallagher JJ. Supraventricular tachycardia with reentry in accessory pathways. In: Kastor JA, ed, *Arrhythmias*. Philadelphia: WB Saunders, 1994:262–96.

92 Miles WM, Klein LS, Rardon DP, Mitrani RD, Zipes DP. Atrioventricular reentry and its variants: Mechanisms, clinical features, and management. In: Zipes DP, Jalife J, eds, *Cardiac electrophysiology: from cell to bedside*, 2nd edn. Philadelphia: WB Saunders, 1995: 638–55.

93 Packer DL, Zipes DP. Anatomical and physiological substrates for antidromic reciprocating tachycardia. In: Zipes DP, Jalife J, eds, *Cardiac electrophysiology: from cell to bedside*, 2nd edn. Philadelphia: WB Saunders, 1995:655–66.

94 Yee R, Klein GJ, Guiraudon GM. The Wolff–Parkinson–White syndrome. In: Zipes DP, Jalife J, eds, *Cardiac electrophysiology: from cell to bedside*, 2nd edn. Philadelphia: WB Saunders, 1995:1199–214.

95 Haissaguerre M, Clémenty J, Warin J-F. Catheter ablation of atrioventricular reentrant tachycardia. In: Zipes DP, Jalife J, eds, *Cardiac electrophysiology: from cell to bedside*, 2nd edn. Philadelphia: WB Saunders, 1995:1487–99.

96 Guiraudon GM, Klein GJ, Yee R, Thakur RK, Guiraudon CM. Surgery for the Wolff-Parkinson-White syndrome. In: Zipes DP, Jalife J, eds, *Cardiac electrophysiology: from cell to bedside*, 2nd edn. Philadelphia: WB Saunders, 1995:1553–63.

97 Wit AL, Janse MJ. *The ventricular arrhythmias of ischemia and infarction: Electrophysiological mechanisms.* Mt Kisco, NY: Futura, 1993.

98 CAST Investigators. Preliminary Report. Effect of encainide and flecainide on mortality in a randomized trial of arrhythmia suppression after myocardial infarction. *N Engl J Med* 1989;**321**:406–12.

99 CAST-II. Effect of the antiarrhythmic agent moricizine on survival after myocardial infarction. *N Engl J Med* 1992;**327**:227–33.

100 Flaker GC, Blackshear JL, McBride R, Kronmal RA, Hart RG. Antiarrhythmic drug therapy and cardiac mortality in atrial fibrillation. *J Am Coll Cardiol* 1992;**20**:527–32.

101 Grant AO. Mechanisms of action of antiarrhythmic drugs: From ion channel blockage to arrhythmia termination. *PACE* 1997;**20**; 432–4.

102 Spach MS, Boineau JP. Micofibrosis produces electrical load variations due to loss of side-to-side cell connections. *PACE* 1997;**20**:397–413.

103 Weber KT, Spach MS, Starmer MF. Chaos in the hall of mirrors. Cardiovasc Res 1995;**30**:336–44.

104 Whalley DW, Wendt DJ, Grant AO. Basic concepts in cellular cardiac electrophysiology: Part II: Block of ion channels by antiarrhythmic drugs. *Pace* 1995;**18**:1686–704.

105 Van Bogaert P-P, Goethals M. Pharmacological influence of specific bradycardic agents on the pacemaker current of sheep cardiac Purkinje fibres. A comparison between three different molecules. *Eur Heart J 1987*;**8**(suppl L):35–42.

106 Whitcomb DC, Gilliam FR 3rd, Starmer CF, Grant AO. Marked QRS complex abnormalities and sodium channel blockade propoxyphene reversed with lidocaine. *J Clin Invest* 1989;**84**:1629–43.

107 Zipes DP. Management of cardiac arrhythmias: Pharmacological, electrical, and surgical techniques. In: Braunwald E, ed, *Heart disease*, 5th edn. Philadelphia: WB Saunders, 1997:593–639.

108 Duff HJ, Roden D, Primm RK, Oates JA, Woosley RL. Mexiletine in the treatment of resistant ventricular arrhythmias: Enhancement of efficacy and reduction of dose related side effects of combination with quinidine. *Circulation* 1983;**67**:1124–8.

109 Kim SG, Mercondo AD, Tom S. Combination of disopyramide and mexiletine for better tolerance and additive effects for treatment of ventricular arrhythmias. *J Am Coll Cardiol* 1989;**13**:659–64.

110 Singh B. Controlling cardiac arrhythmias by lengthening repolarization: Historical overview. *Am Heart J* 1993;**72**:18F-24F.

111 Mason JW. A comparison of seven antiarrhythmic drugs in patients with ventricular tachyarrhythmias. *N Engl J Med* 1993;**329**:452–8.

112 Vaughan Williams E. Classification of antiarrhythmic drugs. In: Sandoe E, Flensted-Jensen E, Olesen K, eds, *Cardiac arrhythmias.* Sodertaljie, Sweden: AB Astra, 1971:449–72.

113 Harrison D, Winkle R, Sami M, Mason J. Encainide: a new and potent antiarrhythmic agent. In: Harrison D, ed, *Cardiac arrhythmias: a decade of progress.* Boston: GK Hall, 1981:315–30.

114 Stambler BS, Wood MA, Ellenbogen KA, Perry KT, Wakefield LK, VanderLugt JT, and the Ibutilide repeat dose study Investigators. Efficacy and safety of repeated intravenous doses of ibutilide for rapid conversion of atrial flutter or fibrillation. *Circulation* 1996;**94**:1613–21.

115 Hondeghem LM, Snyders DJ. Class III antiarrhythmic agents have a lot of potential but a long way to go. *Circulation* 1990;**81**:686–90.

116 Carmeliet E. K$^+$ channels and control of ventricular repolarization in the heart. *Fundam Clin Pharmacol* 1993;**7**:19–28.

117 Jurkiewicz NK, Sanguinetti MC. Rate-dependent prolongation of cardiac action potentials by a methanesulfonanilide Class III antiarrhythmic agent. *Circ Res* 1993;**73**:75–83.

118 Colatsky TJ. Potassium channel blockers: Synthetic agents and their antiarrhythmic potential. In: Weston AH, Hamilton TC, eds, *Potassium channel modulators: pharmacological, molecular and clinical aspects.* London: Blackwell Scientific Ltd, 1992:304–40.

119 Carmeliet E. Use-dependent block and use-dependent unblock of the delayed rectifier K$^+$ current by almokalant in rabbit ventricular myocytes. *Circ Res* 1993;**73**:857–68.

117

120 Hondeghem LM. Development of Class III antiarrhythmic agents. J Cardiovasc Pharmacol 1992;**20** (suppl 2):S17-22.
121 Atlee JL. Halothane: cause or cure for arrhythmias? *Anesthesiology* 1987;**67**:617–18.

4: Coronary physiology

HANS-JOACHIM PRIEBE

A thorough knowledge of normal coronary physiology is required to understand the mechanisms involved in coronary pathophysiology and, thus, for the optimal care of the patient with coronary artery disease. The heart, unlike any other organ, not only provides flow to the entire organism, but also has to generate its own perfusion pressure. This poses an extraordinary metabolic load on the coronary circulation. Complicating matters further, unlike any other regional circulation, the coronary circulation is subjected to marked variations in extravascular compressive forces related to the cardiac cycle.

Such unique physiology requires a highly specialised circulation if metabolic requirements are to be met. Consequently, the coronary circulation is composed of different kinds of vessels, each with distinct physiological, anatomical, and pharmacological characteristics.[1] [2]

The myocardium is almost entirely dependent on aerobic metabolism. Thus, there is little capacity to accumulate an oxygen (O_2) debt, and O_2 demand must be met on a beat-to-beat basis. As myocardial O_2 extraction is about 70% even at rest, increased myocardial O_2 consumption ($M\dot{V}o_2$) is principally met by increases in coronary blood flow (CBF). This results in a linear relationship between CBF and $M\dot{V}o_2$ (Fig 4.1). As a consequence, coronary sinus O_2 tension (18–20 mm Hg or 2·4–2·7 kPa) and saturation (25–30%) remain remarkably constant, O_2 delivery in excess of demand (so called "luxury" perfusion) is not usually observed, and inadequate O_2 supply in relation to demand will rapidly cause myocardial ischaemia.

Obviously, matching of O_2 delivery to O_2 demand is the essential task of the coronary circulation. The anatomical, physical, and biochemical factors responsible for this precise matching are discussed below. This provides the basis for understanding the pathophysiology of the diseased coronary circulation.

Coronary anatomy

The right and left coronary arteries provide the entire blood supply to the myocardium. They arise from the coronary ostia in the sinuses of Valsalva,

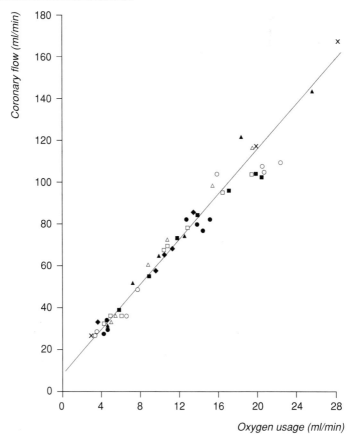

Fig 4.1 Relationship between coronary blood flow and myocardial oxygen consumption in conscious dogs. Each dog is represented by a separate symbol. A close correlation between the two variables over a wide range is evident. (Reproduced with permission from Khouri EM, Gregg DE, Rayford CR. Effect of exercise on cardiac output, left coronary flow and myocardial metabolism in the unanesthetized dog. *Circ Res* 1965;**17**:427–37.)

located at the aortic root above the anterior and left posterior cusps of the aortic valve. The anatomical arrangement between valve leaflets and coronary ostia ensures CBF even during systole. The two main coronary arteries run along their respective atrioventricular grooves where they branch repeatedly.

The left coronary artery divides into the anterior interventricular (also called the left anterior descending) and the circumflex artery. Branches of the anterior interventricular artery supply the anterior walls of the left and right ventricles, part of the left lateral wall, and most of the interventricular

120

septum. The circumflex artery supplies the left atrium, parts of the lateral and posterior left ventricular wall, and, in about 45% of hearts, the sinus node. It also perfuses the anterior papillary muscle of the left ventricle, whereas the posterior papillary muscle is perfused by branches of both right and left coronary arteries.

The right coronary artery supplies the remainder of the right ventricle and, in 90% of hearts, the atrioventricular node through its posterior interventricular branch. In about 55% of hearts, the sinus node artery originates from the right coronary artery. An extensive network of collateral and communicating vessels between branches of right and left coronary arteries encircles the epicardial surface of the heart. These vessels play an important role in maintaining some degree of regional perfusion when coronary occlusion develops.

The term "dominant" refers to that particular coronary artery from which the posterior interventricular artery originates. This branch supplies the lower (apical) part of the interventricular septum and the diaphragmatic surface of the left ventricle. The vast majority of normal human hearts (80–85%) have a dominant right coronary system. Of the remaining 15–20% of individuals, half demonstrate a left dominant coronary circulation and the other half a balanced circulation in which right and left coronary arteries contribute to septal and left ventricular diaphragmatic perfusion.[3] When comparing results of different studies, it is important to realise that significant species differences exist in regard to the dominant coronary system. Porcine hearts – like human hearts – have a dominant right coronary system, whereas the canine heart has a dominant left coronary system.

The myocardial wall is supplied by branches that arise from the large epicardial coronary arteries. These branches penetrate the ventricular wall in an almost perpendicular fashion. Within the myocardium there is further division of these branches into extensive networks of small arteries and arterioles, which give rise to the myocardial capillary bed. Certain branches from the epicardial vessels arborise in the subepicardium whereas others plunge deep into the myocardial wall to form a dense subendocardial network of vessels. Control of vasomotor tone differs between these two types of vessels, which enables changes in transmural flow distribution.[1] Coronary angiography can only visualise arterial segments that are larger than 500 μm in diameter. Visualisation of coronary microvessels between 15 and 500 μm requires highly specialised microvascular imaging techniques.

Most of the coronary vascular bed lies within the myocardial wall. As a result of easier accessibility, however, much of our knowledge of the coronary circulation is based on studies of the large epicardial vessels. Although they are the most frequent site of atherosclerotic alterations in coronary artery disease, they are mostly not representative of coronary physiology in general.

121

Morphologically, the major coronary vascular resistance (CVR) lies in arterioles smaller than 450 μm in diameter.[4] Almost half of the total CVR resides in vessels 100–450 μm in diameter, and the rest in arterioles of less than 100 μm. Whereas the small resistance vessels constitute the major resistance to flow, the large conductance vessels determine the quantity of blood arriving at the resistance vessels.

After passage through the capillary beds, most of the venous blood returns to the right atrium through the coronary sinus. Of coronary sinus outflow, 90–95% is derived from the left coronary artery. Most of the venous return from the right ventricle drains into the anterior cardiac veins that empty directly into the right atrium. A small amount of venous drainage of the heart drains via Thebesian veins directly into the left atrium, and the right and left ventricles, so contributing to the physiological arteriovenous shunt. A striking feature of the coronary venous system is the abundance of large anastomoses between all major veins,[5] which may result in considerable fluctuations in coronary sinus outflow.

The outer layer (adventitia) of small coronary arteries contains nerves. Although they do not penetrate the media, release of transmitter substances from nerve varicosities close to the smooth muscle layer is likely. Circumferentially arranged smooth muscle cells constitute the media. Layers of smooth muscle cells number between six in vessels that are 300 μm in diameter, and one in arterioles that are 30–50 μm in diameter. The smooth muscle cells behave electrically like a syncytium. The luminal surface of the coronary vessels is lined by endothelial cells which penetrate into the media. Through this contact with the smooth muscle cells, the vascular endothelium plays a key role in the control of coronary vasomotor tone (see below).

Coronary microcirculation

The microcirculation regulates terminal arterioles and capillaries that are responsible for the exchange of O_2 from blood to myocardial tissue. Capillary flow is determined less by the morphological properties of the capillary itself than by the tone of the feeder arteriole.

Of the more than 2000 capillaries/mm^3, usually only 60–80% are open. The normal intercapillary distance is about 17 μm (Table 4.1). During hypoxaemia, the intercapillary distance decreases to 14·5 μm as a result of recruitment of additional capillaries. Recruitment occurs by relaxation of precapillary sphincter tone. During prolonged hypoxaemia, the intercapillary distance decreases even further to 11 μm (Table 4.1).

Recruitment of coronary capillaries with subsequent reduction in intercapillary distance is an important compensatory mechanism to meet

Table 4.1 *Recruitment of coronary capillaries*

	Distances (μm)	
	Intercapillary	Diffusion
Normal	17	8·5
Exercise (estimated)	14	7·0
Hypoxia	14·5	7·3
Prolonged anoxia	11	5·5
Maximal recruitment	6·5	3·3

Adapted with permission from Opie LH. *The heart*, 3rd edn. Philadelphia: Lippincott-Raven, 1998:270.

increased M$\dot{V}o_2$. Augmentation of CBF alone at times of elevated O_2 demands would be insufficient compensation.

Coronary collateral circulation

Collateral vessels are accessory vascular channels which provide perfusion distal to an obstructed native coronary artery. Even in the normal myocardium, inter- and intracoronary collaterals exist at all levels of vessel sizes except the capillaries.[6] In certain species (for example, humans and dogs), they are present even in the neonatal heart. In the unstimulated state, collaterals are 40 μm in diameter and often only one cell layer thick. In the stimulated state, they may have diameters as large as 1 mm, and histologically they are similar to a myocardial arteriole.

There are considerable species differences in localisation and extent of intercoronary collaterals, which have to be taken into account when comparing results of different studies. The dog and the guinea pig have a relatively well developed collateral circulation. Pigs (similar to humans without coronary artery disease) have practically no anatomically demonstrable collaterals. Consequently, acute coronary occlusion leads very quickly to transmural infarction.

There are species differences not only in native (pre-existent) collaterals but also in transformed (developed) collaterals. In the human and porcine heart, collaterals develop predominantly in the subendocardium, and these look histologically like abnormally thin-walled arteries. By contrast, collaterals in canine hearts develop only in a narrow subepicardial zone around the edge of the zone that is potentially ischaemic. These collaterals generally exhibit significantly higher resistance than the vessels that they have replaced, although they are not nearly as flow limiting as the collaterals that develop in humans with ischaemia.

The factors that induce the transformation from the unstimulated to the stimulated state are largely unknown. Ischaemia seems to be a very powerful stimulus for the development of coronary collaterals.[7] Several experimental findings would, however, suggest that ischaemia of the cardiac myocyte may not necessarily be a prerequisite for the stimulation of collateral growth:[7 8] (1) growing segments of collaterals that are relatively far removed from areas of tissue hypoxia; (2) progressive ameroid induced coronary artery stenosis leading to the development of collaterals in the surrounding subepicardium even though subepicardial perfusion is not necessarily impaired; and (3) lack of defined time or spatial relationship between presumed ischaemia and collateral growth.

There is evidence that an inflammatory response may be the primary stimulus for collateral growth.[8] As a result of the lack of preformed arteriolar connections between superficial and deeper vascular territories in humans, a progressive stenosis of large epicardial vessels is likely to cause ischaemia-induced local micronecroses. The subsequent inflammatory response produces angiogenic mitogens mediated by macrophages/monocytes that trigger collateral growth. Thus, in humans (unlike the dog and like the pig) development of subendocardial collateral plexus appears to be a result of true angiogenesis. Reduction in arterial inflow at rest may be the predominant trigger mechanism. Other factors such as coronary occlusion, anaemia, and hypoxia have also been shown to stimulate collateral growth.[9]

Well developed canine collateral vessels do not vasoconstrict in response to α-adrenergic agonists. Sympathetic activation is therefore unlikely to cause collateral vasoconstriction. There is, however, thromboxane A_2 mediated vasoconstriction induced by platelet activating factor (PAF) in mature canine coronary collaterals.[10] As myocardial ischaemia can rapidly increase lyso-PAF (the precursor of PAF) by as much as 50%,[11] collateral dependent myocardial areas may well be susceptible to PAF-induced vasoconstriction and decrease in blood flow.

Although the protective role of coronary collaterals in humans has been debated in the past, prospectively collected data provide evidence that the collateral circulation limits the degree of ischaemia and improves survival during controlled intracoronary balloon occlusion, and after coronary artery spasm, acute myocardial infarction and post-coronary artery bypass graft closure.[9] Thus, in humans the coronary collateral circulation appears to constitute an important alternative source of blood supply to "jeopardised" myocardium.

Regulation of coronary blood flow

As with flow in any other vascular bed, CBF varies with perfusion pressure and vasomotor tone (that is, vascular resistance). Three major factors regulate coronary vascular tone: (1) the vascular endothelium, (2) local metabolism, and (3) the neurohumoral system.

Endothelial control of coronary vascular tone

The coronary vascular endothelium plays a major role in regulating vasomotor tone in health and disease.[12] It modulates the contractile activity of the underlying smooth muscle through the secretion and synthesis of substances with different biological activities in response to a variety of pharmacological agents (for example, acetylcholine, substance P, catecholamines) and physical stimuli (for example, blood flow, pulsatile flow, shear stress).

Endothelium-derived relaxing factors

Since the initial observation that an intact endothelium is necessary for acetylcholine-induced vasodilation,[13] many physiological stimuli have been shown to cause vasodilation by stimulating the release of powerful vasodilators such as endothelium-derived relaxing factor (EDRF), nitric oxide, prostacyclin, and endothelium-derived hyperpolarising factor (EDHF) (Fig 4.2). (By contrast, adenosine and the nitrovasodilators nitroglycerine and nitroprusside are endothelium-independent vasodilators.)

Nitric oxide – For practical purposes, EDRF is identical to nitric oxide (NO). NO is formed in endothelial cells from L-arginine by oxidation of its guanidine–nitrogen terminal. The catalysing enzyme involved is endothelial NO synthase (eNOS). It is calcium sensitive,[14] constitutively expressed, and exists in several isoforms in endothelial cells, vascular smooth muscle cells, platelets, macrophages, and the brain.

An inducible form of NO synthase (iNOS) exists in vascular smooth muscle, endothelium, and macrophages. This enzyme is calcium-independent, and can produce large amounts of NO. It is induced by cytokines such as endotoxin, interleukin-1β, and tumour necrosis factor (TNF).

Nitric oxide formation can be pharmacologically inhibited by the administration of L-arginine analogues such as L-N^G-monomethyl arginine (L-NMMA) or L-nitroarginine methyl ester (L-NAME). These compounds compete with the natural precursor L-arginine at the catalytic site of NOS.

Nitric oxide travels from the endothelium to the vascular smooth muscle where it stimulates guanylate cyclase to produce vasodilatory cGMP. NO has a very short half life (in the order of seconds or smaller), and thus just acts at the site where it is formed. Physiological stimuli that cause release of NO include acetylcholine, increased flow (via shear force), bradykinin,[15] hypoxia, and (somewhat surprisingly) endothelin.[16] Damage to the endothelium (for example, mechanical insult, formation of free radicals, early

125

atheroma) results in inhibition of NO release. In addition, in the presence of a non-intact endothelium, acetylcholine causes vasoconstriction (by a direct effect on vascular smooth muscle), and angiotensin II, platelet-derived growth factor, free radicals, and thrombin stimulate the release of vasoconstrictory endothelin.

Coronary vasodilation after intracoronary infusion of substances known to stimulate endothelial NO production (for example, acetylcholine, substance P, and serotonin) have provided indirect evidence of a role for NO in the human coronary circulation. The role of NO in the regulation of basal coronary vasomotor tone, however, remains controversial. Although several studies seem to indicate that basal formation of NO exerts a tonic dilator influence on the resting coronary circulation,[17 18] inhibition of NO synthesis does not consistently decrease basal CBF.[19 20] When compared with wild type rats, basal CBF (as well as reactive hyperaemic response to

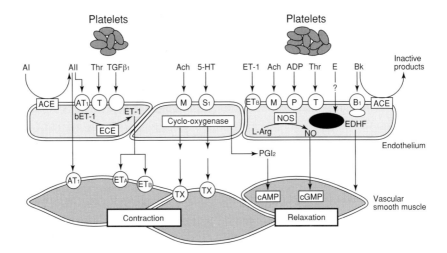

Fig 4.2 Endothelium-derived vasoactive substances (left contracting factors; right relaxing factors). AI = angiotensin I; AII = angiotensin II; ACE = angiotensin converting enzyme; Ach = acetylcholine; ADP = adenosine diphosphate; Bk = bradykinin; cAMP/cGMP = cyclic adenosine/guanosine monophosphate; E = oestrogen; ECE = endothelin converting enzyme; EDHF = endothelium-derived hyperpolarising factor; bET-1 = big endothelin-1; ET-1 = endothelin-1; 5-HT = 5-hydroxytryptamine (serotonin); L-Arg = L-arginine; NO = nitric oxide; NOS = nitric oxide synthase; O_2^- = superoxide; PGH$_2$ = prostaglandin H$_2$; PGI$_2$ = prostacyclin; TGFβ_1 = transforming growth factor β_1; Thr = thrombin; TXA-$_2$ = thromboxane A$_2$. Circles represent receptors: AT$_1$ = angiotensinergic; B$_2$ = bradykinergic; ET$_{A/B}$ = endothelin-A/B receptor; M = muscarinic; P = puriner-gic; S$_1$ = serotoninergic; T = thrombin receptor; TX = thromboxane/prostaglandin H$_2$ receptor. (Reproduced with permission from Wight E, Noll G, Lüscher TF. Regulation of vascular tone and endothelial function and its alterations in cardiovascular disease. *Baillière's Clin Anaesthesiol* 1997;**11**:531–60.)

short term ischaemia, and responses to intracoronary administration of adenosine and acetylcholine) was not different in endothelial NO synthase knockout mice.[21] Even combined NO synthase inhibition and adenosine receptor blockade failed to decrease resting CBF.[22] The combined evidence would suggest that under resting conditions NO is not essential to maintain basal CBF.

By contrast, NO formation is apparently the major pathway involved in the dilatation of large epicardial coronary arteries that is caused by elevated shear stress and by acetylcholine.[23] Residual dilatation of coronary conductance arteries to acetylcholine is, however, commonly observed even after blockade of NO formation by arginine analogues. The relative contribution of NO may well depend on the underlying stimulus. Whereas in shear stress-induced (that is, flow-dependent) vasodilation NO is the major mediator, in acetylcholine-induced (that is, receptor-operated) dilatation mediators other than NO seem to be involved. One such intermediate may be EDHF.[24] This EDHF could be a cytochrome P450 metabolite of arachidonic acid.[25 26]

In contrast to conductance vessels, dilatation to acetylcholine that is resistant to arginine analogues does not occur in coronary resistance vessels.[26] This would suggest that NO is the principal mediator of both flow-dependent and receptor-operated vasorelaxation in the resistance vessels of the coronary circulation.

During high $M\dot{V}o_2$, deficiencies in NO release by the coronary endothelium may be balanced by powerful metabolic stimuli. Adenosine release apparently compensates for diminished NO release.[27] Only block-ade of both NO synthase and adenosine receptors prevents an adequate increase in CBF during stress.[27] Activation of ATP-sensitive K^+ channels (K_{ATP}^+ channels) may also compensate for diminished NO release.[22] Thus, although NO contributes to coronary vasodilation during exercise, a redundancy of vasodilatator mechanisms apparently compensates for a loss of NO release in the otherwise normal heart.

Nitric oxide synthase inhibition decreases total reactive hyperaemic flow.[28] Combined blockade of K_{ATP}^+ channels, adenosine receptors, and NO synthase does not, however, fully block reactive hyperaemia.[22] Other vasodilators such as prostacyclin, EDHF, or metabolic alterations (that is, decreased pH and increased CO_2 tension or PCO_2) could contribute to the residual vasodilation. In general, the respective response to any NO inhibition will vary with species, baseline vasomotor tone, state of consciousness (awake versus anaesthetised), and experimental model.

Prostaglandins – The first vasoactive endothelium-derived substance discovered was prostacyclin, or prostaglandin I_2. Prostacyclin (PGI_2) is the major breakdown product of cyclo-oxygenase and the major vasodilatory prostaglandin. It is released from the endothelium in response to shear stress, pulsatile flow, hypoxia, and several other substances that also release

NO, such as adenosine diphosphate (ADP), adenosine triphosphate (ATP), serotonin, and thrombin. In most blood vessels, however, its platelet inhibitory effects are probably more important than its vasodilatory ones.

Bradykinin – Increased shear forces as a result of an increased blood flow stimulate the formation of bradykinin in vascular endothelium.[15] Bradykinin binds to two types of endothelial receptors: the B_1- and B_2-receptor. B_2-receptors are more sensitive to bradykinin than B_1-receptors. Their stimulation results in the release of the two powerful vasodilators EDRF/NO and PGI_2. Local formation of bradykinin may, therefore, be important in the mechanism of flow-induced vasodilation.

Endothelium-derived contracting factors

Endogenous (for example, arachidonic acid, noradrenaline, thrombin) and pharmacological substances (for example, calcium, nicotine, high potassium), and physicochemical stimuli (shear stress, mechanical stress, hypoxia) can stimulate endothelium-dependent vasoconstriction.[15 16] Major endothelium-derived vasoconstrictors are endothelin, thromboxane A_2, and prostaglandin H_2 (see Fig 4.2)

Endothelin – Endothelin is a peptide composed of 21 amino acids. It is a potent vasoconstrictor in disease states. When physiologically released in small amounts, however, it may function as a vasodilator, possibly by stimulating endothelium-dependent release of NO and PGI_2 (which in turn inhibit endothelin production via a negative feedback mechanism).

Of the three isoforms endothelin-1, endothelin-2, and endothelin-3, endothelial cells produce exclusively endothelin-1. It is derived from pre-pro-endothelin and pro(big)-endothelin, which is converted to the biologically active peptide endothelin-1 by the endothelin converting enzymes (ECE-1 and ECE-2). The main pathophysiological stimuli for the release of endothelin-1 are thrombin, platelet-derived transforming growth factor β_1 (TGF β_1), angiotensin II, noradrenaline, adrenaline, vasopressin, interleukin-1, hypoxia, ischaemia, O_2-derived free radicals, and shear stress.[29]

All three isoforms of endothelin bind to two types of endothelin receptors: the ET_A and the ET_B receptors. ET_A receptors are expressed on vascular smooth muscle cells and mostly mediate the constrictor effects. ET_B receptors are predominantly located on the endothelial cell surface and mostly mediate vasodilation by facilitating the release of NO and PGI_2.

Whereas endothelin-1 causes vasodilation at very low concentrations, it becomes the most potent endogenous vasoconstrictor at higher concentrations, eventually leading to myocardial ischaemia, cardiac arrhythmias, and death.[30] The exact role of endothelin in the regulation of coronary vasomotor tone is not fully understood.

Prostanoids – The major endothelium-derived vasoconstrictor prostanoids are thromboxane A_2 (TXA_2) and prostaglandin H_2 (PGH_2). Both promote platelet aggregation. They activate thromboxane receptors on vascular smooth muscle cells and platelets, this way counteracting the protective effects of NO and PGI_2 on both cell types.

Mechanical forces (for example, shear stress) or pharmacological agonists (for example, acetylcholine) cause the endothelial co-release of vasodilatory NO and PGI_2 on the one hand, and of vasoconstrictory TXA_2 and PGH_2 on the other. The final vascular response will depend on the net balance between released vasodilating and vasoconstricting factors. Decreased release of relaxing factors combined with an increased formation of contracting factors (as in ageing or hypertension) will attenuate endothelium-dependent relaxation. Vasoconstriction after platelet aggregation and damage is the result of smooth muscle cell activation by platelet-derived TXA_2 (and serotonin).

EDRFs and EDCFs in disease states

Normal coronary arteries exhibit endothelium-dependent dilatation in response to both local acetylcholine and increased flow. These physiological responses are lost in humans with advanced coronary artery disease.[31] Oxidised low density lipoproteins and hypoxia or anoxia inhibit the release of EDRF. Ischaemia and reperfusion induce impairment in endothelium-dependent relaxation to most EDRF/NO agonists.[32] Although such studies underscore the potential clinical relevance of impaired release of EDRF/NO in ischaemic syndromes, a potentially important role for endothelin is also possible. Hypoxia,[33] and decreased flow and shear stress[34] may induce endothelin gene expression and secretion. After global myocardial ischaemia and reperfusion during cardiopulmonary bypass, not only is there impaired release of EDRF in the coronary artery, but the ischaemic event may also increase the production of an endothelium-derived contracting factor (EDCF).[35]

The impaired release of EDRF will suppress coronary vasodilation in areas of jeopardised myocardium, and will facilitate platelet adhesion and aggregation as well as platelet-induced coronary vasoconstriction. The stimulated release of endothelin (induced by vascular injury, impaired release of EDRF, ischaemia, and decreased shear stress) will, in turn, also promote vasoconstriction. The finding of augmented vasoconstrictor actions of endothelin in the presence of simultaneous inhibition of EDRF synthesis[36] supports the hypothesis that the endogenous EDRF system serves as a functionally important modulator of the vasoconstrictor actions of endothelin. When the delicate balance between endothelium-mediated vasodilation and vasoconstriction is disturbed in disease states associated with injured endothelium (for example, coronary atherosclerosis), the attenuated release of EDRF and stimulated secretion of endothelin will facilitate vasoconstriction, thrombosis, and smooth muscle cell proliferation. An intact endothelium protects the vasculature from a variety of potentially vasoconstrictory stimuli. In turn, endothelial damage can convert usually vasodilatory stimuli into vasoconstrictory ones.

All of the presented data indicate that the endothelial system cannot be viewed as simply an inert lining of blood vessels, but rather it must be regarded as a highly active endocrine organ that serves a wide variety of biological functions including synthesis, metabolism, and binding of various vasoactive and non-vasoactive substances. Impaired endothelial function is likely to contribute significantly to the pathophysiology of coronary artery disease and myocardial ischaemic syndromes. Endothelial dysfunction of the coronary arteries is found across a broad spectrum of conditions in patients free of angiographic evidence of coronary athero-sclerosis, including advanced age,[37] hypertension,[38] left ventricular hypertrophy,[38] hyperlipidaemia,[39] diabetes mellitus,[40] and chronic tobacco use.[41]

Metabolic control of coronary vascular tone

Relationship between CBF and MV̇o$_2$

CBF and MV̇o$_2$ are closely coupled because the myocardium depends almost completely on aerobic metabolism (see Fig 4.1) As baseline coronary venous O$_2$ saturation is only 25–30%, additional O$_2$ extraction is limited. Coronary vascular resistance therefore responds within a second to changes in MV̇o$_2$. The precise mediators responsible for the tight coupling between myocardial demand and supply still need to be identified.[42] As matching of O$_2$ supply to metabolic demands remains almost unaffected when neurohumoral factors are eliminated,[43] there is general agreement that CBF is metabolically regulated.[44] Alterations in the level of myocardial energy use,[45] or in the balance of O$_2$ supply and demand cause production of vasodilator substances that restore the supply/demand balance and, thus, maintain myocardial function.

Various substances (for example, adenosine, NO, prostaglandins, CO$_2$, H$^+$) have been investigated in this context.[46] Changes in their concentra-tions in the perivascular space are small, however, and their significance in controlling steady state coronary vascular resistance has been ques-tioned.[47]

Adenosine

When ATP utilisation exceeds resynthesis by myocardial cells, adenosine monophosphate (AMP) will be produced. Adenosine is formed from AMP by the enzyme 5'-nucleotidase. Adenosine (and its metabolites inosine and hypoxanthine) can enter the interstitial space and appear in the coronary sinus effluent.

As a purine compound, adenosine acts on purinergic receptors. These are subdivided into adenosine-sensitive P$_1$-receptors and ATP-sensitive P$_2$-receptors. The P$_1$-receptors can, in turn, be further subdivided into myocardial A_1- and vascular A_2-receptors. Vascular A_2-receptors are located on vascular smooth muscle cells, and promote coronary vasodilation by stimulating production of cAMP.

Adenosine is a potent coronary vasodilator.[48] In addition, the coronary circulation appears to be more sensitive to adenosine than the peripheral circulation.[49] The exact role of adenosine in this context, however, remains inconclusive. Adenosine has been hypothesised to be the major metabolite that regulates CBF.[50] According to this hypothesis, adenosine is released from myocardial cells as cellular O_2 tension decreases. It traverses the interstitial space and acts on coronary vascular smooth muscle to cause vasodilation. The subsequent increase in CBF restores myocardial O_2 tension. Data exist both to support[51] and to reject the hypothesis[52] that adenosine is the principal metabolic regulator of CBF.

For example, the production of adenosine increases during myocardial O_2 supply/demand mismatch, and the interstitial concentration correlates with CBF. Furthermore, uncoupling of increases in CBF from increases in myocardial metabolism has been demonstrated. Adenosine receptor blockade almost abolished the hyperaemia associated with dobutamine-induced increases in cardiac work, and it dramatically exaggerated the reduction in CBF associated with intracoronary vasopressin infusion. These findings would suggest a role for adenosine as a mediator of CBF changes.

On the other hand, physiological and pathological conditions as diverse as resting CBF, exercise-induced coronary dilatation, reactive hyperaemia, and rapid atrial pacing are largely unrelated to the release of adenosine. Overall evidence would suggest that adenosine is probably involved to some extent in the metabolic control of myocardial perfusion. It does not, however, appear to be the primary mediator of the close coupling between flow and metabolism.

ATP-sensitive K^+ channel

There is considerable evidence that opening of ATP-sensitive K^+ channels (K_{ATP}^+ channels) is the principal mechanism of metabolic coronary vasodilation. When this channel opens, K^+ leaves the cell resulting in hyperpolarisation of the cell membrane. Such hyperpolarisation closes Ca^{2+} channels. Consequently, cytosolic Ca^{2+} decreases and vascular smooth muscle relaxes. K_{ATP}^+ channels are opened either by receptor activation (for example, by adenosine or acetylcholine) or by metabolic factors (for example, by a decrease in ATP as in hypoxia or severe ischaemia). This constitutes an important mechanism for metabolic coronary vasodilation.[53]

Blockade of K_{ATP}^+ channels lowers CBF both at rest and during exercise.[22] Infusion of pinacidil, a K_{ATP} channel opener, induces coronary vasodilation comparable to that observed during the peak reactive flow response.[54] With

K_{ATP}^+ channels intact, NO and adenosine are not essential for maintaining resting CBF or for coronary vasodilation during exercise.[22] Blockade of adenosine receptors after K_{ATP}^+ channel blockade does not further decrease resting CBF but reduces the exercise induced increase in CBF by more than half.[55] This finding emphasises the importance of adenosine in causing metabolic vasodilation after K_{ATP}^+ channel blockade. Additional NOS inhibition (after blockade of K_{ATP}^+ channels and adenosine receptors) entirely abolishes coronary vasodilation during exercise.[55] This finding implies that NO contributes to coronary vasodilation during exercise when other vasodilator systems are blocked. Blockade of any one of the three vasodilator mechanisms alone does not blunt the increase in CBF during exercise. Hypoxia may cause vasodilation by opening K_{ATP}^+ channels.[56]

Neurohumoral control of coronary vascular tone

Autonomic control

The coronary arteries are richly innervated by adrenergic and parasympathetic nerves.[57] Superior, middle, and inferior cervical and the first four sympathetic ganglia supply the heart with sympathetic, and the vagi with parasympathetic innervation. Sympathetic innervation is present at all coronary microvascular segments, but the density of innervation may differ among various vascular levels.[58] Rather than increasing concentrations of circulating levels of catecholamines, cardiac efferent sympathetic signals seem to account for the increase in CBF in response to activation of the sympathetic nervous system.[59] The increase in CBF appears to correlate with the magnitude of regional stores of noradrenaline (norepinephrine) in cardiac sympathetic nerve terminals.[59]

The role of cholinergic nerves in the regulation of CBF is controversial.[60] Although parasympathetic stimulation seems to dilate small coronary arteries,[57] the response is weak and transitory. Coronary vasodilation that normally follows parasysmpathetic stimulation may be dependent on the release of EDRF.[61]

α-Adrenergic control

α_1- and α_2-adrenergic receptors exist throughout the coronary circulation. They are not, however, uniformly distributed.[2] The α_1-receptors seem to predominate in large epicardial vessels, whereas α_2-receptors predominate in vessels that are less than 100 μm in diameter.[1,2]

Activation of both α_1- and α_2-adrenergic receptors produces coronary vasoconstriction.[2] In accordance with the non-uniform distribution of the receptor subtypes, the α-adrenergic responses of the coronary circulation to various physiological and pharmacological interventions seem to vary between vessel segments of different morphology and location. For example, α_1- and α_2-receptors are both involved in the vasoconstriction of resistance vessels. In contrast, larger coronary arteries mainly respond to α_1-receptor activation, and mature coronary collaterals do not respond to α-receptor stimulation.[62]

Paradoxically, in vitro coronary arterioles are refractory to α-adrenergic agonists.[63] This is puzzling, because isolated coronary venules[63] and large coronary arteries (> $500\,\mu m$ in diameter)[64] do constrict on α_1- and α_2-adrenergic stimulation. It has recently been shown that α_1-adrenergic stimulation causes in vivo coronary arteriolar constriction by stimulating cardiac myocytes to release a vasoconstrictor, possibly endothelin-1.[65] It thus appears that cardiac myocytes have a requisite role in mediating α_1-adrenergic coronary arteriolar constriction.

There is evidence for baseline α-adrenoceptor-mediated coronary vasoconstriction in humans.[66] Cardiac denervation decreases coronary vascular resistance, lowers arteriovenous O_2 extraction, and raises coronary venous O_2 content, indicating direct vasodilation. α-Adrenoceptor blockade also reduces coronary vascular resistance.

Under physiological conditions, increased sympathetic activity causes dilatation of coronary resistance vessels and, subsequently, increases myocardial blood flow. This vasodilator response appears to be partly mediated by endothelial function.[67] It may result from the direct stimulation of α_2-adrenergic receptors in intact endothelial cells, and from the release of NO, possibly through activation of local kinin synthesis.[68] In fact, removing the vascular endothelium enhances the vasoconstrictor response to noradrenaline,[69] and inhibition of NO synthesis in coronary arteries potentiates α-adrenergic vasoconstriction.[70]

During neurohumoral adrenergic stimulation, α-adrenergic stimulation competes with metabolic vasodilation.[66] Although under physiological conditions the net result of α-adrenergic stimulation is always an increase in CBF, such stimulation nevertheless attenuates the increase in CBF by 20–30%. Such attenuation of CBF in the presence of increased myocardial O_2 demand seems paradoxical. α-Adrenoceptor-mediated vasoconstriction may, however, have beneficial effects on the transmural blood flow distribution.[71] An α-blockade during myocardial hypoperfusion results in redistribution of CBF from the subendocardium to subepicardium.[72] This would suggest that α-receptor-mediated vasoconstriction during hypoperfusion exhibits an "anti-steal" effect by limiting perfusion to the subepicardium and improving that to the subendocardium. The postulated mechanism of this beneficial effect is that α-adrenoceptor-mediated vasoconstriction preferentially "stiffens" coronary vessels that are larger than $100\,\mu m$ in diameter. This will reduce intramyocardial vascular capacity and, subsequently, to-and-fro oscillation of CBF during the cardiac cycle.[73]

133

Although there is little evidence for a physiological role of α-adrenergic coronary vasoconstriction under normal conditions, controversy continues about the importance of α-adrenergic receptor stimulation during myocardial hypoperfusion. No doubt, sympathetic stimulation activates vasoconstricting α-adrenoceptors in coronary arteries. The physiological role of such α-adrenoceptor-mediated vasoconstriction still has, however, to be determined.[71]

β-Adrenergic control

Contrary to what might be expected from other vascular beds, coronary β-adrenoceptors are not only of the non-cardiac β_2 subtype. Whereas β_2-receptors may regulate coronary vascular resistance (CVR) in small vessels, β_1-receptors dominate in large human coronary arteries.[74] There appears to be a segmental distribution of β-adrenergic receptors, with a higher density of β-receptors in resistance vessels than in large vessels. The resistance vessels may contain both β_1- and β_2-receptor subtypes, whereas large epicardial vessels have predominantly β_1-receptors. Coronary vasodilation mediated by β_1- and β_2-adrenoceptors of both large and small coronary vessels,[43 75 76] and of mature canine collaterals[77] has been demonstrated.

At first it would seem paradoxical that administration of noradrenaline causes simultaneous α-adrenoceptor-mediated coronary vasoconstriction and β-adrenoceptor-mediated vasodilation.[76] These seemingly opposing effects may, however, be of benefit. α-adrenoceptor-mediated vasoconstriction of large and medium sized coronary arteries possibly lessens the to-and-fro oscillation of flow from subendocardium to subepicardium during systole and diastole, thus preserving flow.[78] On the other hand, direct β-adrenoceptor-mediated vasodilation probably occurs mostly in small arteries, and serves to match blood flow and myocardial metabolism. It may thus be postulated that α-adrenoceptor-mediated vasoconstriction serves to adjust phasic coronary impedance, which preserves left ventricular subendocardial perfusion, whereas β-adrenoceptor-mediated vasodilation prevents large decreases in myocardial tissue P_{O_2}.[76]

Inhibition of NO synthesis by L-NAME antagonises isoproterenol-induced coronary vasodilation.[79] This would suggest that β-adrenergic dilatation of resistance vessels involves an endothelium-dependent mechanism that is linked to the L-arginine/NO pathway.

Cholinergic control

Acetylcholine is a powerful coronary vasodilator when given intravenously. Cholinergic stimulation consistently results in coronary dilatation.[80] Whereas in patients with angiographically normal coronary arteries intracoronary acetylcholine causes dilatation,[81] in atherosclerotic segments it elicits constriction.[82] Intracoronary acetylcholine binds to endothelial muscarinic receptors and stimulates the release of EDRF.

Peptidergic control

It is generally thought that neural control depends primarily on the release of noradrenaline and acetylcholine from sympathetic and para-sympathetic nerve terminals, respectively. It is now recognised, however, that, in addition to the classic neurotransmitters, other putative trans-mitters (including several vasoactive peptides) may also be involved in regulating coronary vasomotor tone. Such peptides identified in nerves associated with coronary vessels include neuropeptide Y (NPY), vasoactive intestinal polypeptide (VIP), calcitonin gene-related peptide (CGRP), and tachykinins such as substance P and neuropeptide K.[83]

Human epicardial coronary arteries are supplied by numerous, peptide-containing, perivascular nerve populations.[83] The number of peptide-containing nerve fibres varies with vessel size, with the distal segments of epicardial coronary arteries being more densely innervated than the proximal segments. NPY immunoreactive nerve fibres seem to be the most abundant of the peptide-containing nerve populations identified in human epicardial coronary arteries. They appear to have a distribution pattern similar to that of nerves containing the catecholamine-synthesising enzyme tyrosine hydroxylase.[83] Most NPY-containing nerves in the heart represent postganglionic sympathetic neurons originating in the stellate and other paravertebral ganglia. This supports the extracardiac origin of this neuropeptide.

Neuropeptide Y has generally been regarded as a vasoconstrictor peptide.[84] Its vasomotor activity appears, however, to vary with vessel size and location. NPY does not seem to elicit a vasoconstrictor response in epicardial coronary arteries, but it induces some constriction of intra-myocardial resistance vessels.[85] Its vasomotor action is possibly mediated by specific Y_1 and Y_2 receptors.[86] NPY is co-stored and co-released with noradrenaline from sympathetic nerve terminals. Sympathetic stimulation increases the ratio of NPY to noradrenaline release. NPY is concentrated around coronary arteries and is a potent vasoconstrictor; it possibly contributes to coronary vasoconstriction during profound sympathetic stimulation. Although the functional significance of NPY in the regulation of coronary vasomotor tone still has to be defined, it may well play a role in modulating the effect of other vasoactive substances.[87]

Substance P and CGRP immunoreactive nerve fibres are rare in the proximal region of epicardial coronary arteries and increase in number distally.[83] Substance P and CGRP produce a marked relaxation of epicardial coronary arteries[88 89] but exert only a weak vasodilatory effect on intramyocardial resistance vessels.[89 90]

Vasoactive intestinal peptide is present in post-ganglionic parasympa-thetic (vagal) and intrinsic cardiac nerve fibres of humans.[83] Cardiac VIP nerve fibres are predominantly found in coronary arteries, sinoatrial and atrioventricular nodes, the atria, and the right ventricle.[91] Within the coronary arteries, VIP nerve fibres are present in the epicardial vessels and to a lesser extent in the arterioles.

Various findings suggest that VIP has a direct vasodilator effect on the coronary arteries.[92] VIP appears to have a more potent effect on large epicardial vessels than on resistance vessels. The increase in CBF during administration or release of VIP is not the result of an increase in $M\dot{V}o_2$ and cardiac metabolism.[92]

Although the exact physiological role of VIP in the control of the coronary circulation is still uncertain, VIP may well be important in the regulation of CBF. Vagal nerve stimulation releases VIP which, in turn, directly dilates coronary arteries and increases CBF to the left ventricle.[92] The phenomenon of post vagal tachycardia (although not directly reflecting changes in CBF) is thought to be the result of VIP release from cardiac vagal nerves after intense vagal stimulation.[93]

In summary, a network of neuropeptide-containing nerve fibres located in the adventitia and at the adventitial–medial border supplies human coronary arteries.[83] Neuropeptides appear to modify CBF either directly or indirectly by modifying the effects of other vasoactive substances.

Opposing vasodilatory and vasoconstrictory mechanisms

Final vasomotor tone is the net result of opposing vasodilatory and vasoconstrictory mechanisms operating at various levels and modifying each other (Table 4.2). As a result of such opposing and interacting mechanisms, the final effect of each individual mechanism on vasomotor

Table 4.2 *Opposing vasodilatory and vasoconstrictory mechanisms in the regulation of vascular smooth muscle tone*

Site	Vasodilation	Vasoconstriction
Autonomic nervous system	Cholinergic neurons (ACh) Adrenal medulla (A)	Adrenergic neurons (NA)
Nerve terminal receptor	α_1-Adrenoceptors Muscarinic receptors	β_2-Adrenoceptors Angiotensin II receptors
Vascular receptor	β_2 Adenosine Endothelin B (ET_B)	α_1 and α_2 Angiotensin II Endothelin A (ET_A)
Endothelium	EDRF/NO Prostacyclin (PGI_2) Endothelin (low concentration)	Endothelin (high concentration)
Vascular ion channel	K^+_{ATP} channel K^+_{Ca} channel	Ca^{2+} channels (ROC, VOC)

ACh, acetylcholine; NA, noradrenaline; A, adrenaline; EDRF, endothelium-derived relaxing factor; NO, nitric oxide; K^+_{ATP} channel, ATP-sensitive potassium channel; K^+_{Ca} channel, calcium-activated potassium channel; ROC, receptor-operated channel; VOC, voltage-operated channel.
(Adapted from Opie LH. *The heart*. 3rd edn. Philadelphia: Lippincott-Raven, 1998:255.)

tone is difficult to predict in vivo. Whereas the in vitro effect can be described clearly, the in vivo effect will vary with baseline conditions (for example, baseline autonomic tone, baseline concentrations of vasoactive substances, endothelial responsiveness), species, and vascular bed. In addition, activation of one mechanism normally results in immediate activation of counterbalancing mechanisms to maintain homoeostasis.

There is complex interaction of the autonomic nervous system, vascular smooth muscle cell receptor, and endothelium (Fig 4.3). Release of noradrenaline from the nerve terminal (as a result of sympathetic activation) stimulates postsynaptic vasoconstrictory α_1- and α_2-receptors. A variety of hormones and autonomic signals modulates vasomotor tone by modifying the release of noradrenaline. The parasympathetic transmitter acetylcholine decreases noradrenaline release by stimulation of presynaptic muscarinic receptors. Circulating adrenaline (epinephrine) can exert dual action: it may indirectly cause vasoconstriction by increasing the release of noradrenaline through stimulation of presynaptic β_2-receptors; or it may cause direct vasodilation by stimulation of postsynaptic β_2-receptors. Angiotensin II promotes vasoconstriction, either directly by acting on postsynaptic angiotensin II receptors, or indirectly by increasing the release of noradrenaline via stimulation of presynaptic angiotensin II receptors.

A couple of interactions at the endothelial level may serve as examples of opposing and modifying mechanisms. Endothelin may stimulate NO release via ET_B receptors, thereby limiting its vasoconstrictory effect.[29] Part of NO-induced vasodilation may result from concomitant inhibition of endothelin production by NO. Like NO, PGI_2 may exert a negative feedback inhibition on endothelin production. In porcine coronary arteries, PGI_2 potentiates the relaxing activity of NO by stimulating its release. Certain stimuli (for example, shear stress, acetylcholine) cause the concomitant release of vasodilatory NO and cyclo-oxygenase-derived contracting factors, such as TXA_2, PGH_2, and superoxide radical, which all attenuate the relaxing effects of NO.[94] The final vascular response will depend on the type and degree of interactions (which are related to amounts and potency of factors released); these are likely to differ between vascular beds. Vasomotor tone is thus under the triple control of autonomic tone, activity of vascular smooth muscle cell receptors, and endothelial function.

Autoregulation

Autoregulation has been defined as "the intrinsic tendency of an organ to maintain constant blood flow despite changes in arterial perfusion pressure".[95] Using a more operational definition, autoregulation is a proportional change in vascular resistance in response to a change in perfusion pressure. This active change in vascular resistance constitutes an

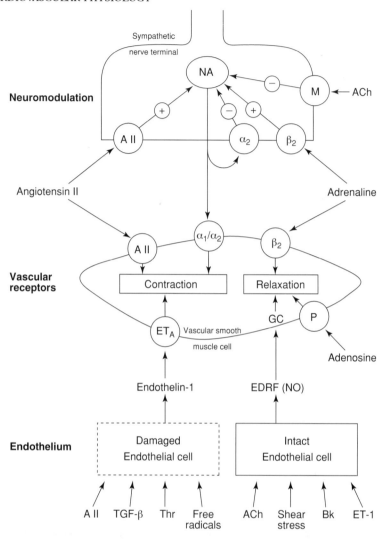

Fig 4.3 Regulation of vasomotor tone by neuromodulation, vascular receptors, and endothelium. NA = noradrenaline. A II = angiotensin II. TGF-β = transforming growth factor β. Thr = thrombin. Ach = acetylcholine. Bk = bradykinin. ET-1 = endothelin-1. EDRF = endothelium-derived relaxing factor. NO = nitric oxide. GC = guanylyl cyclase. Circles represent receptors: ET$_A$ = endothelin-A receptor. M = muscarinic. P = purinergic. $\oplus$ = Excitatory effect. $\ominus$ = Inhibitory effect.
(Modified from Opie LH. *The heart*, 3rd edn. Philadelphia: Lippincott-Raven, 1998: 270.)

intrinsic mechanism that is independent of extrinsic neurohumoral factors.

Perfusion is autoregulated mainly by arterioles that are larger than 150 μm in diameter. As perfusion pressure continues to decline, however, smaller arterioles are recruited.[96] There are lower and upper limits of autoregulation beyond which CBF will (pressure-dependently) decrease or increase, respectively.

Such a mechanism requires immediate adjustment of vasomotor tone in response to alterations in perfusion pressure. Autoregulatory changes in coronary vasomotor tone behave in a dynamic fashion. If metabolic demand is kept constant, a sudden change in coronary perfusion pressure results in an immediate directionally identical change in CBF which returns to normal over 10–30 s[46] (Fig 4.4). As, at rest, the coronary vasculature appears to be under greater vasoconstrictor tone than other vascular beds, this greater vasodilatory reserve provides the capacity to increase flow remarkably.

The definition of autoregulation assumes that organ metabolism and venous pressure do not change as arterial perfusion pressure is altered. As aortic pressure is a major determinant of left ventricular afterload, and as developed left ventricular systolic pressure correlates with left ventricular $M\dot{V}o_2$,[97] it is impossible to study coronary autoregulation simply by

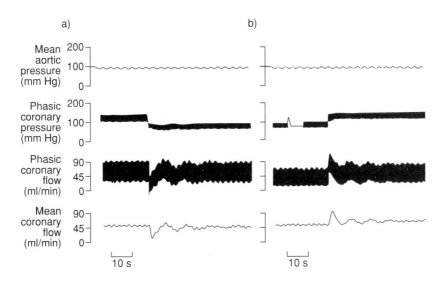

Fig 4.4 Dynamic coronary flow response to a sudden change in perfusion pressure in the left circumflex artery in the dog. (a) Flow response to a step decrease in pressure; (b) response to a step increase in pressure. (Reproduced with permission from Dole WP. Autoregulation of the coronary circulation. *Prog Cardiovasc Dis* 1987;**29**:293–323.)

changing aortic pressure because this would lead to marked changes in myocardial metabolism. This problem can be overcome by cannulating a coronary artery and perfusing it with a pump. Nevertheless, low perfusion pressures may cause myocardial ischaemia with subsequent decreases in myocardial metabolism and increases in venous pressure. On the other hand, higher than normal perfusion may increase cardiac contractility and myocardial metabolism, secondary to the increase in CBF. Doubling of the resting CBF may increase the strength of cardiac contraction by 15%.[98] This phenomenon is referred to as the "Gregg effect", after its discoverer[99] (see below). Either increasing CBF by increasing cannulated coronary artery pressure or increasing it by pharmacological vasodilation at constant coronary perfusion pressure will elicit this effect, thus changing myocardial metabolism simultaneously. As autoregulation constitutes a flow response to changes in perfusion pressure, a Gregg effect will always be involved in autoregulatory investigations. Such simultaneous changes in $M\dot{V}o_2$ will complicate the interpretation of acquired data on autoregulation.

Adenosine

The precise mechanism(s) responsible for maintaining CBF in the presence of decreasing coronary perfusion pressure remain(s) controversial.[46 100] Autoregulation is largely unrelated to the release of adenosine.[101] Furthermore, intracoronary infusion of adenosine deaminase or adenosine receptor antagonists that blunt reactive hyperaemia does not affect coronary autoregulation,[47 101] and interstitial levels of adenosine do not change with decreases in coronary perfusion pressure within the autoregulatory range.[47] These data would suggest that adenosine plays at best a minor role in coronary autoregulation.

EDRF/NO

Endothelium-dependent production of NO in coronary vessels appears to be an important mechanism in the regulation of myocardial perfusion only during hypoperfusion.[102] Inhibiting NO synthase with L-NAME increased the critical pressure at which myocardial ischaemia began (lower autoregulatory break point) from 45 ± 3 mm Hg under control conditions to 61 ± 2 mm Hg after L-NAME (Fig 4.5). In addition, both the slope of the coronary pressure–flow relation below the autoregulatory point, and the peak reactive hyperaemic flow response were reduced, reflecting impaired capability to minimise coronary vascular resistance. On the other hand, flow recruitment in response to increased metabolic demand (that is, a twofold increase in heart rate) was not affected by L-NAME. These findings would suggest that both initial autoregulatory adjustments to decreases in

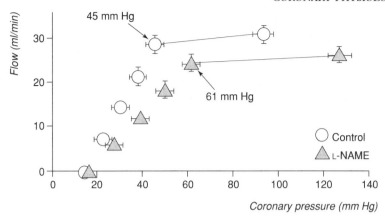

Fig 4.5 Plots summarising pressure–flow relationships under control conditions (open circles) and following inhibition of nitric oxide synthesis by N_ω-nitro-L-arginine (L-NAME) (hatched triangles). L-NAME had no significant effect on flow regulation over the autoregulatory plateau. The lower autoregulatory break point (arrows) as well as the pressure–flow relationship during ischaemia were, however, shifted to the right after inhibition of nitric oxide production. (Reproduced with permission from Smith TP, Canty JM Jr. Modulation of coronary autoregulatory responses by nitric oxide. *Circ Res* 1993;**73**:232–40.)

coronary perfusion pressure and flow recruitment in response to increased metabolic demand are probably mediated by metabolic factors independent of NO production. During hypoperfusion, however, endothelium-dependent production of NO is importantly involved in minimising coronary vascular resistance.

O_2 and CO_2 tension

Changes in myocardial O_2 and CO_2 tensions may mediate coronary autoregulation.[103 104] There appears to be a strong inverse relationship between coronary venous O_2 tension and coronary autoregulation. Good autoregulation was observed when coronary venous O_2 tension was 25 mm Hg(3·3 kPa) and autoregulation was lost when venous O_2 tension was more than 32 mm Hg(4·3 kPa).[104] This, again, would indicate that the dominant mechanism of coronary autoregulation is metabolic. The normal resting coronary sinus P_{O_2} of 18–25 mm Hg(2·4–3.3 kPa) indicates a tight coupling between $M\dot{V}_{O_2}$ and myocardial O_2 delivery.

Changes in $P_{a_{O_2}}$ (arterial O_2 tension) itself induce variations in coronary vasomotor tone, independent of O_2 content and metabolic regulation of CBF. A high $P_{a_{O_2}}$ constricts coronary arteries, possibly mediated by closure of K^+_{ATP} channels.[105]

Although possibly involved in the phenomenon of autoregulation, the effect of CO_2 tension is probably small at venous O_2 tension (PV_{O_2}) of more than 20 mm Hg(2·7 kPa).[103] It remains unclear whether coronary autoregulation is mediated directly by changes in tissue O_2 tension or by some mediating factors, such as K^+_{ATP} channels.

ATP sensitive K^+ channels

Glibenclamide, a putative blocker of K^+_{ATP} channels, abolishes autoregulation in the canine heart perfused with blood in situ.[106] K^+_{ATP} channels open when intracellular ATP concentration falls in myocardial and vascular smooth muscle cells.[53 56 107] It has been suggested that a decrease in myocardial tissue O_2 tension may be sensed by the vascular smooth muscle cell. By regulation of the generation of ATP, this decrease may subsequently lead to an opening of K^+_{ATP} channels in vascular smooth muscle cells.[53] This is consistent with the previous finding that coronary autoregulation is coupled strongly to tissue O_2 tension rather than to $M\dot{V}_{O_2}$.[104] It is, however, also conceivable that other tissue factors modify coronary autoregulation because K^+_{ATP} channel activity is also affected by tissue concentrations of ADP, lactate, and extracellular cations.[108] It is interesting to note that adenosine-induced coronary vasodilation is in part mediated by K^+_{ATP} channels.[56 109]

Myogenic control

Vascular smooth muscle contracts in response to increased distending force (referred to as "stretch-induced contraction"). This mechanism may form the basis for the myogenic control of perfusion. It might contribute to coronary autoregulation, particularly in arterioles that are less than 100 μm in diameter.[42] How this mechanism works is unknown; stretch activated channels may be involved. Increased intraluminal pressure causes arteriolar smooth muscle to contract. The subsequent increase in resistance tends to normalise blood flow despite an elevated perfusion pressure. This mechanism is called myogenic control. It seems to be more important in arterioles smaller than 100 μm, compared with larger arterioles, and in subepicardial compared with subendocardial arterioles.[110]

Studies in isolated coronary resistance arterioles that are uncoupled from metabolic mediators of vascular tone have shown that both myogenic and flow-mediated, endothelium-dependent mechanisms may be involved in local blood flow regulation throughout much of the coronary microcirculation.[111] There seem to be transmural differences in the potential for myogenic dilatation. In subendocardial arterioles, myogenic dilatation was maximal at pressures of 60 cm H_2O, whereas in subepicardial arterioles myogenic dilatation was present up to pressures as low as 40 cm H_2O.[112] The changes in vessel diameter over the pressure range studied were, however, only modest (<10% of resting values). In contrast, flow-dependent influences on coronary vasomotor tone increased arteriolar diameter by up to 25% of resting value.[111]

Thus, although myogenic responses have been observed in isolated coronary vessels, their demonstration in vivo has been difficult, probably because of the predominance of the metabolic control of CBF. Although some argument can be made for a myogenic component in coronary reactive hyperaemia,[113] overall there is little experimental evidence for myogenic effects in the coronary circulation.

Left ventricular autoregulation

Subendocardial flow of the left coronary artery (LCA) begins to decline at 37 mm Hg, and subepicardial flow at 25 mm Hg.[114] Down to a LCA perfusion pressure of 40 mm Hg (that is, almost a 50% decrease), LCA autoregulation remains preserved. In anaesthetised animals with stable myocardial metabolism, CBF stays rather constant over a pressure range of 60–160 mm Hg.[103] Increasing myocardial metabolism results in an upward shift of the autoregulatory curves.[104]

Autoregulatory capacity of the subendocardium is considerably less than that of the subepicardium. Whereas in the awake animal subepicardial autoregulation was preserved until the perfusion pressure reached 25 mm Hg, subendocardial autoregulation was impaired at 40 mm Hg.[114] Such reduced subendocardial vasodilator reserve explains the well known greater vulnerability of the left ventricular subendocardium to ischaemia when compared with the subepicardium.[115]

Experimental conditions and extent of cardiac work influence the lower limits of autoregulation. At a heart rate of 100 beats/min, perfusion pressure can decrease to 38 mm Hg before subendocardial ischaemia develops, but ischaemia develops at 61 mm Hg if the heart rate is 200 beats/min.[116] Even during tachycardia and at pressures as low as 33 mm Hg, subepicardial flow was maintained.

What could be the explanation for the lower subendocardial vasodilator reserve? The pressure–flow relationship during a long diastole would suggest that pressure at zero flow (P_{zf}) is higher in the subendocardium than in the subepicardium.[117] P_{zf} is, however, unlikely to be high in any myocardial layer, and unlikely to be higher in the subendocardium by more than 2–3 mm Hg.[118] This excludes the possibility that different diastolic myocardial compressive forces account for the differences in regional vasodilator reserve.

During systole, compressive forces are greatest in the subendocardium, resulting in higher vascular resistance. With the start of diastole, flow follows first the path of lowest vascular resistance (that is, the large subepicardial vessels) before reaching the higher resistance subendocardial vessels. This hypothesis of an interaction between systole and diastole has

143

been proposed as a possible explanation for the lower subendocardial vasodilator reserve.[118]

Right ventricular autoregulation

Absence of effective right coronary artery (RCA) pressure–flow autoregulation (that is, variation of RCA flow with RCA perfusion pressure) has been a consistent finding.[119] However, when the change in right ventricular $M\dot{V}o_2$ (accompanying changes in RCA flow) is taken into account, the "corrected" RCA autoregulatory gain is comparable to the LCA autoregulatory gain (gain being a measure of autoregulatory potency).[120] RCA autoregulation in conscious dogs fails at approximately 42 mm Hg,[120] a pressure somewhat higher than for failure of LCA autoregulation.[114] Anaesthesia does not seem to depress RCA autoregulatory gain, but attenuates the range.[120] Right ventricular myocardial performance is preserved in both conscious and anaesthetised animals until RCA perfusion pressures fall below 50 mm Hg.[120] Above 50 mm Hg, right ventricular function does not seem to be coupled to RCA blood flow. Probably related to low right ventricular systolic pressures, inner and outer layers of the right ventricle have similar lower limits of autoregulation.

Conclusion

The precise activating signals and mediators of autoregulation still have to be defined. At the lower range of autoregulation, NO formation[102] and opening of K^+_{ATP} channels[106] may be involved. It is possible that O_2 tensions within a critical range may be the initial metabolic stimulus for coronary autoregulation. Although adenosine does not appear to be essential for autoregulation, it is probably reasonable to speculate that compensatory mechanisms other than adenosine exist in the myocardium, which gain importance once the action of adenosine is prevented. It is rather unlikely that a highly oxidative organ such as the heart depends on just one "host defence" mechanism to preserve the balance between supply and demand. Furthermore, the mechanisms involved in the control of coronary vasomotor tone may well be distributed in a way that metabolic, flow-dependent, or myogenic control mechanisms predominate in different classes of arteriolar vessel. Furthermore, each of the mediators may have differing physiological relevance under differing conditions.

Variations in myocardial perfusion

Blood supply to the heart is affected by ventricular contraction and relaxation. Any myocardial stress is expected to alter underlying myocardial geometry and, in turn, geometry of intramyocardial vessels. This may affect vascular resistance and flow. Forces acting on a myocardial segment may include interactions between myofibres and adjacent vessels, intramyocardial tissue (fluid) pressure, cavity pressure transmitted as radial stress, myofibre force transmitted tangentially, and pericardial pressure. Intramyocardial tissue pressure possibly constitutes a major component of coronary vascular resistance. It differs between right and left ventricular wall, atrial and ventricular chambers, and epicardial and endocardial layers, and it varies with systole and diastole.

During systole, the myocardial fibre bands that encircle both ventricles exert lateral shearing forces on the perpendicularly penetrating intramyocardial branches of the large epicardial vessels. This may entirely abolish flow to certain regions of the myocardium.[121] At the same time, however, those intramyocardial vessels running parallel to the muscle fibres are compressed during systole which propagates blood further downstream. Coronary venous blood is drained almost entirely in systole partly as a result of this squeezing effect of myocardial contraction. This in itself promotes coronary arterial inflow.[122]

Resting myocardial perfusion

Although mean resting myocardial blood flow in all larger mammals is consistently 0·6–1·0 ml/min per g,[58] local flow distribution is remarkably heterogeneous varying between 20% and 200% of the mean value.[123] Such flow heterogeneity most probably reflects local differences in aerobic metabolism.[124] Thus, high flow areas do not represent a state of luxury perfusion, but rather reflect higher local O_2 demands. They should be as susceptible to hypoperfusion as low flow areas.

Phasic myocardial perfusion

Intermittently high and low extravascular resistances during systole and diastole are responsible for the phasic pattern of coronary perfusion (Fig 4.6). In the left ventricle, extravascular compression during systole is so great that normally only 20–30% of left coronary artery flow occurs during systole.[125] As a result of considerably lower systolic and, thus, intramyocardial pressure generated by the thin-walled right ventricle, right coronary arterial systolic flow constitutes a much greater proportion of total coronary inflow (30–50%)(Fig 4.6). Systolic myocardial compression increases with rises in heart rate, afterload, preload, and contractility. The relative contribution of each of these factors to the regulation of myocardial perfusion remains controversial.[126] When coronary perfusion pressure is increased experimentally, systolic and diastolic components of epicardial flow increase, with diastolic flow dominating.[127]

The effects of contraction on phasic flow pattern seem to vary with the contractile state of the myocardium. During uniform global contraction, local intramyocardial forces rather than transmitted forces (that is, cavity

145

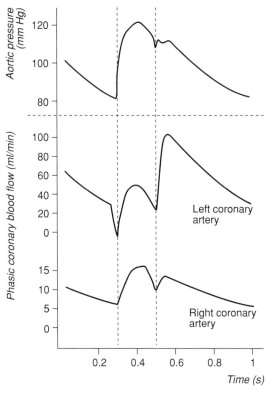

Fig 4.6 Phasic blood flows of right and left coronary arteries in relation to aortic pressure. Whereas right coronary artery flow exists throughout the cardiac cycle, left coronary flow is largely confined to diastole. (Reproduced with permission from Berne RM, Levy MP. *Cardiovascular physiology*, 5th edn. St Louis: CV Mosby, 1986:200.)

pressure) are primarily responsible for the phasic flow variation.[128] In a non-contracting region of myocardium, however, left ventricular pressure becomes a major determinant of phasic flow pattern.[128]

This dependence of flow characteristics on the contractile state may be explained by differences in myocardial behaviour during systole. During normal contraction, the myocardium stiffens and then becomes resistant to deformation by externally transmitted stress such as cavitary pressure. When contraction is absent, however, the respective myocardial segment fails to stiffen, and the intramyocardial vessels are now prone to deformation by externally applied forces.

Normal intramyocardial and peripheral epicardial coronary arteries exhibit almost exclusive forward flow during diastole. Reverse flow is frequently observed during systole.[129] With coronary artery stenosis, systolic reverse flow increases whereas diastolic forward flow decreases.[130] Reduced back pressure to systolic reverse flow as a result of decreased post-stenotic distal pressure, and increased coronary arterial capacitance resulting from a pressure-dependent capacitance change[131] may both serve as explanation.

Transmural myocardial perfusion

During the cardiac cycle, transmural flow distribution is non-uniform. Normally, subendocardial flow exceeds subepicardial flow by about 10%, resulting in an endo-/epicardial perfusion ratio of 1·1. As systolic intramyocardial compressive forces are greatest in the subendocardium, but low in the subepicardium, it was postulated that the subepicardium was perfused throughout the cardiac cycle, whereas the subendocardium received blood only during diastole. However, findings of possibly very little flow to the subepicardium even during systole argue against such a mechanism.[118]

During normal contraction, primarily subendocardial vessels are compressed,[132] and a steep transmural gradient of intramyocardial pressure persists in an empty beating heart. When a beating heart is arrested, subendocardial flow has been shown to increase but subepicardial flow to decrease.[78] Thus, contraction appears to augment subepicardial perfusion. It has been proposed that during cardiac contraction blood is squeezed out of subendocardial vessels and translocated in a retrograde fashion to superficial layers of the myocardium. In this way, the subepicardial vessels represent a low pressure and low resistance "sink" for any translocation of blood from deep to superficial layers. It is to be expected that the amount of retrograde flow will depend on the transmural pressure gradient. Consequently, absent global[78] or regional contraction[128] causes marked changes in phasic inflow to the myocardium and in transmural flow distribution, most probably by altering the transmural pressure gradient. When contraction is absent, left ventricular pressure becomes a powerful determinant of transmural flow distribution and, subsequently, the subendocardial/subepicardial flow ratio more than doubles, indicating favoured subendocardial perfusion.[128]

The left ventricular subendocardium is more susceptible to hypoperfusion than the epicardium, for two major reasons: (1) coronary vessels penetrate the ventricular wall from outside to inside, so that the inner layers are further away from the epicardial conduit arteries; and (2) systolic compressive force is greater in the subendocardium than in the epicardium.[133] Whereas subendocardial arterioles narrow by about 20% during systole, subepicardial arteriolar diameter changes little during the cardiac cycle.[134] It has been postulated that systole and diastole create a to-and-fro oscillation of blood flow in the coronary vessels that penetrates the myocardial wall from outside to inside.[78 135] The oscillating flow only fills and empties intramyocardial arteries and arterioles, without providing nutritive flow to the subendocardial capillaries. At the end of diastole, blood flows from the aorta through the coronary vascular tree to all layers of the myocardium. At the start of systole, cardiac contraction produces retrograde flow in penetrating coronary arteries. Part of the retrograde flow originates at the subendocardial layers, and is diverted to the outer epicardial layers that are less compressed than the inner layers.[78 134] At the onset of diastole, forward flow refills the intramyocardial vessels that had been compressed and emptied during the preceding systole. Only then does nutritive flow through the capillaries of the subendocardium begin. As a result of the oscillatory coronary flow pattern, the outer layer of the myocardium (the epicardium) is perfused throughout the cardiac cycle, but the inner layer (the subendocardium) is perfused only during diastole.

Tachycardia and intense adrenergic activation of the heart (as during maximal exercise) pose a particular threat to the subendocardium because: (1) the duration of diastole becomes very short, whereas systole hardly shortens; (2) $M\dot{V}o_2$ increases; and (3) intramyocardial blood volume increases as a result of metabolically-induced coronary vasodilation. Increased intramyocardial capacitance will contribute to a proportionally greater oscillatory flow, which encroaches on nutritive flow to the subendocardium. In other words, when intense cardiac stress results in high $M\dot{V}o_2$ and CBF, in tachycardia, and in compromise of local metabolic vasodilator reserve, the mechanical effects of systolic compression and oscillating transmural flow may lead to subendocardial hypoperfusion.

Thus, opposing factors such as wall stiffness, regional contractility, and cavity pressure influence phasic inflow and transmural flow distribution. The net result on myocardial perfusion will depend on their interactions during specific conditions. With changes in baseline conditions, the relative importance of each of the factors will also change. During uniform global contraction, local tissue–vessel interactions and/or intramyocardial fluid pressure caused by active contraction appear to play a dominant role in determining myocardial perfusion. When regional contraction is abolished, left ventricular pressure assumes a more prominent role. This, however, does not imply that the effects of intramyocardial forces caused by contraction are simply removed when myocardial stiffness is low. Rather, changes in underlying conditions will result in complex changes in the spatial and temporal course of forces that act on intramyocardial vessels. Such considerations may help us to understand mechanisms governing myocardial perfusion under clinical conditions of regional myocardial dysfunction (such as myocardial ischaemia and "stunned" myocardium).

Coronary vascular resistance

Vascular tone of coronary arterioles larger than 100 μm in diameter is regulated primarily by myogenic and local metabolic factors.[136] Adenosine and dipyridamole produce their vasodilator effects mainly in vessels of this size. Up to 40% of total coronary resistance resides, however, in small arteries that are 100–400 μm in diameter.[137] Vasomotor tone in these small coronary arteries is controlled by endothelial, humoral, and neural autonomic influences.[138] Although these small vessels are not under direct metabolic control, they may, nevertheless, influence maximal coronary blood flow importantly. When vasodilation of the arterioles causes an increase in flow, the resultant increase in endothelial shear stress will augment NO production and, subsequently, cause vasodilation of the small arteries.[22 136] Thus, arteriolar vasodilation leads to dilatation of the small resistance arteries by way of endothelium-dependent flow/shear-mediated NO release. In hyperlipidaemia, such endothelium-dependent, flow-mediated vasodilation of the small arteries may be impaired or abolished.[139]

The principal functions of the resistive vessels are: (1) to match myocardial blood flow to $M\dot{V}o_2$ when metabolic demand varies; and (2) to maintain myocardial perfusion (proportionate to metabolic demand) when perfusion pressure varies. Under pathological conditions, dilatation of the resistance vessels compensates for the increase in resistance of the conduit arteries caused by stenoses. In experimental animals, as well as in humans, normal epicardial arteries vasodilate in response to increases in blood flow. This response is endothelium-dependent, because removal of the endothelium abolishes the flow-mediated vasodilation. Metabolic vasodilation of the coronary resistance vessels during exercise or pacing also causes flow-mediated vasodilation of the epicardial arteries.[18]

For a better understanding of vasomotor dysregulation which may lead to myocardial ischaemia, it is helpful to distinguish functionally between two components within the resistive coronary vasculature, which are arranged in series (Fig 4.7): (1) more proximal, "prearteriolar" vessels in which vasomotor tone and flow are not metabolically regulated because of the epicardial position or thickness of the vessel wall; and (2) more distal, "arteriolar" vessels in which major pressure reductions occur, and in which tone and flow are metabolically regulated.[140] As no anatomical differentiation is possible between the two segments, functional differentiation is expected to be vague.[141]

The continuous matching of flow to demand by the resistive vessels is so precise that myocardial O_2 extraction remains practically constant over a wide range of metabolic demand and coronary perfusion pressure. The site of action and the mechanisms involved may differ, however, when flow is varied either in response to changes in metabolic demands at constant aortic pressure, or when flow is maintained in the presence of changes in aortic pressure at constant metabolic demand.

Reduction of coronary perfusion pressure to 40 mm Hg causes dilatation of vessels smaller than 100 μm in diameter, but constriction of larger

149

vessels.[96] Two possible explanations exist for such a heterogeneous response: (1) large reductions in coronary perfusion pressure cause metabolically-induced dilatation of arteriolar vessels but a passive, low, distending, pressure-induced reduction in prearteriolar vessel diameter; or (2) reduced flow-mediated release of EDRF/NO causes prearteriolar constriction.

When CBF increases in response to metabolically-mediated arteriolar vasodilation, one would expect a proportionate increase in pressure drop across the prearteriolar vessels unless they respond with compensatory flow-mediated vasodilation. If this does not occur (as with endothelial dysfunction in coronary artery disease), pressure at the origin of the maximally dilated arterioles may decrease to an extent that impairs

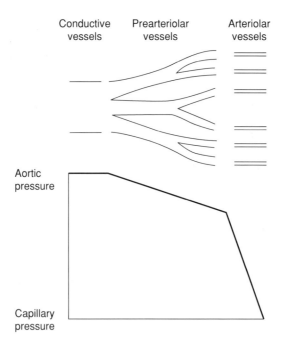

Fig 4.7 Schematic representation of pressure reduction from the aorta to capillaries. Three components of the coronary circulation can be identified: (1) conductive vessels with negligible pressure drop; (2) prearteriolar vessels with moderate pressure drop; and (3) arteriolar vessels with greatest pressure drop. (Reproduced with permission from Maseri A, Crea F, Cianflone D. Myocardial ischemia caused by distal coronary vasoconstriction. *Am J Cardiol* 1992;**70**: 1602-5.)

subendocardial perfusion.[135] Thus, during metabolically-induced arteriolar vasodilation adequate perfusion pressure at the origin of the arterioles can be maintained only if there is an appropriate change in vasomotor tone at the prearteriolar level. Flow-mediated vasodilation on the basis of a tonic release of endothelial NO and/or other endothelium-derived relaxing factors may be primarily involved in the adaptation of prearteriolar vessel size to changes in flow.

Coronary blood flow varies little over a wide range of aortic pressures (see Autoregulation). This requires constant changes in coronary vasomotor tone and vascular resistance. Depending on the initiating stimulus, the adaptive mechanisms maintaining CBF may differ. An increase in aortic pressure may primarily trigger prearteriolar constriction, thus maintaining optimal pressure at the origin of the arterioles. On the other hand, when aortic pressure decreases metabolically-induced arteriolar dilatation, in addition to flow-mediated prearteriolar dilatation may be required to maintain CBF.

It is the traditional view that myocardial ischaemia in coronary artery disease is caused by a fixed or dynamic obstruction of large conduit coronary arteries resulting in a critical reduction in perfusion pressure at the origin of fully dilated arterioles. Clinical studies suggest, however, that myocardial ischaemia can also be the result of constriction of small, distal, resistive coronary vessels.[142] Such small vessel constriction can result from dysfunction of either prearteriolar or arteriolar vessels. The mechanisms of the abnormal behaviour of the distal resistive vessels resulting in myocardial ischaemia can be multiple, and may involve different sites.[143 144]

The concept that coronary vascular resistance resides in large conduit arteries and, primarily, in small resistance vessels practically ignores the contribution of the venous system to total coronary vascular resistance. Whereas under control conditions only 7% of the total coronary vascular resistance resides in veins that are more than $150 \mu m$ in diameter, under conditions of vasodilation with dipyridamole the total contribution of the venous component increases to 31%.[145] Thus, during coronary vasodilation the coronary venous system may considerably modify myocardial perfusion. Furthermore, by affecting ventricular distensibility related to changes in myocardial blood volume,[146] alterations in venous reactivity may also have an impact on diastolic cardiac function.

Isolated coronary venules dilate in response to an increase in flow.[147] This flow-induced vasodilation is endothelium-dependent and mediated by the release of a nitrovasodilator. Endothelial disruption results in flow-induced constriction, suggesting that shear stress may directly act on the vascular smooth muscle.[147] Whereas the additive effects of flow-induced dilatation and possibly myogenic relaxation of arterioles can maximise myocardial oxygen delivery during elevated $M\dot{V}o_2$, the flow-induced venular dilatation may possibly contribute to a reduction in postcapillary resistance.

Pressure-flow relationships

Flow (*F*) across a resistance (*R*) is determined by the difference between pressures upstream and downstream of the resistance (*P*), according to the equation:

$$F = P/R.$$

The driving pressure, *P*, is the coronary perfusion pressure. Whereas upstream pressure can clearly be defined as the pressure at the aortic root, definition of what constitutes downstream pressure is still somewhat controversial.[148] [149] For Fig 4.8, the downstream pressure is taken as the coronary sinus pressure or left ventricular end diastolic pressure, and the

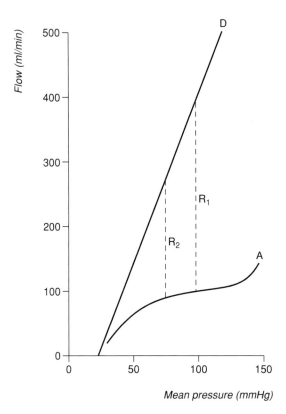

Fig 4.8 Schematic presentation of coronary pressure–flow relationships in the normal left ventricle during autoregulated flow (A), and during maximal vasodilation (D). R_1 and R_2 denote coronary vascular reserves at mean coronary perfusion pressures of 100 (R_1) and 75 mm Hg (R_2) (Reproduced with permission from Hoffman JIE. Maximal coronary flow and the concept of coronary vascular reserve. *Circulation* 1984;70:153–9.)

(apparent) coronary perfusion pressure is the difference between down-stream and mean aortic diastolic pressure.

The normal pressure–flow relationship (A, Fig 4.8) has three separate regions of interest: (1) a high pressure region, where flow increases with coronary perfusion pressure; (2) an intermediate pressure range, where flow changes little with changes in coronary perfusion pressure (referred to as "autoregulation"); and (3) a low pressure region, where flow decreases with decreasing coronary perfusion pressure.

The controversy surrounding the downstream value for coronary perfusion pressure centres around the extrapolation of the low pressure region to zero flow (Fig 4.9). It is accepted that the coronary pressure–flow relationship always has a positive intercept.[148 150 151] It had been suggested that myocardial perfusion stopped at pressures considerably higher than coronary sinus pressure.[117] The pressure at which flow stopped was termed "critical closing pressure" or "zero flow pressure" (P_{zf} or $P_{f=0}$) (Fig 4.9). This would imply that the effective downstream pressure for the calculation of coronary vascular resistance would be P_{zf} rather than the much lower coronary sinus or left ventricular end diastolic pressure. Results were, however, obtained on the basis of measurements on large proximal epicardial vessels, and it now seems that flow through intramural coronary vessels actually continues after large superficial vessel flow has already ceased. Furthermore, it has been shown that forward movement of red blood cells in arterioles that are $20\,\mu m$ in diameter continues until perfusion pressure is only a few millimetres of mercury higher than

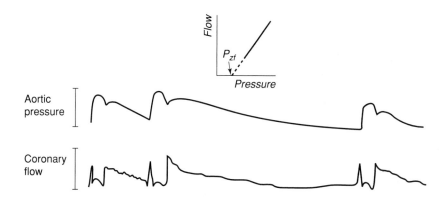

Fig 4.9 Graphic presentation of the concept of critical closing pressure (P_{zf}). During a long diastole, pressure in the aortic root or coronary artery, and flow through an epicardial coronary artery are recorded simultaneously (solid line in pressure–flow plot). The pressure at which flow through the (epicardial) coronary artery is zero (P_{zf}) is either determined directly or derived by linear extrapolation (dashed line). (Reproduced with permission from Sethna DH, Moffitt EA. An appreciation of the coronary circulation. *Anesth Analg* 1986;**65**:294–305.)

coronary sinus pressure.[152] Thus, the initial findings of a considerably higher P_{zf} than coronary sinus pressure can probably be explained on the basis of arterial collateral flow[153] and coronary capacitance.[154]

An increase in coronary sinus pressure can shift the entire pressure–flow relationship to a higher P_{zf} without affecting its slope.[150 151] This way, coronary sinus pressure may become a determinant of CBF and transmural flow distribution. There appear to be regional differences in the response of the pressure–flow relationship to an increase in coronary sinus pressure: whereas the subepicardial pressure–flow relationship behaves like the total relationship, in the subendocardium neither the pressure–flow relationship nor intramyocardial tissue pressures changed in response to high coronary sinus pressure.[151] Such transmural differences in intramyocardial pressures and P_{zf} support the existence of a vascular waterfall mechanism in the myocardium.[155]

The concept of P_{zf} remains controversial, and the clinical relevance of changes in P_{zf} in response to interventions remains questionable. For clinical purposes, coronary perfusion pressure in normal coronary arteries can be defined as the difference between (mean) aortic diastolic and coronary sinus or left ventricular end diastolic (or even right atrial) pressures.

Flow–function relationship

Tennant and Wiggers[156] first reported in 1935 that myocardial performance is closely coupled to perfusion. The degree of transmural flow reduction required to impair contractile function, however, varies considerably. As the right ventricle differs importantly from the left ventricle in O_2 extraction, $M\dot{V}o_2$, and transmural pressure, differences in the flow–function relationship between the two ventricles are to be expected.

Right and left ventricular functions are well maintained as perfusion pressures are reduced to 50 mm Hg.[114 120] Whereas left ventricular perfusion remained unchanged,[114] RCA flow decreased by 34% as perfusion pressure declined.[120] As the right ventricle has a greater O_2 extraction reserve than the left,[157] moderate right ventricular hypoperfusion might be compensated for by increasing O_2 extraction. Alternatively, right ventricular internal cardiac work and, thus, right ventricular $M\dot{V}o_2$ decreases as the reduction in coronary perfusion pressure reduces intravascular volume and, thus, right ventricular systolic stiffness.[158] For these reasons, a highly effective autoregulation is less important for the right than for the left ventricle to maintain myocardial performance above a perfusion pressure of 50 mm Hg.

Gregg was the first to note that coronary perfusion pressure independently affects $M\dot{V}o_2$ and contractile performance.[99] The exact mechanism of this so called "Gregg phenomenon" is still unknown. It is possible that the two aspects of the Greggs' phenomenon are based on different mechanisms: the increase in $M\dot{V}o_2$ may be related to an augmentation in CBF, and the increase in contractility may be secondary to changes in vascular shear stress induced by perfusion pressure,[159] possibly at the capillary level.[160]

The increase in $M\dot{V}o_2$ correlates with an increase in coronary vascular volume.[161] Such expanded volume could result in a more rigid coronary hydraulic "skeleton", which, in turn, requires more energy (that is, greater $M\dot{V}o_2$) for systolic contraction.[158] This is in agreement with the finding that perfusion-induced changes in $M\dot{V}o_2$ and contractility are greatest during poor coronary autoregulation, when coronary vascular volume is also greatest.[158 161]

When the increase in CBF is caused by an elevation in perfusion pressure, this phenomenon is termed the "garden hose effect", because the resultant coronary distension is thought to cause an increase in myocyte sarcomere length, thereby augmenting cardiac performance by the Frank–Starling mechanism. Increases in CBF without a change in perfusion pressure have a similar effect.[158]

Coronary flow reserve

The pressure–flow relationship during maximum coronary vasodilation is almost straight (D, Fig 4.8). Maximum flow at any given pressure is determined primarily by the cross–sectional area of the resistance vessels. The difference between autoregulated (A, Fig 4.8) and maximally dilated (D, Fig 4.8) flow is the reserve capacity for vasodilation. Coronary flow reserve (CFR) is defined as the ratio of CBF during maximal coronary vasodilation to CBF under resting conditions.[162] Depending on the technique used (that is, nuclear techniques, transoesophageal echocardiography, coronary catheterisation, intracoronary Doppler wire), normal values for CFR have been reported from as low as 1·8 to as high as 5·5.[163] A value of 3·0 or more is, however, generally considered to be normal.[163]

Three principal factors determine CFR: (1) a vascular factor (reflecting coronary vascular resistance); (2) an extravascular factor (reflecting myocardial compressive forces); and (3) a rheological component (reflecting blood composition). As CFR presents a ratio, its value will depend substantially on the baseline coronary flow rate. Age, myocardial hypertrophy, and elevated heart rate and blood pressure may increase resting coronary flow, thus "falsely" lowering the CFR.[163]

In general, CFR values of less than 3·0 suggest microvascular disease on the basis of functional or structural anomalies. In routine clinical practice, maximal vasodilation of the resistance vessels is best achieved pharmacologically (for example, by adenosine). Physical exercise or cardiac pacing is less suitable.

155

Coronary flow reserve may be reduced principally by elevation of the autoregulatory line or depression of the line for maximally attainable flow. Anaemia, left ventricular hypertrophy, or increased $M\dot{V}o_2$ lead to higher resting CBF, thus elevating the autoregulation line (A_2, Fig 4.10). If the maximally attainable flow at any given pressure remains unchanged, coronary flow reserve will decrease (R_1–R_2, Fig 4.10). Concomitant hypertension will, however, preserve CRF (R_3, Fig 4.10).

Coronary artery disease, tachycardia, polycythaemia, and marked increases in left ventricular end diastolic pressure or contractility all

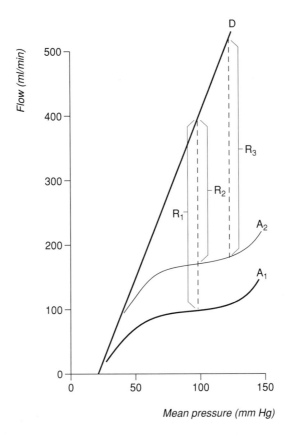

Mean pressure (mm Hg)

Fig 4.10 Diagram of pressure–flow relationships during autoregulation in the normal (A_1) and in the left ventricle with anaemia or increased contractility or hypertrophy (A_2). As pressure–flow relationships during maximal vasodilation remain about the same (D), coronary vascular reserve will be lower in the abnormal (R_2) than in the normal (R_1) left ventricle. Elevation of coronary perfusion pressure (as in hypertension) may restore or even increase absolute coronary vascular reserve (R_3). (Reproduced with permission from Hoffman JIE. Maximal coronary flow and the concept of coronary vascular reserve. *Circulation* 1984;**70**:153–9.)

156

decrease the slope of the line for maximally attainable flow (D, Fig 4.10), so reducing the CFR (R_1-R_2, Fig 4.10). In the case of coronary artery disease, this reflects a decrease in total cross sectional area of the coronary vascular bed.

Many studies have estimated CFR from the reactive myocardial hyperaemia that follows transient total coronary occlusion. If there is no hyperaemia, coronary vascular reserve is deemed to have been exhausted by having to compensate for a stenosis in the supply vessel, and the supply vessel is deemed to be "critically constricted".[164] Reactive hyperaemia is, however, the result of complex interactions between vasodilator metabolites, myogenic relaxation, and coronary capacitance.[165] It is difficult to standardise because it varies with the duration of occlusion, basal $M\dot{V}o_2$, coronary perfusion pressure, sympathetic tone, and reactivity of adenosine receptors.[165] Pharmacological vasodilators such as adenosine or dipyridamole may lower resistance much more than ischaemic stimuli[166] (Fig 4.11). During maximal exercise in humans, CBF may increase by two or four times the control values, but with dipyridamole, increases of three to

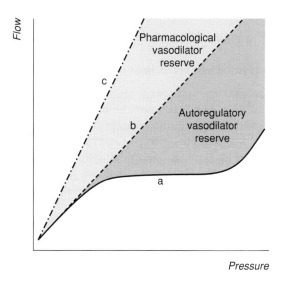

Fig 4.11 Autoregulation and coronary vasodilator reserve. Traditionally, it was thought that the coronary pressure–flow relationship below the autoregulatory range (line a) was identical with the pressure–flow relationship in the maximally dilated bed (line b), indicating exhausted coronary vasodilator reserve. Considerable flow reserve well below the autoregulatory range has, however, been demonstrated in response to intracoronary application of vasodilation (line c). Thus, pharmacological vasodilator reserve (c–a) may be preserved at times of exhausted (physiological) autoregulatory vasodilator reserve. (Reproduced with permission from Dole WP. Autoregulation of the coronary circulation. *Prog Cardiovasc Dis* 1987;**29**:293–323.)

157

five times the control have been described.[167] Thus, endogenous (ischaemic) stimuli may not be as effective in revealing true (maximal) coronary flow reserve as potent pharmacological vasodilators (Fig 4.11).

The overall evidence seems to indicate that the degree of CFR provides potentially valid information on what might happen during maximal stress, as long as other factors that might modify maximally attainable and autoregulated flows are controlled for (or accounted for if changes do occur during the study). Determination of CFR using maximal pharmacological vasodilation has been used to assess the physiological significance of coronary stenoses, and the results of coronary angioplasty and coronary bypass surgery.

Methods to determine coronary/myocardial blood flow

Correct interpretation of coronary circulatory behaviour in response to a given intervention is critically dependent on reliable determination of perfusion. Contradictory findings may at times reflect differences in methodology employed to measure perfusion. All methods of measuring blood flow have technical limitations.[168]

Radioactive microsphere technique

This has become the standard technique to evaluate transmural myocardial blood flow distribution in the experimental animal.[169] It is an extraction method that rests on the assumptions that microspheres injected into the bloodstream are distributed like red blood cells, and that basically all microspheres are trapped in tissues on their first passage. Under such conditions, blood flow should be proportional to radioactivity per tissue mass.

Microspheres are denser and larger, and stream more centrally than red cells. They are, therefore, not distributed in quite the same way as native blood. As subendocardial shunting (non-entrapment) of $9 \mu m$ spheres is somewhat greater than shunting of $15 \mu m$ spheres, endo-/epicardial flow ratios determined with $9 \mu m$ spheres tend to be lower than those determined with $15 \mu m$ spheres. In general, endo-/epicardial values are lower in open chest preparations than in conscious dogs.[58] The necessity of obtaining multiple myocardial tissue samples requires sacrifice of the animal and prohibits its use in humans.

Inert gas clearance technique

By determining the arteriocoronary sinus difference in gas saturation, CBF can be calculated from equations originally developed by Kety and Schmidt.[170] For this technique to be accurate, several requirements must be fulfilled:[171] (1) the indicator must be physiologically inert; (2) partition coefficients for the gas in the myocardium, fat, red cells, and plasma must be known; (3) venous blood from the entire myocardial region of interest must be sampled; (4) during the period of saturation and desaturation (5–20 min), the CBF must be stable; and (5) the entire washout curve must be analysed.

The principal disadvantages of the inert gas clearance technique (particularly when using non-radioactive tracers) include: (1) poor spatial resolution; (2) length of time required for making measurements; (3) variations in venous drainage patterns distorting results; and (4) the inability to determine right ventricular and atrial flows because venous blood from those areas cannot be sampled. Although the introduction of radioactive xenon^{-133}(^{133}Xe) has added spatial resolution to the inert gas clearance technique,[172] transmural blood distribution cannot be determined, the temporal resolution remains limited (requiring stable flow during measurements), only a limited number (two to five) of flow determinations is possible (as a result of xenon's eight times greater solubility in fat than in myocardium), and only flow rates below 200 ml/min per 100 g can be measured with reasonable accuracy.[173] Therefore, determination of flow rates during maximal coronary vasodilation is probably not possible.

Electromagnetic flow meters

The principle of this technique is based on Faraday's induction law which states that a conductor moving in a magnetic field generates electric current. When blood flows through the vessel, electrical voltage proportional to the rate of the flow is generated, and this voltage is recorded by an appropriate flow meter apparatus. Use of accurate, non-occlusive (electronic) zero that can be used at any time and compared with occlusive (mechanical) zero, automatic flow ranging (autoranging) that provides an instantaneous readout of blood volume flow, and precalibration during flow probe production that eliminates the need for time consuming flow calibration have made it possible to provide immediate, reliable determinations of blood flow.

The principal drawbacks of this technique include the relatively large sized flow probes (limiting its application to major epicardial vessels), its inability to determine transmural blood flow distribution, and its invasiveness (requiring thoracotomy and coronary artery dissection). Variability in contact between flow probe and vessel may result in major errors in measurement.

Ultrasonic Doppler techniques

This technique is based on the Doppler principle that states that, when sound waves are reflected from a moving structure, the frequency of the reflected wave is shifted to a higher or lower frequency (Doppler shift). In the case of blood vessels, the Doppler shift is caused by ultrasonic waves that reflect off moving red blood cells. Coronary flow velocity can be measured by several Doppler techniques: Doppler flow meter, Doppler catheter,[174] Doppler guidewire,[175 176] an epicardial probe,[177] a trans-oesophageal probe,[178] and a transthoracic Doppler probe.[176] Guide wires as small as 0·36 mm in diameter, tipped with a 15 MHz piezoelectric ultrasound transducer, allow reliable velocity measurements even in poststenotic areas of coronary arteries.[176] Intracoronary Doppler measurements can be affected by positioning of the wire, tortuous segments, and areas of varying luminal dimensions or configurations.[179] Non-invasive flow velocity measurement using transthoracic Doppler echocardiography, under the guidance of colour Doppler flow mapping correlates well with measurements obtained invasively by an intracoronary Doppler catheter.[176]

The temporal resolution of this technique is ideal, allowing continuous online measurements of changes in velocity. The principal drawback of this technique is the fact that velocity rather than flow is measured. For the correct interpretation of results, it is crucial to have precise knowledge of the magnitude and direction of any change in coronary cross sectional area in response to a given intervention. Otherwise, statements regarding changes in absolute flow are not valid.

Thermodilution technique

This technique is based on the principle that a change in temperature of a downstream fluid–blood mixture is proportional to blood flow. A fluid indicator (saline) with a known temperature (lower than that of blood) is infused (upstream) into the coronary sinus or great cardiac vein. Although coronary sinus thermodilution is still being used for the estimation of myocardial blood flow,[180] it has almost been forgotten that the initial studies validating this technique were performed in animals under very rigid conditions, which cannot be reproduced in humans (catheter tied into position in coronary sinus; assurance of adequate mixing of blood and tracer; normal coronary arteries and myocardium).

The technique has very crude spatial and only modest temporal resolution. Wide variations in coronary venous drainage patterns make direct comparisons of flow between patients impossible. Even slight variations in catheter position in the coronary sinus may have major effects on flow determination. This practical limitation will make it difficult to interpret results obtained during interventions that are likely to affect cardiac size, and it will make comparison of data gained on different occasions almost impossible (even in the same patient).

As a result of both fundamental and practical deficiencies, thermodilution should be used only in very special circumstances. At present, only large changes (>30%) in coronary sinus or great cardiac vein flow, in patients with no evidence of coronary artery disease, should be accepted as semiquantitative indices of directional changes in CBF.[171]

Positron emission tomography

With this technique the essential features of myocardial perfusion, function, metabolism, and viability can be examined.[181] Positron emission tomography (PET) in humans uses either [^{13}N]ammonia[7] or ^{15}O-labelled water[182] as indicators of myocardial blood flow. Dynamic imaging assesses uptake and retention of the tracer ^{13}NH$_3$ or H$_2$^{15}O. The uptake phase depends on blood flow, and the later (myocardial) retention phase depends on the conversion of NH$_3$ into glutamine. The conversion rate is considered to be constant, and can thus be dealt with mathematically. As positrons emitted per unit mass constitute the mass factor that is incorporated into the rate constant for the delivery of the tracer into the myocardium, myocardial blood flow is reported as millilitres/100 grams per minute (ml/100 g per min).

At present, PET is the only method that allows non-invasive quantification of myocardial blood flow in humans.[183] The correlation with the reference technique (that is, microsphere technique) is excellent ($r = 0.97$) over a wide flow range.[184] PET measures actual myocardial nutritive tissue perfusion. Its major disadvantages are great expense, and limited spatial and transmural resolution.[185]

Thallium-201 scintigraphy

Thallium-201(^{201}Tl) is an analogue of potassium. Its myocardial distribution is the result of two processes. The initial distribution phase reflects myocardial blood flow distribution. The following (redistribution) phase reflects the uptake of ^{201}Tl by the myocardial cell. Uptake of the tracer depends on the same Na$^+$/K$^+$ pump (Na$^+$/K$^+$ ATPase) that transports potassium. Tl binds faster, however, and to more sites than potassium. In hypoperfused but viable myocardium, both the uptake and washout of ^{201}Tl are delayed. Whereas initially there is a difference in radioactivity between normally and hypoperfused areas of myocardium (referred to as a "filling defect" when comparing the intensity of radioactivity of the hypoperfused with that of the normally perfused area), levels of radioactivity in both areas tend to equalise in time (referred to as "redistribution", an actual misnomer because there is no redistribution in the sense of the word). In infarcted areas of myocardium, there is no uptake of ^{201}Tl, and no equalisation of radioactivity between various areas can take place, that is, the "filling defect" persists. Thallium scintigraphy cannot assess absolute blood flow, acute changes in flow, and transmural flow distribution.

Myocardial contrast echocardiography

This technique involves intracoronary injection of microbubbles with a mean size of 10 μm or less under echocardiographic monitoring.[186] Contrast enhancement indicates adequate perfusion, whereas contrast defects are consistent with areas of myocardial hypoperfusion.[186 187] Myocardial contrast echocardiography enables assessment of the spatial distribution of microvascular perfusion. It requires coronary artery catheterisation, and does not allow quantification of blood flow.

Conclusion

All methods (with the exception of PET) are invasive. They require either venous access or surgical dissection of vessels (electromagnetic flow probes), or they involve catheter manipulation in coronary arteries (intracoronary Doppler ultrasonography, xenon-133 clearance). In addition, most methods expose the patient to ionising radiation. At present, no technique is available for clinical use that would allow determination of absolute myocardial perfusion with high temporal and spatial resolution.

In general, methods that use tracers have a poor temporal resolution because they require at least one circulation time for tracer distribution, or 5–20 minutes for inert gas saturation or desaturation to occur. In contrast, methods that assess arterial blood velocity or venous drainage have good temporal but poor spatial resolution. Newer techniques such as magnetic resonance imaging, contrast echocardiography, and ultrafast X-ray computed tomography have theoretically a sufficent spatial resolution to distinguish variation in transmural perfusion.[168]

1 Chilian WM. Adrenergic vasomotion in the coronary microcirculation. *Basic Res Cardiol* 1990;**85**(suppl I):111–20.

2 Chilian WM. Functional distribution of α_1- and α_2-adrenergic receptors in the coronary microcirculation. *Circulation* 1991;**84**:2108–122.

3 Bittl JA, Levin DC. Coronary arteriography. In: Braunwald E, ed, *Heart disease*, 5th edn. Philadelphia: WB Saunders, 1997:240–72.

4 Sonntag M, Deussen A, Schultz J, Loncar R, Hort W, Schrader J. Spatial heterogeneity of blood flow in the dog heart. I. Glucose uptake, free adenosine and oxidative/glycolytic enzyme activity. *Pflügers Arch* 1996;**432**:439–50.

5 Hutchins GM, Moore GW, Hatton EV. Arterial–venous relationships in the human left ventricular myocardium. Anatomic basis for countercurrent regulation of blood flow. *Circulation* 1986;**74**:1195–202.

6 Schaper W, Görge G, Winkler B, Schaper J. The collateral circulation of the heart. *Prog Cardiovasc Dis* 1988;**31**:57–77.

7 Cohen MV. Myocardial ischemia is not a prerequisite for the stimulation of coronary collateral development. *Am Heart J* 1993;**126**:847–55.

8 Schaper W. New paradigms for collateral vessel growth (Editorial). *Basic Res Cardiol* 1993;**88**:193–8.

9 Charney R, Cohen M. The role of the coronary circulation in limiting myocardial ischemia and infarct size. *Am Heart J* 1993;**126**:937–45.

10 Kinn JW, Bache RJ. Effect of platelet activation on coronary collateral blood flow. *Circulation* 1998;**98**:1431–7.

11 Leong L, Sturm M, Taylor R. The lyso-precursor of platelet activating factor (lyso-PAF) in ischemic myocardium. *J Lipid Mediat* 1991;4:277–88.

12 Pearson PJ, Vanhoutte PM. Vasodilator and vasoconstrictor substances produced by the endothelium. *Rev Physiol Biochem Pharmacol* 1993;**122**:1–67.

13 Furchgott RF, Zawadzky JV. The obligatory role of endothelial cells in the relaxation of arterial smooth muscle by acetylcholine. *Nature* 1980;**288**:373–6.

14 de Belder AJ. Radomsky MW. Nitric oxide in the clinical arena (Editoral). *J Hypertens* 1994;**12**:617–24.

15 Lüscher TF, Boulanger CM, Yang Z. Interactions between endothelium-derived relaxing and contracting factors in health and cardiovascular diseases. *Circulation* 1993;87(suppl V):V36–44.

16 Yanagisawa M. The endothelin system. A new target for therapeutic intervention. *Circulation* 1994;**89**:1320–22.

17 Losano G, Pagliaro P, Gatullo D, Marsh NA. Control of coronary blood flow by endothelial release of nitric oxide. *Clin Exp Pharmacol Physiol* 1994;**21**:783–9.

18 Quyyumi AA, Dakak N, Andrews NP, Gilligan DM, Panza JA, Cannon RO. Contribution of nitric oxide to metabolic coronary vasodilation in the human heart. *Circulation* 1995;**92**:320–6.

19 Duncker DJ, Bache RJ. Inhibition of nitric oxide production aggravates myocardial hypoperfusion during exercise in the presence of a coronary artery stenosis. *Circ Res* 1994;**74**:629–40.

20 Bernstein RD, Ochoa FY, Xu X, et al. Function and production of nitric oxide in the coronary circulation of the conscious dog during exercise. *Circ Res* 1996;**79**:840–8.

21 Gödecke A, Decking UKM, Ding Z, et al. Coronary hemodynamics in endothelial NO synthase knockout mice. *Circ Res* 1998;**82**:186–94.

22 Ishibashi Y, Duncker DJ, Zhang J, Bache RJ. ATP-sensitive K^+-channels, adenosine, and nitric oxide-mediated mechanisms account for coronary vasodilation during exercise. *Circ Res* 1998;**82**:346–59.

23 Bassenge E. Endothelium-mediated regulation of coronary tone. *Basic Res Cardiol* 1991;**86**(suppl 2):69–76.

24 Cohen RA, Vanhoutte PM. Endothelium-dependent hyperpolarization: beyond nitric oxide and cyclic GMP. *Circulation* 1995;**92**:3337–49.

25 Campbell WB, Gebremedhin D, Pratt PF, Harder DR. Identification of epoxyeicosa-trienoic acids as endothelium-derived hyperpolarizing factors. *Circ Res* 1996;**78**:415–23.

26 Ming Z, Parent R, Lavallée M. Nitric oxide-independent dilation of conductance coronary arteries to acetylcholine in conscious dogs. *Circ Res* 1997;**81**:977–87.

27 Matsunaga T, Okumura K, Tsunoda R, Tayama S, Tabuchi T, Yasue H. Role of adenosine in regulation of coronary flow in dogs with inhibited synthesis of endothelium-derived nitric oxide. *Am J Physiol* 1996;**270**:H427–34.

28 Altmann JD, Kinn J, Duncker DJ, Bache RJ. Effect of inhibition of nitric oxide formation on coronary blood flow during exercise in the dog. *Cardiovasc Res* 1994;**28**:119–24.

29 Wight E, Noll G, Lüscher TF. Regulation of vascular tone and endothelial function and its alterations in cardiovascular disease. *Ballière's Clin Anaesthesiol* 1997;**11**:531–60.

30 Clozel J-P, Clozel M. Effects of endothelin on the coronary vascular bed in open-chest dogs. *Circ Res* 1989;**65**:1193–200.

31 Cox DA, Vita J, Treasure CB, et al. Atherosclerosis impairs flow-mediated dilation of coronary arteries in humans. *Circulation* 1989;**80**:458–65.

32 Warren JB, Pons F, Brady AJB. Nitric oxide biology: implications for cardiovascular therapeutics. *Cardiovasc Res* 1994;**28**:25–30.

33 Kourembanas S, Marsden PA, McQuillan LP, Faller DV. Hypoxia induces endothelin gene expression and secretion in cultured human endothelium. *J Clin Invest* 1991;**88**:1054–7.

34 Sharefkin JB, Duamond SL, Eskin SG, McIntire LV, Dieffenbach CW. Fluid flow decreases preproendothelin mRNA levels and suppresses endothelin-1 peptide release in cultured human endothelial cells. *J Vasc Surg* 1991;**14**:1–9.

35 Pearson PJ, Lin PJ, Schaff HV. Production of endothelium-derived contracting factor is enhanced after coronary reperfusion. *Ann Thorac Surg* 1991;**51**:788–93.

36 Lerman A, Sandok EK, Hildebrand FL Jr, Burnett JC Jr. Inhibition of endothelium-derived relaxing factor enhances endothelin-mediated vasoconstriction. *Circulation* 1992;**85**:1894–8.

37 Celermajer DS, Sorensen KE, Spiegelhalter DJ, Georgakopoulos D, Robinson J, Deanfield JE. Aging is associated with endothelial dysfunction in healthy men years before the age related decline in women. *J Am Coll Cardiol* 1994;**24**:471–6.

38 Treasure CB, Klein JL, Vita JA, et al. Hypertension and left ventricular hypertrophy are associated with impaired endothelium-mediated relaxation in human coronary resistance vessels. *Circulation* 1993;**87**:86–93.

39 Zeiher AM, Drexler H, Saurbier B, Just H. Endothelium-mediated coronary blood flow modulation in humans: effects of age, atherosclerosis, hypercholesterolemia, and hypertension. *J Clin Invest* 1993;**92**:652–62.

40 Johnstone MT, Creager SJ, Scales KM, Cusco JA, Lee BK, Creager MA. Impaired endothelium-dependent vasodilation in patients with insulin dependent diabetes mellitus. *Circulation* 1993;**88**:2510–16.

41 Quillen JE, Rossen JD, Oskarsson HJ, Minor RL, Lopez AG, Winniford MD. Acute effect of cigarette smoking on the coronary circulation: constriction of epicardial and resistance vessels. *J Am Coll Cardiol* 1993;**22**:642–7.

42 Muller JM, Davis MJ, Chilian WM. Integrated regulation of pressure and flow in the coronary microcirculation. *Cardiovasc Res* 1996;**32**:668–87.

43 Bassenge E, Heusch G. Endothelial and neuro-humoral control of coronary blood flow in health and disease. *Rev Physiol Biochem Pharmacol* 1990;**116**:77–165.

44 Bardenheuer H, Schrader J. Supply-to-demand ratio for oxygen determines formation of adenosine by the heart. *Am J Physiol* 1986;**250**:H173–80.

45 Olsson RA, Bünger R. Metabolic control of coronary blood flow. *Prog Cardiovasc Dis* 1987;**29**:369–87.

46 Dole WP. Autoregulation of the coronary circulation. *Prog Cardiovasc Dis* 1987;**29**:293–323.

47 Hanley F, Grattan MT, Stevens MB, Hoffman JIE. Role of adenosine in coronary autoregulation. *Am J Physiol* 1986;**250**:H558–66.

48 Olsson RA, Pearson JD. Cardiovascular purinoceptors. *Physiol Rev* 1990;**70**:761–845.

49 Glover DK, Ruiz M, Yang JY, et al. Pharmacological stress thallium scintigraphy with 2-cyclohexylmethylindenehydrazino adenosine (WRC-0470). *Circulation* 1996;**94**: 1726–32.

50 Berne RM. The role of adenosine in the regulation of coronary blood flow. *Circ Res* 1980;**47**:807–13.

51 Martin SE, Lenhard SD, Schmarkey LS, Offenbacher S, Odle BM. Adenosine regulates coronary blood flow during increased work and decreased supply. *Am J Physiol* 1993;**264**:H1438–46.

52 Rossen JD, Oskarsson H, Minor RL Jr, Talman CL, Winniford MD. Effect of adenosine antagonism on metabolically mediated coronary vasodilation in humans. *J Am Coll Cardiol* 1994;**23**:1421–6.

53 Nichols CG, Lederer WJ. Adenosine triphosphate-sensitive potassium channels in the cardiovascular system. *Am J Physiol* 1991;**261**:H1617–86.

54 Imamura Y, Tomoike H, Narishige T, Takahashi T, Kasuya T, Takeshita T. Glibenclamide decreases basal coronary blood flow in anesthetized dogs. *Am J Physiol* 1992;**263**:H339–404.

55 Duncker DJ, van Zon ND, Pavek TJ, Herrlinger SK, Bache RJ. Endogenous adenosine mediates coronary vasodilation in response to exercise after K^+_{ATP} channel blockade. *J Clin Invest* 1995;**95**:285–95.

56 Daut J, Maier-Rudolph W, Von Beckerath N, Mehrke G, Günther K, Goedel-Meiner L. Hypoxic dilation of coronary arteries is mediated by ATP-sensitive potassium channels. *Science* 1990;**247**:1341–44.

57 Young MA, Vatner SF. Regulation of large coronary arteries. *Circ Res* 1986;**59**:579–96.

58 Feigl EO. Coronary physiology. *Physiol Rev* 1983;**63**:1–206.

59 DiCarli MF, Tobes MC, Mangner T, et al. Effects of cardiac sympathetic innervation on coronary blood flow. *N Engl J Med* 1997;**336**:1208–15.

60 Cox DA, Hintze TH, Vatner SF. Effects of acetylcholine on large and small coronary arteries in conscious dogs. *J Pharmacol Exp Ther* 1983;**225**:764–9.

61 Feigl EO. EDRF - a protective factor? *Nature* 1988;**331**:490–1.

62 Harrison DG, Sellke FW, Quillen JE. Neurohumoral regulation of coronary collateral vasomotor tone. *Basic Res Cardiol* 1990;**85** (Suppl I): 121–9.

63 Jones CJH, deFily DV, Kuo L, Davis MJ, Chilian WM. α-Adrenergic responses of isolated canine coronary microvessels. *Basic Res Cardiol* 1995;**90**:61–9.

64 Chilian WM, Harrison DG, Haws CW, Snyder WD, Marcus ML. Adrenergic coronary tone during submaximal exercise in the dog is produced by circulating catecholamines: evidence for adrenergic denervation supersensitivity in the myocadium but not in coronary vessels. *Circ Res* 1986;**58**:68–82.

65 Tiefenbacher CP, DeFily DV, Chilian WM. Requisite role of cardiac myocytes in coronary α_1-adrenergic constriction. *Circulation* 1998;**98**:9–12.

66 Lorenzoni R, Rosen SD, Camici PG. Effect of α_1-adrenoceptor blockade on resting and hyperemic myocardial blood flow in normal humans. *Am J Physiol* 1996;**271**:H1302–6.

67 Zeiher AM, Drexler H. Wollschläger H, Just H. Endothelial dysfunction of the coronary microvasculature is associated with coronary blood flow regulation in patients with early atherosclerosis. *Circulation* 1991;**84**:1984–92.

68 Kichuk MR, Seyedi N, Zhang X, et al. Regulation of nitric oxide production in human coronary microvessels and the contribution of local kinin formation. *Circulation* 1996;**94**:44–51.

69 Cocks TM, Angus JA. Endothelium-dependent relaxation of coronary arteries by noradrenaline and serotonin. *Nature* 1983;**305**:627–30.

70 Berkenboom G, Unger P, Fang ZY, Fontaine J. Endothelium-derived relaxing factor and protection against contraction to norepinephrine in isolated canine and human coronary arteries. *J Cardiovasc Pharmacol* 1991;**17**(suppl 3):S127–32.

71 Baumgart D, Ehring T, Kowallik P, Guth BD, Krajcar M, Heusch G. Impact of α-adrenergic coronary vasoconstriction on the transmural myocardial blood flow distribution during humoral and neuronal adrenergic activation. *Circ Res* 1993;**73**:869–86.

72 Nathan HJ, Feigl EO. Adrenergic coronary vasoconstriction lessens transmural steal during coronary hypoperfusion. *Am J Physiol* 1986;**250**:H645– 53.

73 Morita K, Mori H, Tsujioka K, et al. α-Adrenergic vasoconstriction reduces systolic retrograde coronary blood flow. *Am J Physiol* 1997;**273**:H2746–55.

74 Amenta F, Coppola L, Gallo P, et al. Autoradiographic localization of β-adrenergic receptors in human large coronary arteries. *Circ Res* 1991;**68**:1591–9.

75 Trivella MG, Broten TP, Feigl EO. ß-Receptor subtypes in the canine coronary circulation. *Am J Physiol* 1990;**259**:H1575–85.

76 Miyashiro JK, Feigl EO. Feedforward control of coronary blood flow via coronary ß-receptor stimulation. *Circ Res* 1993;**73**:252–63.

77 Feldman RD, Christy JP, Paul ST, Harrison DG. β-Adrenergic receptors on canine coronary collateral vessels: Characterization and function. *Am J Physiol* 1989;**257**: H1634–9.

78 Flynn AE, Coggins DL, Goto M, Aldea GS, Austin RE, Doucette JW, et al. Does systolic subepicardial perfusion come from retrograde subendocardial flow? *Am J Physiol* 1992;**262**:H1759–69.

79 Parent R, Al-Obaidi M, Lavallée M. Nitric oxide formation contributes to ß-adrenergic dilation of resistance coronary vessels in conscious dogs. *Circ Res* 1993;**73**:241–51.

80 Van Winkle DM, Feigl EO. Acetylcholine causes coronary vasodilation in dogs and baboons. *Circ Res* 1989;**65**:1580–93.

81 Hodgson JMB, Marshall JJ. Direct vasoconstriction and endothelium-dependent vasodilation: Mechanisms of acetylcholine effects on coronary flow and arterial diameter in patients with nonstenotic coronary arteries. *Circulation* 1989;**79**:1043–51.

82 Ludmer PL, Selwyn AP, Shook TL, et al. Paradoxical vasoconstriction induced by acetylcholine in atherosclerotic coronary arteries. *N Engl J Med* 1986;**315**:1046–51.

83 Gulbenkian S, Opgaard OS, Ekman R, et al. Peptidergic innervation of human epicardial coronary arteries. *Circ Res* 1993;**73**:579–88.

165

84 Tseng C-J, Robertson D, Light RT, Atkinson JR, Robertson RM. Neuropeptide Y is a vasoconstrictor of human coronary arteries. *Am J Med Sci* 1988;**296**:11–16.

85 Clarke JG, Davies GJ, Kerwin R, et al. Coronary artery infusion of neuropeptide Y in patients with angina pectoris. *Lancet* 1987;**i**:1057–9.

86 Sheikh SP, Håkanson R, Schwartz TW. Y$_1$ and Y$_2$ receptors for neuropeptide Y. *FEBS Lett* 1989;**245**:209–14.

87 Gulbenkian S, Edvinsson L, Opgaard OS, Valença A, Wharton J, Polak JM. Neuropeptide Y modulates the action of vasodilator agents in guinea pig epicardial coronary arteries. *Regul Pept* 1992;**40**:351–62.

88 Franco-Cereceda A. Calcitonin gene-related peptide and human epicardial coronary arteries: presence, release and vasodilator effects. *Br J Pharmacol* 1991;**102**:506–610.

89 Yamamoto H, Yoshimura H, Noma M, Kai H, Kikuchi Y. Preservation of endothelium-dependent vasodilation in the spastic segment of the human epicardial coronary artery by substance P. *Am Heart J* 1992;**123**:298–303.

90 Ludman PF, Maseri A, Clark P, Davies GJ. Effects of calcitonin gene-related peptide on normal and atheromatous vessels and on resistance vessels in the coronary circulation in humans. *Circulation* 1991;**84**:1993–2000.

91 Wharton J, Gulbenkian S. Peptides in the mammalian cardiovascular system. *Experientia* 1989;**56**:292–316.

92 Feliciano L, Henning RJ. Vagal nerve stimulation releases vasoactive intestinal peptide which significantly increases coronary artery blood flow. *Cardiovasc Res* 1998;**40**:45–55.

93 Hill MR, Wallick DW, Mongeon LR, Martin PJ, Levy MN. Vasoactive intestinal polypeptide antagonists attenuate vagally induced tachycardia in the anesthetized dog. *Am J Physiol* 1995;**269**:H1467–72.

94 Lüscher TF, Boulanger CM, Dohi Y, Yang ZH. Endothelium-derived contracting factors. *Hypertension* 1992;**19**:117–30.

95 Johnson PC. Review of previous studies and current theories of autoregulation. *Circ Res* 1964;**15**(suppl 1):2–9.

96 Chilian WM, Layne SM. Coronary microvascular responses to reductions in perfusion pressure: Evidence for persistent arteriolar vasomotor tone during coronary hypoperfusion. *Circ Res* 1990;**66**:1227–38.

97 Rooke GA, Feigl EO. Work as a correlate of canine left ventricular oxygen consumption, and the problem of catecholamine oxygen wasting. *Circ Res* 1982;**50**:273–86.

98 Downey JM. Myocardial contractile force as a function of coronary blood flow. *Am J Physiol* 1976;**230**:1–6.

99 Gregg DE. Effect of coronary perfusion pressure or coronary flow on oxygen usage of the myocardium. *Circ Res* 1963;**13**:497–500.

100 Feigl EO. Coronary autoregulation. *J Hypertens* 1989;**7**(suppl 4):S55–8.

101 Dole WP, Yamada N, Bishop VS, Olsson RA. Role of adenosine in coronary blood flow regulation after reductions in perfusion pressure. *Circ Res* 1985;**56**:517–24.

102 Smith TP Jr, Canty JM Jr. Modulation of coronary autoregulatory responses by nitric oxide. Evidence for flow-dependent resistance adjustments in conscious dogs. *Circulation* 1993;**73**:232–40.

103 Broten TP, Feigl EO. Role of myocardial oxygen and carbon dioxide in coronary autoregulation. *Am J Physiol* 1992;**262**:H1231–7.

104 Dole WP, Nuno DW. Myocardial oxygen tension determines the degree and pressure range of coronary autoregulation. *Circ Res* 1986;**59**:202–15.

105 Baron JF, Vicaut E, Hou X, Duvelleroy M. Independent role of arterial O$_2$ tension in local control of coronary blood flow. *Am J Physiol* 1990;**258**:H1388–94.

106 Narishige T, Egashira K, Akatsuka Y, Katsuda Y, Numaguchi K, Sakata M, Takeshita A. Glibenclamide, a putative ATP-sensitive K$^+$ channel blocker, inhibits coronary autoregulation in anesthetized dogs. *Circ Res* 1993;**73**:771–6.

107 Clapp LH, Gurney AM. ATP-sensitive K$^+$ channels regulate resting potential of pulmonary arterial smooth muscle cells. *Am J Physiol* 1992;**262**:H916–20.

108 Miyoshi Y, Nakaya Y, Wakatsuki T, et al. Endothelin blocks ATP-sensitive K$^+$ channels and depolarizes smooth muscle cells of porcine coronary artery. *Circ Res* 1992;**70**:612–6.

109 Aversano T, Ouyang P, Silverman H. Blockade of ATP-sensitive potassium channel modulates reactive hyperemia in the canine coronary circulation. *Circ Res* 1991;**69**:618–23.

110 Rajagopalan S, Dube S, Canty JM Jr. Regulation of coronary diameter by myogenic mechanisms in arterial microvessels greater than 100 microns in diameter. *Am J Physiol* 1995;**268**:H788–93.

111 Kuo L, Davis MJ, Chilian WM. Endothelium-dependent, flow-induced dilation of isolated coronary arterioles. *Am J Physiol* 1990;**259**:H1063–70.

112 Kuo L, Davis MJ, Chilian WM. Myogenic activity in isolated subepicardial and subendocardial coronary arterioles. *Am J Physiol* 1988;**255**:H1558–62.

113 McHale PA, Dube GP, Greenfield JC Jr. Evidence for myogenic vasomotor activity in the coronary circulation. *Prog Cardiovasc Dis* 1987;**30**:139–46.

114 Canty JM Jr. Coronary pressure-function and steady-state pressure-flow relations during autoregulation in the unanesthetized dog. *Circ Res* 1988;**63**:821–36.

115 Hoffman JIE. Transmural myocardial perfusion. *Prog Cardiovasc Dis* 1987;**29**:429–64.

116 Canty JM Jr, Giglia J, Kandath D. Effect of tachycardia on regional function and transmural myocardial perfusion during graded coronary pressure reduction in conscious dogs. *Circulation* 1990;**82**:1815–25.

117 Bellamy RF. Diastolic coronary artery pressure–flow relations in the dog. *Circ Res* 1978;**43**:92–101.

118 Hoffman JIE. Transmural myocardial perfusion. In: Kajiya F, Klassen GA, Spaan JAE, Hoffman JIE, eds, *Coronary circulation - basic mechanism and clinical relevance.* Tokyo: Springer-Verlag, 1990:141–52.

119 Smolich JJ, Weissberg PL, Broughton A, Korner PI. Comparison of left and right ventricular blood flow responses during arterial pressure reduction in the autonomically blocked dog: evidence for right ventricular autoregulation. *Cardiovasc Res* 1988;**22**:17–24.

120 Bian X, Williams AG Jr, Gwirtz PA, Downey HF. Right coronary autoregulation in conscious, chronically instrumented dogs. *Am J Physiol* 1998;**275**:H169–75.

121 Downey JM, Kirk ES. Inhibition of coronary blood flow by a vascular waterfall mechanism. *Circ Res* 1975;**36**:753–60.

122 Goto M, Tsujioka K, Ogasawara Y, et al. Effect of blood filling in intramyocardial vessels on coronary arterial inflow. *Am J Physiol* 1990;**258**:H1042–8.

123 Austin RE Jr, Aldea GS, Coggins DL, Flynn AE, Hoffman JIE. Profound spatial heterogeneity of coronary reserve. Discordance between patterns of resting and maximal myocardial blood flow. *Circ Res* 1990;**67**:319–31.

124 Loncar R, Flesche CW, Deussen A. Coronary reserve of high- and low-flow regions in the dog heart left ventricle. *Circulation* 1989;**98**:262–70.

125 Downey JM, Kirk ES. Distribution of the coronary blood flow across the canine heart wall during systole. *Circ Res* 1974;**34**:251–7.

126 Westerhof N. Physiological hypotheses - intramyocardial pressure. A new concept, suggestions for measurement. *Basic Res Cardiol* 1990;**85**:105–19.

127 Recchia FA, Senzaki H, Saeki A, Byrne BJ, Kass DA. Pulse pressure-related changes in coronary flow in vivo are modulated by nitric oxide and adenosine. *Circ Res* 1996;**79**:849–56.

128 Doucette JW, Goto M, Flynn AE, Austin RE Jr, Husseini WK, Hoffman JIE. Effects of cardiac contraction and cavity pressure on myocardial blood flow. *Am J Physiol* 1993;**265**:H1342–52.

129 Chilian WM, Marcus ML. Effects of coronary and extravascular pressure on intra-myocardial and epicardial blood velocity. *Am J Physiol* 1985;**248**:H170–8.

130 Goto M, Flynn AE, Doucette JW, et al. Effect of intracoronary nitroglycerin administration on phasic pattern and transmural distribution of flow during coronary artery stenosis. *Circulation* 1992;**85**:2296–304.

131 Canty JF, Klocke F, Mates RE. Pressure and tone dependence of coronary diastolic input impedance and capacitance. *Am J Physiol* 1985;**248**:H700–11.

132 Goto M, Flynn AE, Doucette JW, et al. Cardiac contraction affects deep myocardial vessels predominantly. *Am J Physiol* 1991;**261**:H1417–29.

167

133 Heineman FW, Grayson J. Transmural distribution of intramyocardial pressure measured by micropipette technique. *Am J Physiol* 1985;**249**:H1216–H23.

134 Yada T, Hiramatsu O, Kimura A, et al. In vivo observation of subendocardial microvessels of the beating porcine heart using a needle-probe videomicroscope with a CCD camera. *Circ Res* 1993;**72**:939–46.

135 Hoffman JIE, Spaan JAE. Pressure-flow relations in coronary circulation. *Physiol Rev* 1990;**70**:331–90.

136 Komaru T, Lamping KG, Eastham CL, Dellsperger KC. Role of ATP-sensitive potassium channels in coronary microvascular autoregulatory responses. *Circ Res* 1991;**69**:1146–51.

137 Chilian WM, Eastham CL, Marcus ML. Microvascular distribution of coronary vascular resistance in beating left ventricle. *Am J Physiol* 1986;**251**:H779–88.

138 Jones CJH, Kuo L, Davis MJ, Chilian WM. Regulation of coronary blood flow: coordination of heterogeneous control mechanisms in vascular microdomains. *Cardiovasc Res* 1995;**29**:585–96.

139 Yokoyama I, Ohtake T, Momomura S-I, Nishikawa J, Sasaki Y, Omata M. Reduced coronary flow reserve in hypercholesterolemic patients without overt coronary stenosis. *Circulation* 1996;**94**:3232–8.

140 Maseri A, Crea F, Cianflone D. Myocardial ischemia caused by distal coronary vasoconstriction. *Am J Cardiol* 1992;**70**:1602–5.

141 Marcus ML, Chilian WM, Kanatsuka H, Dellsperger KC, Eastham CL, Lamping KG. Understanding the coronary circulation through studies at the microvascular level. *Circulation* 1990;**82**:1–7.

142 Maseri A. Coronary vasoconstriction: visible and invisible. *N Engl J Med* 1991;**325**:1579–80.

143 Maseri A, Crea F. Segmental control of vascular tone in the coronary circulation and pathophysiology of ischemic heart disease. *J Appl Cardiovasc Biol* 1991;**2**:163–73.

144 Maseri A, Crea F, Kaski JC, Crake T. Mechanisms of angina pectoris in syndrome X. *J Am Coll Cardiol* 1991;**17**:499–506.

145 Chilian WM, Layne SM, Klausner EC, Eastham CL, Marcus ML. Redistribution of coronary microvascular resistance produced by dipyridamole. *Am J Physiol* 1989;**256**:H383–90.

146 Watanabe J, Levine MJ, Bellotto F, Johnson RG, Grossman W. Effects of coronary venous pressure on left ventricular distensibility. *Circ Res* 1990;**67**:923–32.

147 Kuo L, Arko F, Chilian WM, Davis MJ. Coronary venular responses to flow and pressure. *Circ Res* 1993;**72**:607–15.

148 Spaan JAE. Coronary diastolic pressure–flow relation and zero-flow pressure explained on the basis of intramyocardial compliance. *Circ Res* 1985;**56**:293–309.

149 Klocke FJ, Mates RE, Canty JM Jr, Ellis AK. Coronary pressure–flow relationships. Controversial issues and probable implications. *Circ Res* 1985;**56**:310–23.

150 Bellamy RF, Lowensohn HS, Ehrlich W, Baer RW. Effect of coronary sinus occlusion on coronary pressure–flow relations. *Am J Physiol* 1980;**239**:H57–64.

151 Cantin B, Rouleau JR. Myocardial tissue pressure and blood flow during coronary sinus pressure modulation in anesthetized dogs. *J Appl Physiol* 1992;**73**:2184–91.

152 Kanatsuka H, Ashikawa K, Suzuki T, Komaru T, Suzuki T, Takishima T. Diameter change and pressure–red blood cell velocity relations in coronary microvessels during long diastoles in the canine left ventricle. *Circ Res* 1990;**66:**503–10.

153 Messina LM, Hanley FL, Uhlig PN, Baer RW, Grattan MT, Hoffman JIE. Effects of pressure gradients between branches of the left coronary artery on the pressure axis intercept and the shape of steady state circumflex pressure–flow relations in dogs. *Circ Res* 1985;**56**:11–19.

154 Mates RE, Klocke FJ, Canty JM Jr. Coronary capacitance. *Prog Cardiovasc Dis* 1988;**31**:1–15.

155 Fahri ER, Klocke FJ, Mates RE, et al. Tone-dependent waterfall behavior during venous pressure elevation in isolated canine hearts. *Circ Res* 1991;**68**:392–401.

156 Tennant R, Wiggers CJ. The effect of coronary occlusion on myocardial contraction. *Am J Physiol* 1935;**112**:361.

157 Murakami H, Kim S-J, Downey HF. Persistent right coronary flow reserve at low perfusion pressure. *Am J Physiol* 1989;**256**:H1176–84.

158 Iwamoto T, Bai X-J, Downey HF. Coronary perfusion-related changes in myocardial contractile force and systolic ventricular stiffness. *Cardiovasc Res* 1994;**28**:1331–6.

159 Dijkman MA, Heslinga JW, Sipkema P, Westerhof N. Perfusion-induced changes in cardiac O_2 consumption and contractility are based on different mechanisms. *Am J Physiol* 1996;**271**:H984–9.

160 Dijkman MA, Heslinga JW, Sipkema P, Westerhof N. Perfusion-induced changes in cardiac contractility depend on capillary perfusion. *Am J Physiol* 1998;**274**:H405–10.

161 Bai X-J, Iwamoto T, Williams AG Jr, Fan WL, Downey HF. Coronary pressure–flow autoregulation protects myocardium from pressure-induced changes in oxygen consumption. *Am J Physiol* 1994;**266**:H2359–68.

162 Collins P. Coronary flow reserve. *Br Heart J* 1993;**69**:279–81.

163 Baumgart D, Haude M, Liu F, Ge J, George G, Erbel R. Current concepts of coronary flow reserve for clinical decision making during cardiac catheterization. *Am Heart J* 1998;**136**:136–49.

164 Gould KL, Lipscomb K, Hamilton GW. Physiologic basis for assessing critical coronary stenosis. Am J Cardiol 1974;**33**:87–94.

165 Olsson RA, Bugni WJ. Coronary circulation. In: Fozzard HA, Haber E, Jennings RB, Katz AM, Morgan HE, eds *The heart and cardiovascular system*. Scientific Foundations. New York: Raven Press, 1986:987–1037.

166 Canty JM Jr, Klocke FJ. Reduced regional myocardial perfusion in the presence of pharmacological vasodilator reserve. *Circulation* 1985;**71**:370–7.

167 Brown BG, Josephson MA, Peterson RB, et al. Intravenous dipyridamole combined with isometric handgrip for near maximal acute increase in coronary flow in patients with coronary artery disease. *Am J Cardiol* 1981;**48**:1077–85.

168 Ludman PF, Poole-Wilson PA. Myocardial perfusion in humans: What can we measure? *Br Heart J* 1993;**70**:307–14.

169 Domenech RJ, Hoffman JIE, Nobel MIM, Saunders KB, Henson JR, Subijanto S. Total and regional coronary blood flow measured by radioactive microspheres in conscious and anesthetized dogs. *Circ Res* 1969;**25**:581–96.

170 Kety SS, Schmidt CF. The determination of cerebral blood flow in man by the use of nitrous oxide in low concentrations. *Am J Physiol* 1945;**143**:53–66.

171 White CW, Wilson RF, Marcus ML. Methods of measuring myocardial blood flow in humans. *Prog Cardiovasc Dis* 1988;**31**:79–94.

172 Cannon PJ, Dell RB, Dwyer EM Jr. Measurement of regional myocardial perfusion in man with 133 xenon and scintillation camera. *J Clin Invest* 1972;**51**:964–77.

173 Morgan SM, Fisher JD, Horwitz LD. Validation of regional myocardial flow measurements with scintillation camera detection of xenon-133. *Invest Radiol* 1978;**13**:132–7.

174 Yoshikawa J, Akasaka T, Yoshida K, Takagi T. Systolic coronary flow reversal and abnormal diastolic flow patterns in patients with aortic stenosis: assessment with an intracoronary Doppler catheter. *J Am Soc Echocardiogr* 1993;**6**:516–24.

175 Heller LI, Cates C, Popma J, Deckelbaum LI, Joye JD, Dahlberg ST, et al. Intracoronary Doppler assessment of moderate coronary artery disease: comparison with ^{201}Tl imaging and coronary angiography. *Circulation* 1997;**96**:484–90.

176 Hozumi T, Yoshida K, Akasaka T, Asami Y, Ogata Y, Takagi T, et al. Noninvasive assessment of coronary flow velocity and coronary flow velocity reserve in the left descending coronary artery by Doppler echocardiography. Comparison with invasive technique. *J Am Coll Cardiol* 1998;**32**:1251–9.

177 Kenny A, Shapiro LM. Identification of coronary artery stenoses and poststenotic blood flow patterns using a miniature high-frequency epicardial transducer. *Circulation* 1994;**89**:731–9.

178 Stoddard MF, Prince CR, Moriis GT. Coronary flow reserve assessment by dobutamine transesophageal Doppler echocardiography. *J Am Coll Cardiol* 1995;**25**:325–32.

179 Doucette JW, Corl PD, Payne HM, et al. Validation of a Doppler guide wire for intravascular measurement of coronary artery flow velocity. *Circulation* 1992;**85**:1899–911.

180 Ganz W, Tamura K, Marcus HS, Donoso R, Yoshida S, Swan HJ. Measurement of coronary sinus blood flow by continuous thermodilution in man. *Circulation* 1971;**44**:181–95.
181 Hutchins GD, Schwaiger M, Rosenspire KC, Krivokapich J, Schelbert H, Kuhl DE. Noninvasive quantification of regional blood flow in the human heart using N-13 ammonia and dynamic positron emission tomographic imaging. *J Am Coll Cardiol* 1990;**15**:1032–42.
182 De Silva R, Camici PG. Role of positron emission tomography in the investigation of human coronary circulatory function. *Cardiovasc Res* 1994;**28**:1595–612.
183 Uren NG, Melin JA, Bruyne BD, Wijns W, Baudhuin T, Camici PG. Relation between myocardial blood flow and the severity of coronary artery stenosis. *N Engl J Med* 1994;**330**:1782–8.
184 Bol A, Melin JA, Vanoverschelde J, et al. Direct comparison of [^{13}N] ammonia and [^{15}O] water estimates of perfusion with quantification of regional myocardial blood flow by microspheres. *Circulation* 1993;**87**:512–25.
185 Isada L, Marwick TH, MacIntyre WJ. Physiologic evaluation of coronary flow: the role of positron emission tomography. *Cleve Clin J Med* 1993;**60**:19–24.
186 Ito H, Iwakura K. Assessing the relation between coronary reflow and myocardial reflow. *Am J Cardiol* 1998;**81**:8G–12G.
187 Villanueva FS, Glasheen WP, Sklener J, Kaul S. Characterization of spatial patterns of flow within the reperfused myocardium by myocardial contrast echocardiography. Implications in determining extent of myocardial salvage. *Circulation* 1993;**88**: 2569–606.

5: The pulmonary circulation

KEITH SYKES

William Harvey reported the experiments which led him to conclude that blood must flow through the lungs in *De Motu Cordis* in 1628[1] but it was not until 1661 that Malpighi described the microscopic appearance of the pulmonary capillaries which provided the anatomical link between the right and left heart.[2] In 1894 Bradford and Dean[3] reported that the pulmonary artery pressure increased during hypoxia, but it was not until 1946 that von Euler and Liljestrand[4] concluded that this was the result of hypoxic pulmonary vasoconstriction, and suggested that this mechanism might improve the matching of perfusion to ventilation at the alveolar level. Nissel's subsequent demonstration of hypoxic vasoconstriction in the isolated perfused lung confirmed that this was a local response and not mediated by the autonomic system.[5] Meanwhile, the introduction of the cardiac catheter into clinical practice[6] in the 1940s had led to studies of the haemodynamics of the heart and lungs, and to the subsequent development of closed and, later, open heart surgery in the 1950s. The subsequent introduction of radioisotope methods for measuring the distribution of ventilation and blood flow, and the development of practical methods of measuring gas and blood gas tensions, resulted in a vast increase in our understanding of the mechanisms governing gas exchange. Later studies have shown that the pulmonary circulation has three other important roles:

1 It has a regulatory function (for example, as part of the renin–angiotensin system).
2 It takes up or metabolises certain drugs [such as propranolol, lignocaine (lidocaine), and noradrenaline (norepinephrine)].
3 It filters out particulate matter (such as platelet or fat emboli).

The pulmonary circulation is also concerned with the generation of surfactant, which maintains alveolar stability, and with the exchange of water. As anaesthesia, mechanical ventilation, and surgery may produce major changes in the pulmonary circulation, it is important that the anaesthetist should have a clear understanding of the factors that govern the distribution of pulmonary blood flow. Readers interested in the pharmaco-logical aspects of the lung are referred to a review by Bakhle.[7]

The mechanisms affecting the distribution of blood flow in the normal lung will be considered first. This will be followed by a discussion on the effects of posture, haemorrhage, mechanical ventilation, and lung disease. The methods of studying the pulmonary circulation will then be outlined, followed by a brief review of the way in which anaesthetic and related drugs may alter the distribution of blood flow, and so affect the efficiency of gas exchange. Finally, we shall consider the problem of pulmonary hyper-tension, the effects produced by pulmonary vasodilator drugs, and the pathophysiology of pulmonary oedema.

Anatomy and physiology

The pulmonary circulation extends from the right heart outflow to the left atrium. Blood from the right ventricle passes into the thin-walled pulmonary artery which then branches repeatedly in parallel with the bronchi to supply the pulmonary capillary network surrounding the alveoli. The walls of the larger arteries contain more elastic tissue than smooth muscle, but smooth muscle predominates in arteries less than 1 mm in diameter. The pulmonary capillaries are 7–10 μm in diameter and form a dense network around the alveoli. They normally contain about 40% of the pulmonary blood volume, the volume contained in the pulmonary arteries, capillaries, and veins being about 120, 250, and 150 ml respectively, though these values are greatly influenced by the conditions of measure-ment. The blood from the capillaries is collected into the pulmonary veins which run alongside the arteries, bronchi, and lymphatics in the interstitial space, and finally drains into the left atrium. Although there is some autonomic control of the pulmonary circulation, it appears to be relatively unimportant.

There are three requirements for efficient gas exchange:

• the gas exchanging surface between the alveoli and pulmonary capillary blood must have a large area
• the alveolar–capillary membrane must be thin to ensure that there is little hindrance to diffusion
• there must be correct matching of ventilation to perfusion.

To achieve a perfect distribution of blood flow throughout the 30 cm height of the erect adult lung, it would be necessary to have a high pulmonary artery pressure and thick muscular arteries to overcome the effects of gravity. The lung is, however, unique in that it has to receive the whole of the cardiac output, and this may vary from 1–2 l/min in severe shock to 20–25 l/min in exercise. Furthermore, such changes in flow must be accommodated without imposing an undue load on the right heart. These constraints have led to the development of a low pressure, low resistance, pulmonary circulation in which distribution is relatively poorly controlled, but in which increases in flow are accommodated by the recruitment of extra vessels and the distension of vessels that are already open. The increase in flow thus increases the cross sectional area of the vascular bed and so decreases the total pulmonary vascular resistance. So effective is this mechanism that a doubling of flow can be accommodated with a rise of pulmonary artery pressure of only 2–5 mm Hg when the patient is in the erect position.

Gravity and the distribution of pulmonary blood flow

As there is a close anatomical relationship between the pulmonary vasculature and the alveoli, the dimensions of the vessels will be affected by the relationship between the vascular and alveolar pressures, and by changes in lung volume. The effects will depend on the location of the vessels. The large *extrapulmonary vessels* are situated outside the lung and within the mediastinum, and are affected by regional changes in pleural pressure and by local mechanical distortions around the hilum. As these vessels are large, it is unlikely that changes in their geometry will have major effects on flow. The *intrapulmonary vessels* are, however, smaller and their resistance is greatly affected by changes in the surrounding lung. These vessels may be subdivided into three groups according to their anatomical location:

- the alveolar vessels
- the extra-alveolar vessels
- the corner vessels.

The alveolar vessels

The alveolar vessels are the pulmonary capillaries which are compressed when lung volume is increased by an increase in airway pressure. Blood flow through these capillaries depends on the relationship of the alveolar pressure, the pulmonary artery pressure, and the pulmonary venous pressure, and so results in the gravitational distribution of blood flow described by West.[8] In the upright lung (with a height of 30 cm in the adult) three zones may be distinguished.

Zone 1 is the area in the non-dependent part of the lung in which alveolar pressure exceeds pulmonary artery pressure. This results in compression of the capillaries so that there is no blood flow or gas exchange. Continued ventilation of alveoli in this zone contributes to the alveolar dead space. In the supine position, however, the pulmonary artery pressure is usually greater than the vertical distance between the right atrium and the non-dependent part of the lung, so there is usually no zone 1 (Fig. 5.1).

In zone 2 pulmonary artery pressure is greater than alveolar pressure, which is, in turn, greater than pulmonary venous pressure, so capillary blood flow is present and increases linearly down the zone. The cause of the increase in flow is still debated, some workers suggesting that the capillaries behave like a Starling resistor, so that more vessels are recruited in the lower parts of the zone, whereas others claim that the increase in flow down the zone is the result of increased distension of the vessels. It has also been suggested that there are critical opening pressures, as there are in the systemic circulation, and that these must be overcome before blood flow occurs. Others have suggested that there are local control mechanisms which cause different capillary beds to open in sequence.

In zone 3 both pulmonary arterial and venous pressures exceed alveolar pressure. It is believed that all the capillaries are open, and that the small increase in flow down the zone results from further distension. A fourth zone of reduced flow in the most dependent parts of the lung has also been described. The presence of zone 4 was first noted in experimental perfusion preparations and was attributed to the formation of pulmonary oedema; this may well be the explanation for a reduced dependent zone flow in patients with left ventricular failure. Zone 4 has, however, also been demonstrated in normal patients, particularly at low lung volume. The

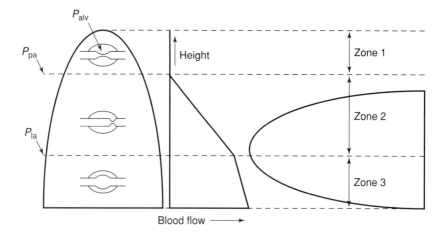

Fig 5.1 The three zone model of the lung. Left: upright lung. Centre: blood flow versus lung height. Right: supine lung. In zone 1 alveolar pressure (P_{alv}) exceeds both pulmonary artery pressure ($P_{\overline{pa}}$) and left atrial pressure (P_{la}) so the capillaries are collapsed and there is no blood flow. In zone 2 pulmonary artery pressure is greater than alveolar pressure, but the alveolar pressure is greater than left atrial pressure, so that the capillaries behave as Starling resistors. In zone 3 both $P_{\overline{pa}}$ and $P_{\overline{la}}$ exceed P_{alv}. All the capillaries are open so that the small increase in flow down the zone is due to further distension. As the height of the supine lung is less than that of the vertical lung, there is usually no zone 1.

reduction in flow could be caused by narrowing of the extra-alveolar vessels resulting from a gravitationally induced decrease in lung volume in dependent zones, or to hypoxic pulmonary vasoconstriction secondary to decreased ventilation caused by airway closure. It could also be caused by the increased vascular resistance resulting from the longer pathway between the hilum and the periphery of the lung.

The extra-alveolar vessels

The extra-alveolar vessels are the arteries and veins that connect the large extrapulmonary vessels to the alveolar-capillary network. They run parallel to the bronchi and are surrounded by an interstitial space which contains fluid, lymphatics, and the fibrous framework of the lung. The transmural pressure, which determines the diameter of these vessels, depends on the intravascular pressure and the interstitial pressure. The pressure in the interstitial space is generated by the elastic recoil of surrounding alveolar units and is believed to approximate to the subatmospheric pleural pressure. In the erect lung at functional residual capacity the pleural pressure is about -1 kPa (-10 cm H_2O) at the apex and -0.25 kPa (-2.5 cm H_2O) at the base, so that the increase in transmural pressure down the lung is less than would have been predicted from the vertical height of the lung (30 cm). When the lung is fully expanded, the extra-alveolar vessels are dilated and so have a minimal effect on the gravitational distribution of blood flow. At residual volume, however, pleural pressure becomes higher than atmospheric at the base of the lung so that vessels in this zone are narrowed. Under these circumstances dependent zone flow may actually equal that in non-dependent zones so the gravitational gradient of flow is abolished.[9]

There may also be regional variations in interstitial pressure caused by differences in regional lung expansion resulting from disease. For example, the reduction in lung volume resulting from an area of atelectasis causes the pleural pressure over that area to be more subatmospheric (that is, to have a lower absolute pressure) than the pressure in the remainder of the pleural space. The resulting increase in transmural pressure may increase the diameter of the extra-alveolar vessels and so decrease the effectiveness of hypoxic vasoconstriction.[10] In general, expansion of the lung will tend to reduce absolute interstitial pressure, so dilating the extra-alveolar vessels, whereas interstitial oedema will tend to increase absolute interstitial pressure and so will narrow them. This may account for the reduced basal blood flow in patients with mitral stenosis.

The corner vessels

The third type of intrapulmonary vessels are the corner vessels. These are small vessels situated at the junction of three alveoli. They are surrounded by an interstitial space, but it is not clear whether this is an extension of the space surrounding the extra-alveolar vessels. The importance of the corner vessels is that they appear to be shielded from the compressive effects of increased alveolar pressure and so permit some flow to occur in zone 1 conditions. It seems probable that this flow only occurs in systole and that it has little effect on gas exchange.

Effects of lung volume on pulmonary vascular resistance

The pulmonary vascular resistance is calculated by dividing the driving pressure (pulmonary artery minus left atrial pressure) by the flow, so it includes the resistance of all the vessels between the right and left heart. The importance of the differentiation between intra- and extra-alveolar vessels is that changes in lung volume exert opposing effects on the two sets of vessels. Expansion of the lung will occur when transpulmonary pressure is increased, whether this is produced by a reduction in absolute pleural pressure or an increase in alveolar pressure, and this will compress the intra-alveolar vessels and so *increase* their resistance to blood flow. These changes will also tend to increase the size of zone 1 and so increase alveolar dead space. On the other hand, expansion of the lung, by whatever means, will increase the diameter of extra-alveolar vessels and so *decrease* their resistance. The diameter of the extrapulmonary vessels will also tend to increase when absolute pleural pressure is decreased, but as these vessels are large the effects on resistance will be relatively small, and these effects may be offset by local distortions of the hilum associated with the expansion of the lung.

As the extra-alveolar vessels are narrow at low lung volumes but expanded at high lung volumes, whereas the pulmonary capillaries are compressed at high lung volumes and open at low lung volumes, the pressure–volume curve for the whole lung is U shaped, the resistance being minimal at the normal end expiratory position or functional residual capacity (Fig. 5.2).

Regional inhomogeneity of blood flow

The gravitational model of the distribution of pulmonary blood flow was derived from radioisotope studies, which measured distribution in relatively large areas of lung. In recent years, methods yielding much higher resolution of the spatial distribution of blood flow have shown that, in humans, there is marked heterogeneity of distribution within an isogravitational plane, and that there is a radial distribution of flow with the greatest flow in the centre of lung lobes.[11][12] There have also been a large number of studies in quadripeds which show: that there is a marked heterogeneity of flow between 1 and 2 cm^2 samples of lung taken from isogravitational planes;[13] that there is a distribution of flow which favours the dorsal regions of lung regardless of posture;[14][15] and that flow distribution changes little when gravitational forces are increased by a factor of three.[16] These studies

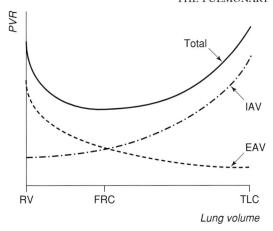

Fig 5.2 The contribution of the resistance of the intra-alveolar (IAV) and extra-alveolar (EAV) vessels to the total pulmonary vascular resistance (PVR) at different lung volumes. Total resistance is minimal at the functional residual capacity (FRC).

suggest that distribution is mainly governed by variations in the resistive properties of the pulmonary vasculature resulting from asymmetrical branching, or other anatomical differences, and that gravity plays a much smaller role than had previously been thought. When considering the animal evidence, it must be remembered that the erect human tends to have a relatively higher lung volume, with distended extra-alveolar vessels, lower smooth muscle tone, and a greater proportion of the serial resistance in the middle (microvascular) segment than the animals studied. Although recent studies have shown that the gravitational gradient of distribution in baboons is decreased when they are held upside down, this finding could be explained by the effects of an alteration in pleural pressure gradient on extra-alveolar vessels. In the absence of firm evidence to the contrary, it seems reasonable to conclude that there is an important gravitational component to distribution in the human, but that there is much more inhomogeneity of distribution than had previously been assumed. How these local variations in pulmonary blood flow can be matched by ventilation distribution to minimise ventilation–perfusion inequalities has yet to be determined.[17] [18]

Clinical implications

Fortunately, the gravitationally induced increase in blood flow down the lung is normally matched by an increase in ventilation. This increase is generated by the interaction between the non-linear pressure–volume curve of the lung and the gravitationally induced gradient of pleural pressure (Fig. 5.3). When the lung is vertical (height 30 cm) the pressure in the pleural space is about -1 kPa (-10 cm H_2O) in the non-dependent areas and about -0.25 kPa (-2.5 cm H_2O) in dependent zones at the normal end expiratory lung volume. The resulting transpulmonary pressure of 1 kPa (10 cm H_2O) at the top of the lung and 0.25 kPa (2.5 cm H_2O) at the base causes the upper alveoli to have a larger resting volume than those at the base. When the transpulmonary pressure is increased by a reduction in absolute pleural pressure during inspiration, however, the lower alveoli will expand more than the upper because they lie on a steeper part of the pressure–volume curve. Thus, under normal conditions, the increase in ventilation down the lung (which is about half that of the increase in blood flow) minimises ventilation–perfusion inequalities (Fig. 5.4). If, however, there is dependent airway closure as a result of a loss of lung elastic recoil or of a reduction in functional residual capacity, there may be no ventilation to dependent zones during the early part of inspiration, so that these zones develop low ventilation–perfusion ratios and arterial P_{O_2} (P_{aO_2}) is reduced.

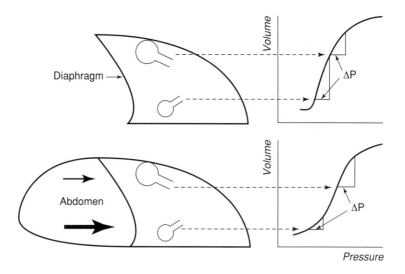

Fig 5.3 Distribution of ventilation. Above: during spontaneous ventilation the gravitationally induced gradient of pleural pressure causes the non-dependent alveoli to lie on the upper, curved part of the lung pressure–volume curve, whereas the dependent alveoli lie on the lower, steep portion. As a result the increase in transpulmonary pressure (ΔP) during inspiration causes more ventilation to enter the dependent zones of the lung. Below: the absence of diaphragmatic activity during controlled ventilation permits the hydrostatic pressure generated by the abdominal contents to influence distribution. The position of the alveoli on the pressure–volume curve of the total respiratory system (that is, lung plus chest wall) now causes ventilation to be preferentially distributed to the non-dependent zones. Note that changes in end expiratory lung volume may modify the distribution by moving the alveoli to different portions of the P/V curves.

During controlled ventilation the distribution of ventilation is determined by the shape of the total respiratory (lung plus chest wall) pressure–volume curve because the inspiratory muscles are no longer active. Furthermore, in the supine position, the hydrostatic pressure produced by the semiliquid abdominal contents exerts an upward pressure on the dependent areas of the diaphragm so that ventilation is preferentially directed into non-dependent zones. As the distribution of blood flow is still gravitationally determined there is gross mismatching of ventilation and perfusion (Figs. 5.3 and 5.4). The situation is exacerbated if there is a decrease in pulmonary artery pressure resulting from a reduction in blood volume, peripheral pooling of blood, or the administration of oxygen or a pulmonary vasodilator drug, because this will result in an increase in zone 1 with a further increase in alveolar dead space. Similar changes may occur if mean alveolar pressure is increased by mechanical ventilation with positive end expiratory pressure (PEEP), or if the emptying of the lung is delayed in patients with increased airway resistance (auto or intrinsic PEEP). When there is an increase in dead space/tidal volume ratio in the spontaneously breathing patient with normal respiratory control mechanisms, minute ventilation will tend to increase to compensate for the increased dead space

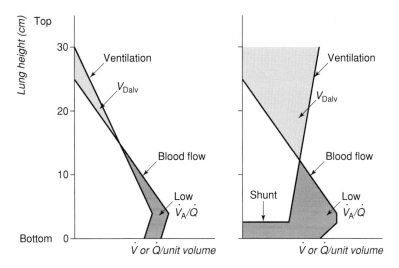

Fig 5.4 Distribution of ventilation ($\dot{V}$) and blood flow ($\dot{Q}$) plotted against lung height during spontaneous respiration (left) and during anaesthesia with controlled ventilation (right). Note that the small alveolar dead space (V_{Dalv}) associated with zone 1 conditions during spontaneous respiration is increased by the greater ventilation to non-dependent zones during controlled ventilation. In elderly people there is often an area with low ventilation–perfusion ($\dot{V}_A/\dot{Q}$) ratios at the base of the lung associated with airway closure. General anaesthesia usually results in the development of a shunt in dependent lung zones as a result of compression collapse.

179

so that P_{CO_2} is maintained at normal levels, but if the minute volume is controlled by a ventilator, P_{CO_2} may increase. If the rest of the lung is normal there will be no effects on Pa_{O_2} other than those arising from any increase in P_{CO_2}.

In most patients undergoing anaesthesia or intensive care there is some alveolar collapse in dependent lung zones and this creates an intrapulmonary right to left shunt.[19] This is usually quantified by expressing the shunt as a percentage of the cardiac output. The Pa_{O_2} resulting from a given shunt depends on the alveolar P_{O_2} (PA_{O_2}) (which in turn depends on the inspired P_{O_2} (PI_{O_2}), the alveolar P_{CO_2} (PA_{CO_2}) and the respiratory exchange ratio) and on the mixed venous P_{O_2} ($P\bar{v}_{O_2}$) (Fig. 5.5). Normally, it is assumed that an increase or decrease in the percentage shunt means that the volume of collapsed lung has increased or decreased. The percentage shunt may, however, change with no alteration of the volume of collapsed lung if the *proportion* of blood flowing through the oxygenated and collapsed zones is changed by an alteration in the pulmonary vascular pressures. For

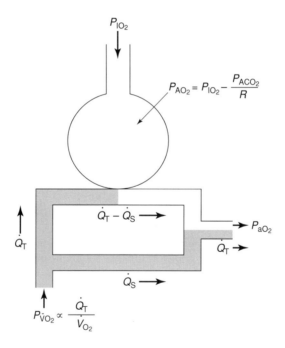

Fig 5.5 Factors governing arterial oxygen tension, PI_{O_2}, PA_{O_2}, PA_{CO_2}, inspired and alveolar gas tensions; R, respiratory exchange ratio (normally 0.8); Pa_{O_2}, $P\bar{v}_{O_2}$, arterial and mixed venous oxygen tensions; $\dot{Q}s$ and $\dot{Q}T$, shunt flow and cardiac output; $\dot{V}_{O_2}$, oxygen consumption per minute. Note that the Pa_{O_2} depends on both the proportion of blood flowing through the shunt and the $P\bar{v}_{O_2}$. $P\bar{v}_{O_2}$ depends on the relationship between $\dot{Q}T$ and $\dot{V}_{O_2}$.

example, blood flow through a collapsed area of lung is maximal when it is in the dependent position but can be reduced by rotating the patient so that the collapsed area is uppermost, with a resultant decrease in shunt and increase in Pa_{O_2}.[20] (The improvement in oxygenation is not, however, usually sustained because collapse soon develops in the areas of lung now made dependent, whereas the collapse in the non-dependent zones disappears.)

The opposite effect can be seen in patients with dependent zone collapse when pulmonary artery pressure and cardiac output are decreased by vasodilator drugs. Under such circumstances the continued flow through the dependent zone with reduced flow to the ventilated area of lung will cause an apparent increase in the *proportion* of shunt, even though the actual flow through the shunt is unchanged (Fig. 5.6). The application of a high peak airway pressure or PEEP will also reduce flow through the ventilated non-dependent zones and so will have a similar effect. Another example is the redistribution of flow which may be seen during anaesthesia for thoracic surgery with a double lumen tube. When the upper lung is collapsed the effects of gravity and hypoxic vasoconstriction in the upper lung decrease the upper lung blood flow so that the shunt is only 20–30% instead of the 45–55% predicted from the relative volume of each lung. If the mean airway

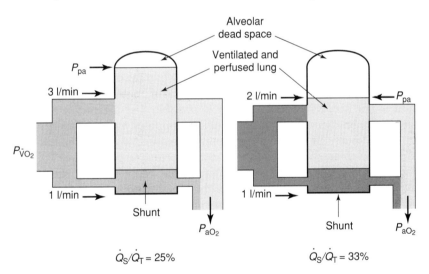

Fig 5.6 The effect of a decrease in pulmonary artery pressure (P_{pa}) resulting from a decrease in cardiac output on percentage shunt in the presence of dependent zone collapse or consolidation. If flow to the ventilated area of lung is decreased from 3 l/min to 2 l/min whilst flow through the shunt remains at 1 l/min the percentage shunt ($\dot{Q}s/\dot{Q}_T$) will increase from 25% to 33%. Note that the resulting fall in arterial Po_2 (Pa_{O_2}) will be accentuated by the decrease in mixed venous Po_2 ($P\bar{v}_{O_2}$) resulting from the decrease in output.

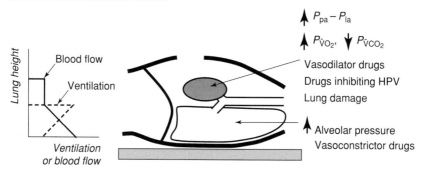

$\uparrow P_{pa} - P_{la}$

$\uparrow P_{\bar{v}O_2}, \quad \downarrow P_{\bar{v}CO_2}$

Vasodilator drugs

Drugs inhibiting HPV

Lung damage

$\uparrow$ Alveolar pressure

Vasoconstrictor drugs

Fig 5.7 Factors that may increase flow through the non-dependent collapsed lung during one lung anaesthesia in the lateral position. The distribution of blood flow and ventilation with lung height is shown on the left of the diagram.

pressure in the dependent lung is increased, however, by the use of high peak or end expiratory pressures, shunt will increase because the compression of capillaries in the dependent lung increases pulmonary artery pressure and so diverts blood flow into the non-dependent collapsed lung (Fig. 5.7). The injection of pulmonary vasoconstrictor drugs will have a similar effect.

Another factor that affects the Pa_{O_2}, even when the areas of shunt are scattered throughout the lung and are not changed by alterations in lung volume, is the direct relationship between shunt and cardiac output. The increase in shunt with cardiac output occurs when the output is changed by altering blood volume or the administration of inotropic drugs but the cause is not properly understood. It is possible that the increase in flow increases pulmonary artery pressure and so opposes hypoxic vasoconstriction. An increase in output will usually increase $P_{\bar{v}O_2}$, and this may also reduce the magnitude of the vasoconstrictor response (see below). Although the increase in $P_{\bar{v}O_2}$ may increase the proportion of shunt it will also increase the oxygen saturation of the blood flowing through the shunt and so tend to offset the effects of the increased percentage shunt on Pa_{O_2}. Obviously, these interactions may lead to very variable effects on Pa_{O_2}.

Factors controlling pulmonary vasomotor tone

As pulmonary vascular tone in the normal human lung is low, vasoconstrictor responses are easily demonstrated, whereas vasodilator responses are small unless the vascular bed has been preconstricted. The major feature that distinguishes the pulmonary circulation from other vascular beds is that it constricts in response to hypoxia. In recent years, it has also become apparent that the endothelium plays a major role in controlling pulmonary vascular tone.

Hypoxic pulmonary vasoconstriction

The response of the pulmonary circulation to hypoxia is characterised by four important features:

- First, the response is present in an isolated perfused lung preparation and in isolated smooth muscle cells from pulmonary arterioles, and so must be controlled by some local mechanism.
- Second, the magnitude of pulmonary vasoconstriction is related to the P_{AO_2}, the response curve of blood flow against P_{AO_2} being sigmoid in shape with the maximum decrease in flow occurring between P_{AO_2} values of 8 and 4 kPa, and a reduction in P_{AO_2} to mixed venous levels resulting in a decrease in flow of about 50%. The apparent anomaly of a reduction in alveolar oxygen tension causing constriction of precapillary vessels (the pulmonary arteries < 300 μm in diameter) has now been explained by the demonstration that these small vessels are completely surrounded by alveoli so that alveolar gases can diffuse directly into the vessel wall.
- Third, the response can also be activated by a reduction in $P_{\bar{v}O_2}$, although a given decrease in $P_{\bar{v}O_2}$ has a smaller effect than a similar decrease in P_{AO_2}. This suggests that the sensor site is situated within the smooth muscle of the arterial wall, but closer to the surrounding alveoli than to the lumen of the vessel.
- The fourth feature that characterises the response is that it occurs rapidly. In humans, blockage of an apical lobe bronchus resulted in an approximately 50% decrease in blood flow within 5 minutes.[21] Recent studies in human volunteers have, however, demonstrated that there is also a slow component to the response; this becomes fully established after two hours of isocapnic hypoxia and persists for at least eight hours.[22]

The exact nature of the constrictor mechanism is still not understood. It is known that hypoxia causes depolarisation of smooth muscle cells from pulmonary arteries, but that it hyperpolarises cells from systemic arteries. Depolarisation results in calcium entry into smooth muscle and vasoconstriction. It appears that depolarisation is caused by closing voltage gated potassium channels in the cell membrane, although it is still not known how the hypoxia is sensed.[23]

Hypoxic vasoconstriction results in a diversion of blood flow away from the hypoxic area of lung, so improving gas exchange.[24] It also produces an increase in pulmonary artery pressure. The magnitude of these effects depends on the volume of lung made hypoxic. If the hypoxic area is large there will be less normal lung to accommodate the diverted flow, so that there will be a greater increase in pressure. As the increase in smooth muscle tone is opposed by the intravascular pressure, there will be less diversion of flow when the rise in pulmonary artery pressure is increased.[25]

183

General factors decreasing hypoxic pulmonary vasoconstriction

Chronic hypoxia
Increased mixed venous P_{O_2} ($P\bar{v}_{O_2}$)
Increased pH
Decreased arterial or mixed venous P_{CO_2} (Pa_{CO_2} or $P\bar{v}_{CO_2}$)
Increased vascular pressures
Increased volume of hypoxic lung
Increased transpulmonary pressures
Hypothermia
Handling or trauma to lung
Endotoxin
Pneumonia
Cirrhosis

Thus hypoxic pulmonary vasoconstriction is least effective when the volume of hypoxic lung is large or when pulmonary vascular pressures are increased by disease, fluid overload, or left heart failure.[26] The magnitude of the response to hypoxia is greatest in the newborn, varies between species and between individuals in any given species, and is reduced by hypothermia, sepsis,[27] trauma to the lung, liver cirrhosis,[28] smoking,[29] and the action of many other drugs. Hypoxia increases the heterogeneity of flow and decreases the central to peripheral gradient of perfusion in lung lobes.[30]

An increase in P_{CO_2} has a more variable effect on pulmonary vascular tone, although it usually augments hypoxic pulmonary vasoconstriction and so increases the response to hypoventilation. A reduction in pH has a similar effect. As collapsed lung equilibrates with mixed venous blood gas tensions, the higher P_{CO_2} augments the diversion of blood flow away from a collapsed area of lung.[31] It now appears that the reduction in blood flow in collapsed lung is almost entirely the result of hypoxic vasoconstriction, and that the mechanical effect produced by narrowing of the extra-alveolar vessels is of only minor importance.

Pa_{CO_2} has a major effect on airway muscle tone, an increase causing bronchodilatation and a decrease bronchoconstriction. Thus alveolar gas concentrations act on both the airways and the pulmonary circulation in a manner that tends to minimise ventilation–perfusion inequalities.

Other factors affecting pulmonary vascular tone

In the early 1970s, it became apparent that the pulmonary endothelium metabolised circulating vasoactive substances. Some, such as bradykinin, were removed, whereas others, such as angiotensin II were produced.

During the next decade it was shown that kinins, peptides, catecholamines, lipoproteins, and many other substances were metabolised in the lung. With the discovery and characterisation of the vasodilator, prostacyclin (PGI_2), and the vasoconstrictor, thromboxane, it became apparent that the endothelium played an important role in controlling the pulmonary circulation itself.[32] In the 1980s it was shown that pulmonary and systemic vessels release a labile endothelium derived relaxing factor (EDRF) which modifies the vasopressor response to various pharmacological agents and to acute hypoxia. It is now clear that EDRF is nitric oxide (NO). The NO is synthesised from L-arginine by nitric oxide synthase. It then diffuses within the cell, or to another cell, where it stimulates soluble guanylyl cyclase or other haem containing proteins. This results in an increase in cyclic guanosine monophosphate (GMP) which produces the physiological effect. For example, in smooth muscle cells cyclic GMP decreases cell calcium which leads to relaxation of the muscle cell and vasodilation. As nitric oxide has a high affinity for haemoglobin with the formation of methaemoglobin, it has a half life measured in seconds. It is also rapidly oxidised to nitrite and nitrate by superoxide radical in the blood vessel wall or by oxygen in free solution.

Vascular tone is controlled by opposing factors which cause constriction or dilatation. Dilatation is induced by acetylcholine, bradykinin, angiotensin converting enzyme inhibitors, and adenine nucleotides, all of which stimulate NO production. It seems likely that pulsatile flow and local shear stress may play an important role in the control of NO release in vivo. There is, however, now evidence that NO may also influence blood pressure by regulating sympathetic nerve activity. Nitric oxide decreases hypoxic vasoconstriction in the lung, and there is evidence that there is either decreased production or increased destruction of NO in systemic and pulmonary hypertension and in ischaemic heart disease. Excessive production of NO may be the cause of the profound vasodilation in septic shock. Nitric oxide also inhibits platelet aggregation. It modulates tubuloglomerular feedback in the kidney, inhibits insulin release, controls the relaxation of sphincters along the gastrointestinal tract, and may also function as a neurotransmitter.[33]

The NO synthase which subserves intercellular communication is Ca^{2+} and cadmodulin dependent, but there is another inducible, Ca^{2+} independent synthase which releases larger quantities of NO over longer periods from activated macrophages, thus causing NO to act as a cytotoxic agent. More recently other NO synthases have been discovered in tissues other than the reticuloendothelial system, so raising the possibility that NO may be implicated in the causation of other types of cell damage.

The rapid inactivation of NO by haemoglobin and the ability to administer the gas by inhalation has enabled NO to be used as a selective pulmonary vasodilator (see page 203).

In 1988 an endothelially derived vasoconstrictor substance termed endothelin was isolated. Subsequently, three peptides have been identified (ET-1, ET-2, and ET-3). These do not appear to be stored in the endothelium but may be released by such diverse factors as shear stress, hypoxia, endotoxin, tumour necrosis factor (TNFα), interferon, adrenaline, angiotensin, thrombin, activated platelets, and some prostanoids. ET-1 is increased in sepsis but it is not yet clear what role these substances play in the mediation of normal vascular tone.

Arachidonic acid metabolites are also released in sepsis. The cyclooxygenase system leads to the formation of prostaglandins, thromboxanes, and PGI_2, whereas the lipo-oxygenase system produces leukotrienes.[32]

Methods of studying the effects of drugs on the pulmonary circulation

Drugs may alter the distribution of pulmonary blood flow by altering the total flow or pulmonary vascular pressures, or by modifying pulmonary vascular tone in the oxygenated or hypoxic areas of lung. Secondary effects may be produced by drugs which affect airway tone and so alter total or regional lung volume.

Most studies of drugs use measurements of pulmonary vascular resistance or changes in the distribution of flow as an index of vascular tone. As a result of the complexity of the pulmonary circulation all the results obtained from these methods must be interpreted with caution. The most commonly used methods are summarised in Table 5.1.

Table 5.1 Control of variables during studies on the pulmonary circulation

Preparation	Variables not controlled	Abnormalities
Isolated perfused lung (constant flow or pressure)	Perfusate P_{O_2}	No neural control or lymph drainage No other organs in circuit
Lobar perfusion (constant flow or pressure)	Left atrial pressure $P\bar{v}_{O_2}$	No neural control or lymph drainage of lobe
Ventilated or collapsed lobe (flowmeters)	Cardiac output, vascular pressures, $P\bar{v}_{O_2}$	No neural control or lymph drainage of lobe
Unilateral hypoxia (radioisotopes, $\dot{V}_{O_2}$, SF_6)	Cardiac output, vascular pressures, $P\bar{v}_{O_2}$	P_{CO_2} decreases with blood flow
Generalised ventilation hypoxia	Cardiac output, vascular pressures, $P\bar{v}_{O_2}$	Arterial hypoxaemia

$P\bar{v}_{O_2}$, mixed venous P_{O_2}; $\dot{V}_{O_2}$, oxygen consumption.

Methods using the concept of pulmonary vascular resistance

Conceptual problems

This measurement is made by dividing the pressure difference across the lung by the flow:

$$\text{PVR} = \frac{P_{\overline{pa}} - P_{\overline{la}}}{\dot{Q}}$$

where PVR is pulmonary vascular resistance, $P_{\overline{pa}}$ and $P_{\overline{la}}$ are mean pulmonary artery and left atrial pressures, and $\dot{Q}$ is the cardiac output. The normal value is approximately 1·5 mm Hg/l per min or 0·1 mm Hg/ml per s. To express the result in CGS units it is necessary to multiply the second figure by 1332, so that the normal value is approximately 100 dyn/s per cm^5. This measurement is useful in that it has conceptual similarities to Poiseuille's law for laminar flow through a parallel sided tube:

$$\text{Resistance} = \frac{\text{Pressure difference}}{\text{Flow}} = \frac{8\eta l}{\pi r^4}$$

This relationship tells us that the resistance increases with increased viscosity (η) of the perfusing fluid, with increasing length (l) of the tube, and is inversely related to the fourth power of the radius (r). Blood is, however, a non-newtonian fluid (with a viscosity that changes with flow), blood flow is pulsatile, and the pulmonary vasculature consists of a branching network of distensible tubes, the cross sectional area of which is augmented by recruitment of extra vessels when flow or pulmonary artery pressure increases. Furthermore, the radius and length of the vessels are affected by changes in transpulmonary pressure and lung volume. It is, therefore, obvious that Poiseuille's equation cannot be applied to the pulmonary circulation and that attempts to do so must frequently yield conflicting results. Nevertheless, the general concept of resistance is of value and the measurement can be used as an index of vascular tone if appropriate precautions are taken to control the variables.

Perfusion preparations

The most reliable measurements are obtained by using one of the various forms of perfused lung preparation in which changes in resistance can be detected by making simultaneous measurements of flow and the pressure difference between pulmonary artery and left atrium. As flow measurement is technically more difficult than pressure measurement, it is usual to measure the changes in pressure across the lung while the lung is perfused at constant flow. With such a preparation, however, changes in intravascular pressure oppose the change in smooth muscle tone, so decreasing the magnitude of the response. Greater sensitivity is obtained

187

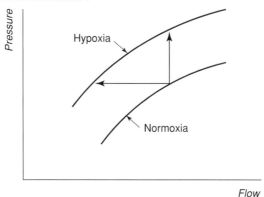

Fig 5.8 Pressure–flow curves obtained when vasomotor tone is normal or increased by hypoxia. The vertical arrow shows the increase in pressure which would be recorded in response to hypoxia during a constant flow perfusion, whereas the horizontal arrow shows the decrease in flow in response to hypoxia with a constant pressure perfusion.

by measuring the changes in flow while the preparation is perfused at constant input and output pressures. Ideally, a number of measurements are made at each stage of the experiment so that pressure–flow curves can be plotted before and after the intervention (Fig. 5.8). A shift of the curve then provides strong evidence of a change in vascular tone provided the other variables have been kept constant. The optimal control of variables is obtained in the isolated perfused lung preparation in which the lungs are either retained in the chest or suspended in a box. The lungs are ventilated at constant tidal volume with 5% carbon dioxide in an oxygen–nitrogen mixture. End expiratory pressure is kept constant and airway pressure is monitored to ensure that there are no changes in lung mechanics. Alveolar hypoxia can then be induced by reducing the inspired oxygen concentration to 3–5%. In the constant flow type of perfusion, blood from a warmed reservoir is pumped by an occlusive pump through a cannula tied into the pulmonary artery. It is then drained through a cannula in the left atrium, which is connected to an overflow system to ensure that left atrial pressure is maintained constant, and both pulmonary artery and left atrial pressures are measured. Flow can be derived from a previous calibration of the pump, or measured by an electromagnetic flowmeter, or by a timed diversion of flow from the atrial cannula into a parallel calibrated reservoir (Fig. 5.9).

In the alternative technique a constant pressure perfusion is effected by pumping the blood up to a reservoir in which the surface is maintained at a constant level by means of an overflow, and flow is again measured by collecting the outflow from the lungs over a measured period, or by using an electromagnetic flowmeter. Both types of preparation are effectively denervated, thus eliminating possible reflex responses, and all the other variables are rigidly controlled. Such preparations are ideally suited to the investigation of agents which are administered by inhalation, or of drugs that are metabolised by the lung. However, there is no bronchial circulation and the normal routes of drug elimination are not included in the circuit. In addition, the ligature round the pulmonary artery occludes the lymphatic drainage so that the preparation tends to become oedematous after several hours of perfusion.

To overcome these problems, many workers use the *in situ* perfused lobe technique. The left lower lobe is usually chosen because it has a long bronchus which can be cannulated easily so that the lobe can be ventilated separately from the rest of the lung. Perfusion of the lobe is achieved by using a constant flow device to pump blood from the right side of the

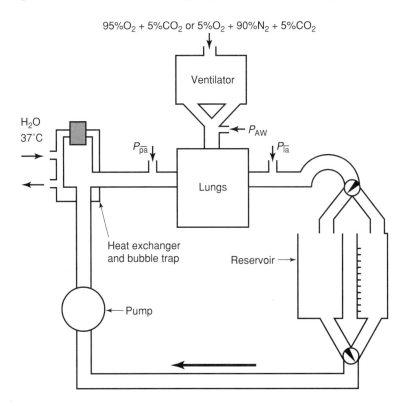

Fig 5.9 Perfusion circuit for isolated perfused lung preparations. The lungs can be ventilated at constant volume with a normoxic or hypoxic gas mixture and the airway (P_{AW}), pulmonary artery ($P_{\overline{pa}}$), and left atrial ($P_{\overline{la}}$) pressures recorded. Blood flow can be measured by diverting the venous outflow into the measuring cylinder for a known time.

heart into a cannula tied into the left lower lobe artery. The blood drains into the left atrium and then circulates normally. The disadvantage of this technique is that left atrial pressure and mixed venous Po_2 cannot be controlled (although they can be monitored). The whole body is, however, perfused normally so that normal detoxification mechanisms are not interfered with. Innervation and lymphatic drainage are destroyed if the cannula is tied in place with a ligature around the pulmonary artery, but these disadvantages can be overcome in larger animals by floating a catheter with a terminal balloon into the appropriate branch of the artery and by ventilating the lobe with a cuffed endobronchial tube.

In vivo studies: errors in the measurement of pulmonary vascular resistance

Most human studies on the effects of drugs have used the concept of pulmonary vascular resistance. As already pointed out there are many disadvantages to this approach. The first is that the measurements are likely to be very inaccurate. It is difficult to measure any vascular pressure with an error less than 1–2 mm Hg and there are many additional sources of error when left atrial pressure is derived from a pulmonary wedge pressure measurement. The accuracy of cardiac output measurement[34] is

Factors affecting measurements of pulmonary vascular resistance (PVR)

"Passive" factors	*Change in PVR*
Pulmonary artery pressure increase	Decrease
Left atrial pressure increase	Decrease
Transpulmonary pressure, increase or decrease from functional residual capacity	Increase
Interstitial pressure increase	Increase
Blood viscosity increase	Increase
"Active" factors	
Blood gases	
Po_2 decrease	Increase
Pco_2 increase	Increase (doubtful in humans)
pH decrease	Increase
Autonomic activity	(Probably negligible in humans)
Endogenous substances	
Catecholamines, angiotensin, histamine	Increase
Acetylcholine, bradykinin, prostacyclin	Decrease

rarely better than $\pm 10\%$ so that the total error in the measurement of resistance may well exceed the change resulting from the experimental intervention. The second disadvantage is that the measured changes may be caused by "passive" or "active" changes in the pulmonary circulation which are not directly related to the action of the drug under test. The major factors that may affect the measurement are shown in the box. From these it may be concluded that a change in pulmonary vascular resistance can only be considered valid if:

1 $(P_{\overline{pa}} - P_{\overline{la}})$ increases or decreases while flow and $P_{\overline{la}}$ are unchanged
2 $(P_{\overline{pa}} - P_{\overline{la}})$ decreases when $P_{\overline{la}}$ decreases or is unchanged and flow decreases or is unchanged
3 $(P_{\overline{pa}} - P_{\overline{la}})$ increases when flow is increased or unchanged and $P_{\overline{la}}$ is increased or unchanged.

One other approach is to construct a pressure–flow curve for each individual by exercising the subject in the supine position (when most of the lung vessels are fully distended). Under these circumstances the curve appears to be linear and so can be defined by two points (Fig. 5.10). If it is assumed that exercise does not in itself alter vasomotor tone, a shift in the curve may be used as an index of vasomotor activity.

It has now been recognised that, although the pressure–flow curves may be reasonably linear in the physiological range of flows, and the extrapolated $(P_{\overline{pa}} - P_{\overline{la}})$/cardiac output plots pass through the origin in

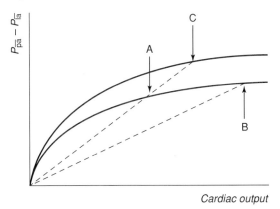

Cardiac output

Fig 5.10 Comparison of single measurements of pulmonary vascular resistance (PVR) made by relating mean pulmonary artery pressure minus mean left atrial pressure $(P_{\overline{pa}} - P_{\overline{la}})$ to cardiac output may be misleading. Thus exercise increases cardiac output from A to B and is associated with a decrease in calculated PVR (slopes of dotted lines from origin to A and B), whereas vasoconstriction (A to C) apparently produces no change in PVR. If, however, the pressure–flow curve (A to B) is defined by exercise, a single measurement (C) may suffice to indicate vasoconstriction.

191

both healthy and diseased lungs under zone 3 conditions, this may not be so when the measurements are made under zone 2 conditions, or when the lung is hypoxic or diseased. Under these circumstances, the convexity towards the pressure axis at low flow rates indicates recruitment of extra vessels as flow is increased, and the intercept of the extrapolated linear portions of the $(P_{\overline{pa}} - P_{\overline{la}})$/cardiac output plots indicates that the effective output pressure from the lung is no longer the left atrial pressure, but results from some external factor narrowing the pulmonary vessels. The critical closing pressure defined by the intercept may be caused by an increase in vasomotor tone, by increased alveolar pressure resulting from high levels of positive and expiratory pressure, by intravascular obstruction, or by an increase in interstitial pressure caused by pulmonary oedema.[35]

Methods using the distribution of flow as an index of pulmonary vascular tone

In human studies it is often possible to reduce the number of variables by studying the regional distribution of blood flow rather than pulmonary vascular resistance. One method of studying the hypoxic response is to measure the redistribution of blood flow in response to unilateral hypoxia induced by the administration of 8–10% oxygen through one limb of a double lumen tube. In the earlier studies the distribution of flow was determined by measuring the oxygen consumption of each lung, because this is directly proportional to blood flow. Attempts were also made to use carbon dioxide output in a similar manner, but this technique proved inaccurate because the carbon dioxide output was also affected by the ventilation to each lung.[36] A much simpler way of measuring the distribution of blood flow is to infuse a solution of a relatively insoluble gas into the pulmonary artery and to measure the concentration evolved into the alveoli on each side. One method is based on the infusion of sulphur hexafluoride and measurement of its concentration in expired gas with infrared analysis.[36] Other methods use a radiolabelled isotope of a relatively insoluble gas such as xenon or krypton.[37] This is dissolved in saline and injected into the right side of the circulation. Most of the radiolabelled isotope is evolved into the alveoli during the first passage of the blood through the lungs so that the count rate is directly related to the blood flow. The radioactivity can either be measured in expired gas or detected by scintillation detectors or a gamma camera placed over the chest. The use of the gamma camera has not only enabled blood flow to be measured in areas of collapsed lung, but has also permitted regional variations in perfusion to be studied. The distribution of flow has also been studied by measuring regional radioactivity after the injection of microspheres or macroaggregates labelled with radioactive isotopes. By using radioisotopes with different energies, up to six sequential injections may be made at different stages of the experiment. As the counting may be delayed for several hours, the method has proved to be of great value when studying the distribution of blood flow in stressful environments such as during zero or exaggerated gravity.

Another method of studying the redistribution of blood flow after the administration of a vasoactive drug is to measure the effects on gas exchange. This can be done by the standard method of calculating percentage shunt and dead space/tidal volume ratio from the oxygen and carbon dioxide tensions in arterial and mixed venous blood, and mixed expired gas. Greater precision is, however, obtained by the Wagner inert gas technique in which a solution of six inert gases of different solubilities is infused into the pulmonary circulation at a constant rate, and the retention/excretion ratios are measured from an arterial and mixed expired gas sample. By using a computer to fit the data to a 50 compartment model of the lung, it is possible to derive values for shunt, dead space, and compartments with intermediate ventilation–perfusion ratios.[38] As with other in vivo measurements it is important to remember that any alterations in the distribution of blood flow which occur may be caused by changes in lung volume or haemodynamics, as well as by changes in vasomotor tone.

It is obvious that the conditions outlined above severely limit the number of useful observations that can be made. Furthermore, as the normal vascular bed has very little tone, the action of pulmonary vasodilator drugs can only be studied after constriction has been induced by some other agent (such as hypoxia). Obviously, vasodilator drugs must also be studied in the patients in whom they are likely to be used, but such studies often produce variable results owing to differences in the aetiology of the pulmonary hypertension in each patient. For these reasons we will first consider the actions of drugs on the normal pulmonary circulation and on hypoxic pulmonary vasoconstriction. In the last section we shall consider the problem of pulmonary hypertension and the effects of vasodilator drugs.

Effect of drugs on the normal pulmonary circulation

It has already been pointed out that the distribution of pulmonary blood flow is primarily controlled by the interrelationship between the pulmonary vascular pressures, the transpulmonary pressure difference, and the effects of gravity, and it has been shown how changes in these variables may affect distribution and gas exchange in the normal and abnormal lung. Many drugs given during anaesthesia have profound haemodynamic effects which will produce major effects on flow distribution. The changes in cardiac output may also affect $P\bar{v}_{O_2}$ which will, in turn, affect the partitioning of blood flow between normoxic and hypoxic areas of lung. A number of these drugs may affect pulmonary vasomotor tone and so further modify the distribution of blood flow. Their effect depends on the pre-existing level of vascular tone. In normoxic areas of lung, pulmonary vascular tone is low so that pulmonary vasodilators have little effect whereas constrictors produce major changes. In areas with hypoxic pulmonary vasoconstriction the reverse is the case. When analysing the effects of drugs on the pulmonary circulation, one must, therefore, consider not only the changes in pulmonary haemodynamics and $P\bar{v}o_2$, but also their effects on vasomotor tone in the normoxic and hypoxic areas of lung (see box).

Anaesthetic drugs

Experimental studies

Although Buckley and colleagues[39] had reported that nitrous oxide increased the pressor response to alveolar hypoxia in dogs, whereas 0·5% halothane decreased it, reversible depression of the hypoxic vasoconstrictor response by inhalational agents such as trichloroethylene, halothane, and ether was not demonstrated in an isolated perfused lung preparation until 1972.[40] Subsequent studies using the isolated perfused lung preparation have demonstrated that halothane decreases vasomotor tone in the normoxic lung and that diethyl ether, halothane, methoxyflurane, enflurane, isoflurane, and sevoflurane produce a dose dependent depression of vasoconstriction in the hypoxic lung. Intravenous anaesthetic agents such as thiopental, pentobarbital, pentazocine, fentanyl, droperidol, ketamine, and diazepam appear to have no effect on hypoxic vasoconstriction.[41–43]

In another series of experiments the left lower lobe was ventilated independently of the rest of the lung and electromagnetic flowmeters used to measure the partition of flow between the lobe and the rest of the lung. Ventilation of the lobe with nitrogen reduced the blood flow by 53% and

---

Drugs affecting hypoxic pulmonary vasoconstriction

Decrease	*Increase*
Inhalational anaesthetic agents	Cyclo-oxygenase inhibitors
β Agonists	Propranolol
Pulmonary vasodilators	Almitrine
α Blockers	Lignocaine (lidocaine)
Sodium nitroprusside	
Nitroglycerine	
Calcium channel blockers	NOS inhibitors
Nitric oxide	

this reduction in flow was approximately halved when isoflurane or fluroxene were added to the nitrogen in a concentration of 2 MAC; 0·3 MAC nitrous oxide produced slight but significant inhibition of the response although halothane and enflurane had little effect (MAC = minimum alveolar concentration). Similar effects were produced when the agent was added to the whole lung while the lobe was hypoxic.[42]

The inhalational agents have also been studied in the intact animal. The hypoxic stimulus was provided by unilateral ventilation hypoxia and the distribution of blood flow between the two lungs measured by radio-isotope methods. In these experiments anaesthetic concentrations of trichloroethylene, ether, and nitrous oxide reduced the magnitude of hypoxic vasoconstriction, whereas 0·5–1·5% halothane had little effect. In intact dogs submitted to whole lung ventilation hypoxia, isoflurane inhibited the pressor response whereas halothane and enflurane had no effect.

The difference in results between the isolated perfused lung experiments and those using in vivo preparations are probably caused by the haemodynamic changes associated with the administration of the anaesthetic agent. Agents such as halothane produce a marked decrease in cardiac output, which may be exaggerated when the animal is made hypoxic. If this causes the intravascular pressure to decrease when vascular tone is decreased by inhibition of hypoxic vasoconstriction, there may be little change in flow through the hypoxic segment. There may also be changes in the hypoxic stimulus as a result of changes in $P\bar{v}o_2$.

Human studies

Studies in the human are subject to many variables and must be interpreted with great caution. The first report of the action of anaesthetic drugs on human pulmonary haemodynamics was published by Johnson in 1951.[44] The first evidence that clinically used concentrations of inhalational anaesthetic agents could inhibit hypoxic vasoconstriction was, however, obtained by Bjertnaes in 1978.[45] He used unilateral hypoxia as the stimulus and administered the agent to the hypoxic lung, the blood flow diversion being measured by the injection of radiolabelled macro-aggregates. Subsequently, Rodgers and Benumof[46] measured Pao_2 before and after the administration of halothane or isoflurane, during one lung anaesthesia that was induced and maintained with either ketamine or methohexital, and concluded that approximately 1 MAC concentrations of halothane or isoflurane do not produce significant depression of hypoxic vasoconstriction in humans. These findings were confirmed by Carlsson and colleagues who measured the diversion of flow in response to unilateral ventilation hypoxia with a continuous infusion of sulphur hexafluoride (a relatively insoluble inert gas). They found that inhaled concentrations of 2% enflurane and 1·0–1·5% isoflurane had no effect on the diversion of flow.[47][48] Subsequent studies[49] suggested that, during a more prolonged period of administration, halothane may indeed cause some depression of hypoxic vasoconstriction. It would seem reasonable to conclude that, although there is a large variation in the effect of inhalational agents on hypoxic vasoconstriction, there is no contra-indication to the use of the inhalational agents in most patients undergoing one lung anaesthesia.

Other drugs

It was Halmagyi and Cotes[50] who first reported the occurrence of arterial hypoxaemia after the administration of bronchodilator drugs such as adrenaline (epinephrine) and aminophylline to patients with asthma. During the next decade similar changes were reported with isoprenaline, salbutamol, and orciprenaline, but it was not clear whether the hypoxaemia resulted from impaired distribution of gas caused by preferential deposition of the aerosol in relatively well ventilated areas of lung, from maldistribution of blood flow secondary to haemodynamic changes, or from impaired hypoxic pulmonary vasoconstriction. Subsequent studies in animals subjected to unilateral ventilation hypoxia showed that bronchodilator drugs such as salbutamol and orciprenaline could inhibit hypoxic vasoconstriction.[51,52] Isoprenaline is known to dilate vessels in both normoxic and hypoxic areas of lung, but the other agents have little effect in normoxia and appear to have a specific action on hypoxic vasoconstriction. These effects have been confirmed by studies using the multiple inert gas elimination method in patients with asthma which have shown that blood flow to low ventilation–perfusion areas was doubled after the administration of nebulised isoprenaline, and that these changes could have accounted for the observed fall in Pao_2.[53]

Two other β agonists, dopamine and dobutamine, are of particular interest because, although both increase blood flow to low ventilation–perfusion areas and decrease Pao_2,[54] they appear to produce their effects by different mechanisms; dobutamine inhibiting the hypoxic vasoconstrictor response, whereas dopamine vasoconstricts the vessels in the oxygenated lung and so decreases the flow diversion from the hypoxic area by increasing the pulmonary artery pressure.[55][56] Protamine also produces pulmonary vasoconstriction and produces hypoxaemia by a similar mechanism.[57]

The vasodilator drugs nitroglycerine (predominantly a venodilator) and sodium nitroprusside (acting mainly on the arterial system) have been shown to produce arterial hypoxaemia in humans, and to depress the diversion of blood flow in response to unilateral hypoxia in the dog.[58] They probably act by releasing nitric oxide. In patients with acute respiratory distress syndrome (ARDS) sodium nitroprusside produced a decrease in pulmonary artery pressure and Pao_2 with an increase in the shunt component measured by the multiple inert gas method.[59] In another study both nitroglycerine and prostaglandin E_1 were found to have similar effects, although PGE_1 administration was accompanied by an increase in cardiac output which increased oxygen delivery.[60] As there was no increase in cardiac output or $P\bar{v}o_2$ with both nitroprusside and nitroglycerine, it seems logical to conclude that the increase in shunt was the result of inhibition of the hypoxic vasoconstrictor mechanism.

The calcium channel blockers also inhibit hypoxic vasoconstriction, although the effects of these drugs in normal humans are somewhat variable.[61] Nifedipine inhibits hypoxic vasoconstriction in experimental preparations[61] and in normal humans.[62] It also reduces pulmonary vascular resistance in patients with primary pulmonary hypertension, or with pulmonary hypertension secondary to chronic obstructive lung disease.[63] Diltiazem has also been shown to decrease Pao$_2$ and to increase shunt in patients with ARDS.

Drugs that augment hypoxic vasoconstriction

It is apparent that many drugs interfere with the hypoxic vasoconstrictor mechanism and so impair gas exchange. This raises the question as to whether any advantage would be gained by the administration of agents which would augment hypoxic vasoconstriction.[64]

The cyclo-oxygenase inhibitors such as aspirin and indometacin have been shown to augment hypoxic vasoconstriction, both in the experimental situation and in patients.[65] Other agents that appear to have similar actions are alcohol, lidocaine, propranolol, and almitrine.[41] Almitrine seems to have a biphasic action, low doses augmenting the response and high doses obtunding it.[66 67] NOS inhibitors have also been shown to increase hypoxic vasoconstriction in sepsis,[68] whereas the combination of the intravenous administration of a NOS inhibitor in the presence of unilateral hypoxia, and NO inhalation to the hyperoxic lung, reduced hypoxic lung blood flow to almost zero.[69] Although augmentation of the response should improve gas exchange, it also increases pulmonary artery pressure, and this may impair right ventricular function and reduce the efficiency of the hypoxic vasoconstrictor mechanism. There appears, therefore, to be little clinical indication for the use of such agents at the present time.

Pulmonary hypertension

Pulmonary hypertension is defined as a chronic increase in pulmonary artery systolic pressure above 30 mm Hg or a mean pressure greater than 20–25 mm Hg. From a consideration of Poiseuille's equation (page 187) it is apparent that pulmonary hypertension may be expected to occur in the following circumstances:

1 When there is a reduction in the number of vessels perfused.

2 When there is a narrowing of the vessels as a result of intimal thickening, muscle hypertrophy, vascular spasm, or a decrease in the transmural pressure holding them open.

3 When there is an increase in the pulmonary venous pressure.

4 When there is an increase in blood viscosity (for example, as a result of polycythaemia).

The clinical conditions that may cause pulmonary hypertension are listed in the box. For convenience these are grouped under five main headings:

• those predominantly associated with a reduction in the size of the vascular bed
• those associated with a narrowing of the vessels
• those associated with an increase in pulmonary venous pressure
• primary or idiopathic (cause unknown)[70]
• diverse aetiology.

It will, however, become apparent that such a categorisation is somewhat artificial for there are often a number of factors contributing to the hypertension in each patient.

Reduction in perfused vascular bed

One obvious cause of a reduction in the pulmonary vascular bed is surgical resection. Even if a pneumonectomy is performed, however, the increase in pulmonary artery pressure is only 5–8 mm Hg provided that the remaining lung is normal. Much greater increases in pressure are seen if the remaining lung is affected by disease. A reduction in the area of perfused vascular bed is also produced by pulmonary embolism. This may result from thromboemboli, amniotic fluid, tumour, fat, or gas bubbles. As the normal pulmonary circulation has a low resistance, thromboembolism leads to little increase in pressure until at least 60% of the pulmonary vessels have been occluded. If, however, pulmonary hypertension is already present (for example, from previous embolisation), right heart failure may be induced by a relatively small embolus. It has been suggested that the release of serotonin (5-hydroxytryptamine) or other endogenous substance may accentuate the hypertension resulting from the obstruction, but there is little evidence that this occurs in humans. Pulmonary embolism results in perfusion defects on the lung scan, and ventilation of these areas of lung increases the alveolar component of dead space. Arterial hypoxaemia is almost invariably present and is caused mainly by an increase in right to left shunt. This could be the result of right to left shunting through a patent foramen ovale, the redistribution of blood flow to collapsed areas of lung, or to the presence of a high pressure pulmonary oedema.

Amniotic fluid embolism typically occurs during or shortly after labour and is commonly fatal. It is believed that the lethal effects of amniotic fluid

---

Clinical causes of pulmonary hypertension

1 Reduction of vascular bed:
  Extensive surgical resection
  Pulmonary embolism
  Emphysema
  Pulmonary fibrosis

2 Narrowing of vessels:
  Chronic increases in blood flow
  Increased vascular tone
    Endogenous vasoconstrictors
    Hypoxia and hypercapnia
  Decreased transmural pressure
    Pulmonary oedema
    Increased alveolar pressure

3 Pulmonary venous hypertension

4 Primary (idiopathic)

5 Other: drugs, toxins, parasites, HIV, portal hypertension

---

emboli result mainly from the thromboses that they induce and from the subsequent development of disseminated intravascular coagulation.

Destruction of the pulmonary vascular bed appears to be the major cause of hypertension in patients with emphysema. There is, however, a poor correlation between the magnitude of the pathological changes and the degree of pulmonary hypertension. It is possible that this is caused by differences in the site of the lesions. For example, right ventricular hypertrophy may occur when as little as 14% of the lung is affected by bronchiolar emphysema, but it rarely develops in patients with panacinar emphysema until 40–70% of the lung is affected.[71]

Large areas of fibrosis occur in the lungs of patients with the pneumoconioses, sarcoidosis, fibrosing alveolitis, and collagen disease such as scleroderma, systemic lupus erythematosus, and rheumatoid arthritis, and these lead to the development of pulmonary hypertension. Pulmonary hypertension has also been reported in patients with advanced tuberculosis and bronchiectasis.

Narrowing of the pulmonary vessels

The presence of pulmonary hypertension in patients with ARDS was first documented in 1977.[72] In the acute phase narrowing of the pulmonary vessels may be caused by endogenous substances, such as thromboxane A_2 or B_2 and prostaglandin E_2, by an increase in interstitial pressure secondary to pulmonary oedema, and by alveolar hypoxia and hypercapnia secondary to respiratory failure. In the later phases of the disease, fibrosis and destruction of the pulmonary vascular bed become important.

Hypoxia and hypercapnia are important causes of pulmonary hypertension in patients with chronic obstructive lung disease and there is now firm evidence that prolonged oxygen therapy has beneficial effects on survival.[73 74] Pulmonary hypertension in patients with chronic bronchitis is increased during acute exacerbations. The administration of oxygen during an acute exacerbation usually results in some reduction in pulmonary artery pressure and an increase in physiological dead space. Although it was originally believed that the increase in Pco_2 associated with the administration of oxygen resulted from a decrease in the hypoxic drive to respiration, it now seems probable that the increase is mainly due to the inability of the patients to increase their minute volume to compensate for the increase in dead space induced by the redistribution of blood flow. Alveolar hypoxia is an important cause of pulmonary hypertension in both the neonatal and adult respiratory distress syndromes and probably accounts for the prevalence of pulmonary hypertension in patients with kyphoscoliosis. Patients with the primary hypoventilation syndrome and those with obstructive sleep apnoea may also develop pulmonary hypertension during sleep. This responds to nocturnal oxygen therapy.

Alveolar hypoxia also appears to be the main cause of pulmonary hypertension in individuals living at high altitude.[75] There is, however, a wide variation in the response between individuals, whether they are normally domiciled at high altitude or are normally domiciled at sea level and then taken to high altitude. In those living constantly at high altitude there is hypertrophy of the media of the muscular pulmonary arteries. When such people are moved to sea level there is an immediate decrease in pulmonary artery pressure, which is probably caused by the release of hypoxic pulmonary vasoconstriction, followed by a more gradual fall, which is probably related to the involution of the muscle fibres.

Sustained high blood flows, such as those resulting from intracardiac shunts, ultimately produce narrowing of the pulmonary vessels and pulmonary hypertension. Initially there is medial hypertrophy in the small pulmonary arterioles, and this is later combined with intimal proliferation, and plexiform and other dilatational lesions. In the more severe cases pulmonary haemosiderosis and fibrinoid necrosis are seen. The hypertension decreases when oxygen is inhaled and the pathological lesions regress if the heart defect is corrected in the earlier stages of the disease, but, if dilatational lesions and plexogenic arteriopathy have developed, the changes are generally irreversible. The time of onset of these changes depends, to a large extent, on the location of the shunt. In patients with pretricuspid shunts (for example, atrial septal defects) the changes tend to develop in young adults or in middle life, whereas patents with posttricuspid shunts (for example, ventricular septal defects) tend to retain the fetal pattern of pulmonary circulation and so have pulmonary hypertension from birth.

Pulmonary blood vessels may also be narrowed by a decrease in transmural pressure caused by a reduction in lung volume or an increase in interstitial pressure resulting from pulmonary oedema. A more common cause of narrowing is an increase in alveolar pressure as a result of an increase in airway resistance. This appears to be an important cause of pulmonary hypertension in patients with asthma and chronic bronchitis.

Pulmonary venous hypertension

Pulmonary venous hypertension may be caused by mediastinal lesions which compress the pulmonary veins, a myxoma or ball-valve thrombus in the left atrium, mitral or aortic valve disease, or left ventricular failure. It may also result from pulmonary veno-occlusive disease.

An acute increase in pressure in the pulmonary venous system results in pulmonary congestion and a corresponding increase in pulmonary artery pressure. If the congestion is severe, pulmonary oedema may result. Chronic increases in venous pressure may lead to pathological changes in the lung but, in contrast to those produced by increases in precapillary pressure, they affect the whole of the pulmonary vasculature. The pulmonary veins and venules show medial hypertrophy, arterialisation, dilatation, and eccentric intimal fibrosis. The microcirculation is characterised by capillary congestion, oedema, dilatation of interstitial and pleural lymphatics, and alveolar haemosiderosis. Pulmonary arterioles are often muscularised and both muscular and elastic arteries may be dilated.[76]

Other causes

There are a number of other clinical conditions in which the cause of the pulmonary hypertension is even more obscure. For example, there was a Swiss epidemic of pulmonary hypertension which appeared to be related to the use of the slimming drug aminorex, and there was another epidemic in Spain associated with the use of contaminated cooking oil. There is an association between portal and pulmonary hypertension, and pulmonary hypertension may occur in patients with schistosomiasis when their ova impact in the lung. Patients with HIV infection may develop pulmonary hypertension, and there is also a condition known as primary or idiopathic pulmonary hypertension in which the aetiology is still far from clear.[70]

Role of pulmonary vasodilators in pulmonary hypertension

The most obvious effect of pulmonary hypertension is that it increases the right ventricular pressure, workload, and oxygen consumption, and so

201

may lead to right ventricular failure. As the blood flow to the right ventricle occurs during both systole and diastole it is important to maintain a high systemic pressure to minimise myocardial ischaemia. A second problem resulting from a high pulmonary artery pressure is that it may cause high pressure pulmonary oedema by increasing the pressure in the precapillary vessels. Pulmonary venous hypertension also causes oedema and in both situations severe arterial hypoxaemia may result. Pulmonary embolism and other conditions causing chronic hypertension may cause a maldistribution of blood flow as a result of changes in arteriolar resistance. Localised reductions in flow result in non-perfused alveoli and an increase in alveolar dead space, but the concomitant increases in pressure may also oppose the effects of hypoxic vasoconstriction, which redistributes flow away from underventilated areas of lung, and so may also increase arterial hypoxaemia.

It will be apparent that there are many causes of pulmonary hypertension, and that a number may be present in any one patient. For example, in chronic obstructive airway disease the hypertension may be caused by alveolar hypoxia and hypercapnia, destruction of the vascular bed, polycythaemia (which increases blood viscosity), gas trapping, and water retention (which increases the static pressure throughout the circulation). Although little can be done to alter the size of the vascular bed, all the other causes are amenable to treatment. The effects of treatment will, however, depend on the magnitude and reversibility of the factors involved in each patient. Similarly in ARDS it seems probable that in the early stages pulmonary hypertension is predominantly caused by vasoconstriction from hypoxia and endogenous mediators, augmented by a reduction in the vascular bed as a result of alveolar collapse, and obstruction of small vessels by leucocytes, although in the later stages medial hypertrophy, thrombosis, and interstitial fibrosis dominate the scene. Again, the relative importance of each factor in the individual patient is difficult to determine. Many of the putative mediators are very short lived and difficult to measure, and there is no good animal model of ARDS. As a number of therapeutic strategies currently employed are designed to reduce pulmonary vasomotor tone, it is necessary to consider some of the implications of this type of therapy.

Pulmonary vasodilator drugs

Conventional vasodilator drugs have three main disadvantages in patients with pulmonary hypertension:

1 Most pulmonary vasodilators also dilate the systemic vascular bed and so decrease aortic pressure. This results in a decrease in coronary perfusion which may lead to myocardial ischaemia when right ventricular stroke work and oxygen consumption are increased by an excessive afterload.

2 The decrease in pulmonary artery pressure may decrease the perfusion of non-dependent zones and so increase alveolar dead space.

3 Inhibition of the hypoxic vasoconstrictor mechanism may increase flow to poorly ventilated areas of lung and so increase arterial hypoxaemia.

These disadvantages, and the failure to document improved survival in adult patients treated with conventional pulmonary vasodilator drugs, suggest that there is little indication for their use in adult practice at the present time. (This is not the case in the neonate where pulmonary vasodilators may play an important role in maintaining pulmonary blood flow in patients with persistent pulmonary hypertension.)

The situation has been radically changed by the recent discovery of the role of nitric oxide as a physiological vasodilator.[77] Nitric oxide is also a bronchodilator.[78] It has now been shown that nitric oxide can vasodilate the pulmonary vascular bed when inhaled in concentrations of 10–80 p.p.m. (parts per million). The advantage of the inhalational route of administration is that the nitric oxide only dilates the pulmonary vessels supplying ventilated alveoli, and does not reach non-ventilated alveoli where vessels are constricted by hypoxia. Furthermore, it has no effect on systemic vessels because it is immediately deactivated by combination with haemoglobin.[79] The inhalation of 18 p.p.m. of nitric oxide decreases pulmonary artery pressure and shunt in patients with ARDS, and the therapy has been continued for many days without apparent toxicity.[80] An even more recent study has demonstrated a significant improvement in oxygenation without any reduction in pulmonary artery pressure when inhaled in concentrations of 60–230 parts per *billion*.[81] Interestingly, this concentration is similar to that produced by endogenous NO production in the nasal mucosa,[82] which is denied the ARDS patient by the use of a tracheal tube! Nitric oxide inhalation has also been used with success in neonates with persistent pulmonary hypertension,[83] but in patients with chronic obstructive lung disease, in which the hypoxaemia is predominantly caused by ventilation–perfusion inequalities, NO may decrease arterial Po_2 because it dilates vessels in areas of lung that had previously been subject to hypoxic pulmonary vasoconstriction.[84] There may also be interactions with anaesthetic agents.[85]

It seems strange that an agent that was once a feared contaminant of nitrous oxide should now be hailed as a therapeutic agent of great promise. However, NO is rapidly oxidised to nitrogen dioxide (NO_2) and requires specially designed apparatus for its administration, together with careful monitoring.[86] As NO is the mediator in so many biological systems, there are many potential side effects of long term administration. This is an exciting new form of treatment which can undoubtedly decrease pulmonary artery pressure and improve arterial oxygenation, but there is no evidence to indicate that it affects mortality from ARDS.

An alternative method of inducing vasodilation in ventilated areas of lung in ARDS is to nebulise prostacyclin.[87-89] Inhaled PGE_1 has, however, been found to be ineffective.[90]

Fluid balance in the lung

No review of the pulmonary circulation would be complete without a brief consideration of its role in the control of water and solute transfer within the lung, and of the mechanisms causing pulmonary oedema.

Electron micrographs show that the basement membranes of the alveolar epithelium and endothelium appear to be fused over the thin portion of the interalveolar septum, where most gas exchange is presumed to take place, but that they are separated in the thick part of the septum by the interstitial space (Fig. 5.11). Although no direct connection between the alveolar interstitial space and the lymphatics surrounding the major conducting airways and blood vessels has been demonstrated, there are lymphatic channels surrounding the small blood vessels and terminal airways which probably drain the alveolar interstitial space into the larger lymphatics. From these, the lymph is pumped into the thoracic duct and so back into the circulation. At the sites where adjacent cells in both the endothelium

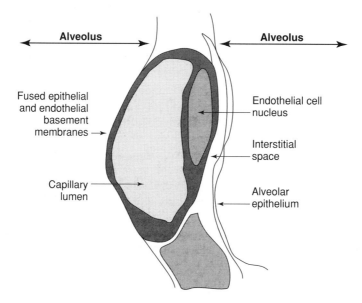

Fig 5.11 Structure of air–blood barrier. The alveolar epithelial and endothelial basement membranes appear to be fused over the thin, gas exchanging, portion of the septum (left), but are separated by the interstitial space in the thick portion of the septum (right).

and alveolar epithelium abut or overlap there are narrow clefts, but, although the clefts between endothelial cells are about 4 nm in diameter, those between alveolar type I and II cells in the epithelium are almost completely fused towards the alveolar spaces. Thus fluids and solutes that move easily between the inside of the capillary and the interstitial space are prevented from passing into the alveolar space. Liquid movements across membranes can occur through cellular junctions or cell membranes, or by endocytosis, and each of these mechanisms can be modelled by "pores" of given dimensions, thus accounting for the differences in permeability of different membranes under different conditions.

The transfer of fluid from the inside of the capillary to the interstitial space ($\dot{Q}$) depends on the balance between the hydrostatic and colloid osmotic pressures. This is traditionally described by the Starling equation:

$$\dot{Q} = K(P_{mv} - P_{pmv}) - \sigma(\pi_{mv} - \pi_{pmv})$$

where K is the capillary filtration coefficient, which describes the permeability characteristics of the endothelial membrane through which exchange occurs, P_{mv} and P_{pmv} are the hydrostatic pressures in the capillary and interstitial space, π_{mv} and π_{pmv} are the colloid osmotic pressures in the microvascular and perimicrovascular compartments, and σ is the reflection coefficient, which is an expression of the permeability of the endothelium to the solute, the most important of which is albumin. A value of unity would indicate that the endothelium was impermeable to albumin, whereas a value of zero would indicate that it was freely permeable. Under the second condition, there would be equal concentrations of solute on both sides of the membrane so there could be no osmotic gradient.

Under normal conditions, pulmonary lymph flow in humans is about 10 ml/h, but it can probably increase tenfold before alveolar flooding occurs. The pulmonary microvascular pressure is between 0 and 20 cm H_2O, depending on the vertical height of the capillary in the lung, and is highest at the proximal end of the capillary. Interstitial pressure around alveolar vessels is difficult to measure but is generally believed to be about 3–5 cm H_2O below atmospheric, whereas interstitial pressure around extra-alveolar vessels is believed to be close to pleural pressure at the same vertical height. The value of σ is about 0·5 and the protein content of lymph is about half that of the plasma, so the colloid osmotic pressure gradient is about $30 - 15 = 15$ cm H_2O. This results in a net pressure gradient favouring filtration, which is greater in dependent zones of the lung, thus accounting for the fact that interstitial oedema usually appears first in dependent zones. The interstitial space can accommodate up to 500 ml of fluid with only a small rise in interstitial pressure, but, when a critical pressure in the interstitial space is exceeded, the fluid may break through the alveolar epithelium, so causing alveolar flooding.[91] This is an all or none phenomenon, so that flooded alveoli may be seen surrounded by apparently normal alveoli.

Causes of pulmonary oedema

There are four major causes of pulmonary oedema: increased hydrostatic pressure, increased capillary permeability, decreased plasma osmotic pressure, and lymphatic obstruction.

Increased capillary hydrostatic pressure may result from overtransfusion, an obstruction to pulmonary venous outflow (for example, caused by left atrial myxoma) or to left heart failure resulting from mitral valve disease or severe dysrhythmias. It may occur when blood flow to a restricted vascular bed is suddenly increased by correction of an anatomical defect (for example, repair of Fallot's tetralogy), and may also be induced by extreme exercise, particularly if the vascular bed is already constricted by hypoxia (as in high altitude pulmonary oedema). High pressure oedema fluid has a low protein content. Extremely high pulmonary capillary pressures (in the region of 30–50 mm Hg) may create what has been termed "stress failure" of the pulmonary vasculature.[92] Discontinuities appear in the bodies of endothelial and type I epithelial cells, whereas the basement membrane often remains intact, and these lesions permit leakage of fluid and protein into the alveoli. Similar abnormalities are believed to occur when the lung is overdistended in mechanically ventilated patients with acute lung injury.[93] Pulmonary oedema has also been described in association with upper airway obstruction, severe laryngospasm, or asthma in children. This is probably caused by large decreases in absolute pleural pressure which increase left ventricular afterload and also increase venous return, so promoting pulmonary congestion and pulmonary oedema.[94]

Increased capillary permeability oedema is seen in situations in which the alveolar capillary membrane is damaged by aspiration of gastric contents, inhalation of toxic agents (smoke, irritant gases), or bacterial or viral agents. It is usually diagnosed when oedema occurs in the face of a pulmonary capillary wedge pressure of less than 18 mm Hg. It is a common complication of generalised sepsis and is the basic feature of lung damage seen in ARDS. The oedema fluid has a protein content that approaches that of plasma and seems to take longer to clear from the lung than high pressure oedema.

Although oedema would be expected to occur frequently in situations where plasma proteins are reduced (for example, in extreme haemodilution), it is not common. This is probably because the decrease in plasma proteins results in an increase in interstitial fluid, which dilutes the protein content of lymph, so restoring the osmotic balance.[95]

Thoracic duct obstruction is a rare cause of decreased lymph drainage. The duct drains into the great veins, however, so that an increase in central venous pressure may increase the likelihood of pulmonary oedema.

Other miscellaneous causes of pulmonary oedema are the neurogenic oedema associated with head injury, the oedema associated with heroin overdose, and that associated with sudden expansion of a collapsed lung.

Measurement of extravascular lung water

The only accurate way of measuring extravascular lung water is by comparing postmortem wet/dry weight ratios after correcting for the residual volume of blood contained in the wet lung. Most of the methods of measuring extravascular lung water that can be used clinically are based on double indicator dilution techniques. Most indicator techniques, however, underestimate lung water because the indicator fails to reach all parts of the lung. Gaseous indicators do not penetrate into collapsed areas of the lung, and intravascular indicators similarly fail to reach non-perfused areas of the lung. Considerable energy has been expended in attempts to improve the double indicator dilution method in which one indicator (usually a dye) is chosen to remain within the circulation, whereas a second indicator (usually "coolth" or tritiated water) diffuses into the extravascular water as well. The extravascular water is then derived from the difference between the two circulation volumes. Compression of extra-alveolar vessels by interstitial oedema, however, inevitably results in localised reductions of pulmonary blood flow, so errors of up to 40% may occur.[96] Thoracic electrical impedance measurements are also subject to large errors. Although measurements using positron emission tomography (PET)[97] and magnetic resonance imaging (MRI)[98] have proved reasonably accurate, the techniques are not suitable for routine use. Computed tomography scans have provided invaluable insights into the pathophysiological changes in ARDS[99] but are not routinely available in the intensive care unit. Most clinicians therefore continue to rely on radiological estimates of the severity of pulmonary oedema, together with measurements of gas exchange, as a guide to therapy.

Conclusions

The low resistance of the pulmonary circulation results in relatively poor control of the distribution of blood flow. Distribution is primarily dependent on the interrelationship of transpulmonary and vascular pressures, but is modified by differences in regional conductance associated with the length of the vascular pathways and the fractal branching pattern of the pulmonary vasculature. Distribution is further modified at alveolar level by the influence of alveolar and mixed venous gas tensions. Pulmonary vascular tone is also influenced by NO and other mediators derived from the endothelium. Drugs may modify the distribution of flow by changing cardiac output and pulmonary vascular pressures, but a number of drugs may alter distribution by altering pulmonary vascular tone in normoxic or hypoxic areas of lung. Drugs that decrease the effectiveness of hypoxic pulmonary vasoconstriction may increase blood flow to underventilated lung regions and so cause arterial hypoxaemia. Selective vasodilation of ventilated lung regions by nitric oxide or PGI_2 may, however, reduce shunt and pulmonary artery pressure. Although the complexity of the system makes it difficult to predict the effects of drugs on gas exchange, a knowledge of the potential mechanisms will enable the clinician to understand many of the phenomena observed in routine clinical practice, and should thus improve the standard of patient care.

1 Harvey W. *An anatomical disssertation concerning the movement of the heart and blood in living creatures.* Translated by G Whitteridge. Oxford: Blackwell Scientific, 1977.
2 Malpighi M. *Duae epistolae de pulmonibus.* Florence, 1661.
3 Bradford JR, Dean HP. The pulmonary circulation. *J Physiol* 1894;16:34–96.
4 Euler US von, Liljestrand G. Observations on the pulmonary arterial blood pressure in the cat. *Acta Physiol Scand* 1946; 12:301–20.
5 Nisell O. Effects of oxygen and carbon dioxide on the circulation of isolated and perfused lungs of the cat. *Acta Physiol Scand* 1948;16:121–7.
6 Cournand A, Ranges HA. Catheterization of right auricle in man. *Proc Soc Exp Biol Med* 1941;46:462–6.
7 Bakhle YS. Pharmacokinetic and metabolic properties of lung. *Br J Anaesth* 1990; 65:79–93.
8 West JB. Blood flow. In: West JB, ed, *Regional differences in the lung.* London: Academic Press, 1977:85–165.
9 Hughes JMB, Glazier JB, Maloney JE, West JB. Effect of lung volume on the distribution of pulmonary blood flow in man. *Respir Physiol* 1968;4:58–72.
10 Chen L, Williams JJ, Alexander CM, Ray RJ, Marshall C, Marshall BE. The effect of pleural pressure on the hypoxic pulmonary vasoconstrictor response in closed chest dogs. *Anesth Analg* 1988; 67:763–9.
11 Amis TC, Jones HA, Hughes JMB. Effect of posture on inter-regional distribution of pulmonary perfusion and VA/Q ratios in man. *Respir Physiol* 1984;56:169–82.
12 Hakim TS, Lisbona R, Dean GW. Gravity-independent inequality in pulmonary blood flow in humans. *J Appl Physiol* 1987;63:1114–21.
13 Glenny RW, Robertson HT. Regional differences in the lung. A changing perspective on blood flow distribution. In: Hlastala MP, Robertson HT, eds. *Complexity in structure and function of the lung.* New York: Marcel Dekker Inc, 1998:461–81.
14 Beck KC, Rehder K. Differences in regional conductances in isolated dog lungs. *J Appl Physiol* 1986;61:530–8.
15 Beck KC, Vettermann J, Rehder K. Gas exchange in dogs in the prone and supine positions. *J Appl Physiol* 1992;72:2292–7.
16 Hlastala MP, Chornuk MA, Self DA, et al. Pulmonary blood flow redistribution by increased gravitational force. *J Appl Physiol* 1998;84:1278–88.
17 Robertson HT. Measurement of regional ventilation by aerosol deposition. In: Hlastala MP, Robertson HT, eds, *Complexity in structure and function of the lung.* New York: Marcel Dekker Inc, 1998:379–99.
18 Swenson ER, Domino KB, Hlastala MP. Physiological effects of oxygen and carbon dioxide on VA/Q heterogeneity. In: Hlastala MP, Robertson HT, eds, *Complexity in structure and function of the lung.* New York: Marcel Dekker Inc, 1998:511–47.
19 Hedenstierna G. Effects of anaesthesia on respiratory function. In: Pearl RG, ed, *The lung in anaesthesia and intensive care. Ballière's Clinical Anaesthesiology* 10.1. London: Ballière Tindall, 1996:1–16.

20 Gattinoni L, Pelosi P, Vitale G, Pesenti A, D'Andrea L, Mascheroni D. Body position changes redistribute lung computed-tomographic density in patients with acute respiratory failure. *Anesthesiology* 1991;**74**:15–23.

21 Morrell NW, Nijran KS, Biggs T, Seed WA. Magnitude and time course of acute hypoxic pulmonary vasoconstriction in man. *Respir Physiol* 1995;**100**:271–81.

22 Dorrington KL, Clar C, Young JD, Jonas M, Tansley JG, Robbins PA. Time course of human pulmonary vascular response to 8 hours of isocapnic hypoxia. *Am J Physiol* 1997;**273**(*Heart Circ Physiol* 42)H1126–34.

23 Barman SA. Potassium channels modulate hypoxic pulmonary vasoconstriction. *Am J Physiol* 1998;**275**:L64–70.

24 Marshall BE, Hanson CW, Frasch F, Marshall C. Role of HPV in pulmonary gas exchange and blood flow distribution. *Intensive Care Med* 1994;**20**:291–7;379–89.

25 Marshall BE, Marshall C, Benumof J, Saidman LJ. Hypoxic pulmonary vasoconstriction in dogs: effects of lung segment size and oxygen tension. *J Appl Physiol* 1981;**51**:1543–51.

26 Benumof JL, Wahrenbrock EA. Blunted hypoxic pulmonary vasoconstriction by increased lung vascular pressures. *J Appl Physiol* 1975;**38**:846–50.

27 Graham LM, Vasil A, Vasil ML, Voelkel NF, Stenmark KR. Decreased pulmonary vasoreactivity in an animal model of chronic *Pseudomonas* pneumonia. *Am Rev Respir Dis* 1990;**142**:221–9.

28 Rodriguez-Roisin R, Roca J, Agusti AG, Mastai R, Wagner PD, Bosch J. Gas exchange and pulmonary vascular reactivity in patients with liver cirrhosis. *Am Rev Respir Dis* 1987;**135**:1085–92.

29 Dupuy PM, Lancon JP, Francoise M, Frostell CG. Inhaled cigarette smoke selectively reverses human hypoxic vasoconstriction. *Intensive Care Med* 1995;**21**:941–4.

30 Mann CM, Domino KB, Walther SM, Glenny RB, Polissar NL, Hlastala MP. Redistribution of pulmonary blood flow during unilateral hypoxia in prone and supine dogs. *J Appl Physiol* 1998;**84**:2010–19.

31 McFarlane PA, Gardaz J-P, Sykes MK. CO_2 and mechanical factors reduce blood flow in a collapsed lung lobe. *J Appl Physiol* 1984;**57**:739–43.

32 Curzen NP, Jourdan KB, Mitchell JA. Endothelial modification of pulmonary vascular tone. *Intensive Care Med* 1996;**22**:596–607.

33 Al-Ali MK, Howarth P. Nitric oxide and the respiratory system in health and disease. *Respir Med* 1998;**92**:710–15.

34 Gómez CMH, Palazzo MGA. Pulmonary artery catheterization in anaesthesia and intensive care. *Br J Anaesth* 1998;**81**:945–56.

35 Leeman M. The pulmonary circulation in acute lung injury: a review of some recent advances. *Intensive Care Med* 1991;**17**:254–60.

36 Carlsson AJ, Hedenstierna G, Blomqvist H, Strandberg A. Separate lung blood flow in anesthetized dogs: a comparitive study between electromagnetometry and SF_6 and CO_2 elimination. *Anesthesiology* 1987;**67**:240–6.

37 Sykes MK, Hill AEG, Loh L, Tait AR. Evaluation of a new method for continuous measurement of the distribution of blood flow between the two lungs. *Br J Anaesth* 1977;**49**:285–92.

38 Hedenstierna G. *Respiratory measurement.* London: BMJ Books, 1998:148–61.

39 Buckley MJ, McLauchlin JS, Fort L, Saigusa M, Morrow DH. Effects of anesthetic agents on pulmonary vascular resistance during hypoxia. *Surg Forum* 1964;**15**:183–4.

40 Sykes MK, Loh L, Seed RF, Kafer ER, Chakrabarti MK. The effect of inhalational anaesthetics on hypoxic pulmonary vasoconstriction and pulmonary vascular resistance in the perfused lungs of the dog and the cat. *Br J Anaesth* 1972;**44**:776–87.

41 Sykes MK. Anaesthetics and the pulmonary circulation. In: Altura BM, Halevy S, eds, *Cardiovascular actions of anaesthetics and drugs used during anaesthesia*, Vol 2. Regional blood flow and clinical consderations. Basel: Karger, 1986:92–125.

42 Eisenkraft JB. Effects of anaesthetics on the pulmonary circulation. *Br J Anaesth* 1990;**65**:63–78.

43 Ishibe Y, Gui X, Uno H, Shiokawa Y, Umeda T, Suekane K. Effect of sevoflurane on hypoxic pulmonary vasoconstriction in the perfused rabbit lung. *Anesthesiology* 1993;**79**:1348–53.

209

44 Johnson SR. Effect of some anaesthetic agents on circulation in man-with special reference to the significance of pulmonary blood volume for the circulatory regulation. *Acta Chir Scand* 1951;suppl158:1–143.

45 Bjertnaes LJ. Hypoxia-induced pulmonary vasoconstriction in man: inhibition due to diethyl ether and halothane anesthesia. *Acta Anaesthesiol Scand* 1978;**22**:570–88.

46 Rogers SN, Benumof JL. Halothane and isoflurane do not decrease Pa_{O_2} during one-lung ventilation in intravenously anesthetized patients. *Anesth Analg* 1985;**64**:946–54.

47 Carlsson AJ, Bindslev L, Hedenstierna G. Hypoxia-induced pulmonary vasoconstriction in the human lung; the effect of isoflurane anesthesia. *Anesthesiology* 1987;**66**:312–16.

48 Carlsson AJ, Hedenstierna G, Bindslev L. Hypoxia-induced pulmonary vasoconstriction in human lung exposed to enflurane anaesthesia. *Acta Anaesthesiol Scand* 1987;**31**:57–62.

49 Benumof JL, Augustine SD, Gibbons JA. Halothane and isoflurane only slightly impair oxygenation during one-lung ventilation in patients undergoing thoractomy. *Anesthesiology* 1987;**67**:910–15.

50 Halmagyi DF, Cotes JE. Reduction in systemic blood oxygen as a result of procedures affecting the pulmonary circulation in patients with chronic pulmonary disease. *Clin Sci* 1959;**18**:475–89.

51 Reyes A, Sykes MK, Chakrabarti MK, Tait A, Petrie A. The effect of salbutamol on hypoxic pulmonary vasoconstriction in dogs. *Bull Eur Physiopathol Respir* 1978;**14**:741–53.

52 Reyes A, Sykes MK, Chakrabarti MK, Carruthers B, Petrie A. Effect of orciprenaline on hypoxic pulmonary vasoconstriction in dogs. *Respiration* 1979;**38**:185–93.

53 Wagner PD, Dantzker DR, Iacovoni VE, Tomlin WC, West JB. Ventilation–perfusion inequality in asymptomatic asthma. *Am Rev Respir Dis* 1978;**118**:511–24.

54 Rennotte MT, Reynaert M, Clerbaux Th, et al. Effects of two inotropic drugs, dopamine and dobutamine, on pulmonary gas exchange in artifically ventilated patients. *Intensive Care Med* 1989;**15**:160–5.

55 Gardaz JP, McFarlane PA, Sykes MK. Mechanisms by which dopamine alters blood flow distribution during lobar collapse in dogs. *J Appl Physiol* 1986;**60**:959–64.

56 Nomoto Y, Kawamura M. Pulmonary gas exchange effects by nitroglycerin, dopamine and dobutamine during one lung ventilation in man. *Can J Anaesth* 1989;**36**:273–7.

57 Kim YD, Michalik R, Lees DE, Jones M, Hanowell S, Macnamara TE. Protamine induced arterial hypoxaemia: the relationship to hypoxic pulmonary vasoconstriction. *Can Anaesth Soc J* 1985;**32**:5–11.

58 D'Oliveira M, Sykes MK, Chakrabarti MK, Orchard C, Keslin J. Depression of hypoxic pulmonary vasoconstriction by sodium nitroprusside and nitroglycerine. *Br J Anaesth* 1981;**53**:11–17.

59 Radermacher P, Huet Y, Pluskwa F, et al. Comparison of ketanserin and sodium nitroprusside in patients with severe ARDS. *Anesthesiology* 1988;**68**:152–7.

60 Radermacher P, Santak B, Becker H, Falke KJ. Prostaglandin E_1 and nitroglycerin reduce pulmonary capillary pressure but worsen ventilation–perfusion distributions in patients with adult respiratory distress syndrome. *Anesthesiology* 1989;**70**:601–6.

61 Naeije R, Mélot C, Mols P, Hallemans R. Effect of vasodilators on hypoxic pulmonary vasoconstriction in normal man. *Chest* 1982;**82**:404–10.

62 Kennedy T, Summer W. Inhibition of hypoxic pulmonary vasoconstriction by nifedipine. *Am J Cardiol* 1982;**50**:864–8.

63 Mélot C, Hallemans R, Naeije R, Mols P, Lejeune P. Deleterious effect of nifedipine on pulmonary gas exchange in chronic obstructive pulmonary disease. *Am Rev Respir Dis* 1984;**130**:612–6.

64 Mélot C, Naeije R, Mols P, Hallemans R, Lejeune P, Jaspar N. Pulmonary vascular tone improves pulmonary gas exchange in the adult respiratory distress syndrome. *Am Rev Respir Dis* 1987;**136**:1232–6.

65 Adnot S, Defouilloy C, Brun-Buisson C, Piquet J, de Cremoux H, Lemaire F. Effects of indomethacin on pulmonary hemodynamics and gas exchange in patients with pulmonary artery hypertension, interference with hydralazine. *Am Revs Respir Dis* 1987;**136**:1243–9.

66 Reyes A, Roca J, Rodriguez-Roison R, Torres A, Ussetti P, Wagner PD. Effect of almitrine on ventilation–perfusion distribution in adult respiratory distress syndrome. *Am Rev Respir Dis* 1988;**137**:1062–7.

67 Mélot C, Deschamps P, Hallemans R, Decroly P, Mols P. Enhancement of hypoxic pulmonary vasoconstriction by low dose almitrine bismesylate in normal humans. *Am Rev Respir Dis* 1989;**136**:111–19.

68 Fischer SR, Deyo DJ, Bone HG, McGuire R, Traber LD, Traber DL. Nitric oxide synthase inhibition restores hypoxic pulmonary vasoconstriction in sepsis. *Am J Respir Crit Care Med* 1997;**156**:833–9.

69 Freden F, Wei SZ, Berglund JE, Frostell C, Hedenstierna G. Nitric oxide modulation of pulmonary blood flow distribution in lobar hypoxia. *Anesthesiology* 1995;**82**:1216–25.

70 Rubin LJ. Primary pulmonary hypertension. *N Engl J Med* 1997;**336**:111–17.

71 Harris P, Heath D. *The human pulmonary circulation*, 3rd edn. Edinburgh: Churchill Livingstone, 1986:511.

72 Zapol WM, Snider MT. Pulmonary hypertension in severe acute respiratory failure. *N Engl J Med* 1977;**296**:476–80.

73 Stuart-Harris C, Bishop JM, Clark TJH, et al. Long term domiciliary oxygen therapy in chronic hypoxic cor pulmonale complicating chronic bronchitis and emphysema. *Lancet* 1981;**i**:681–6.

74 Nocturnal oxygen therapy trial group 1980. Continuous or nocturnal oxygen therapy in hypoxic obstructive airways disease. *Ann Intern Med* 1980;**93**:391–8.

75 Naeije R. Pulmonary circulation at high altitude. *Respiration* 1997;**64**:429–34.

76 Edwards WD. Pathology of pulmonary hypertension. *Cardiovasc Clin* 1988;**18**:321–59.

77 Barnes PJ, Belrisi MG. Nitric oxide and lung disease. *Thorax* 1993;**48**:1034–43.

78 Dupuy PM, Shore SA, Drazen JM, Frostell C, Hill WA, Zapol WM. Bronchodilator action of inhaled nitric oxide in guinea pigs. *J Clin Invest* 1992;**90**:421–8.

79 Frostell C, Fratacci M-D, Wain JC, Jones R, Zapol WM. Inhaled nitric oxide. A selective pulmonary vasodilator reversing hypoxic pulmonary vasoconstriction. *Circulation* 1991;**83**:2038–47.

80 Roissant R, Falke KJ, López F, Slama K, Pison U, Zapol WM. Induced nitric oxide for the adult respiratory distress syndrome. *N Engl J Med* 1993;**328**:399–405.

81 Gerlach H, Pappert D, Lewandowski K, Rossaint R, Falke KJ. Long-term inhalation with evaluated low doses of nitric oxide for selective improvement of oxygenation in patients with adult respiratory distress syndrome. *Intensive Care Med* 1993;**19**:443–9.

82 Gerlach H, Rossaint R, Pappert D, Knorr M, Falke KJ. Autoinhalation of nitric oxide after endogenous synthesis in nasopharynx. *Lancet* 1994;**343**:518–19.

83 Adnot S, Raffestin B, Eddahibi S. NO in the lung. *Respir Physiol* 1995;**101**:109–120.

84 Barbera JA, Roger N, Roca J, Rovira I, Higenbottam TW, Rodriguez-Roisin R. Worsening of pulmonary gas exchange with nitric oxide in chronic obstructive pulmonary disease. *Lancet* 1996;**347**:436–40.

85 Nakamura K, Mori K. Nitric oxide and anesthesia. *Anesth Analg* 1993;**77**:877–9.

86 Young JD, Dyer OJ. Delivery and monitoring of inhaled nitric oxide. *Intensive Care Med* 1996;**22**:77–86.

87 Zwissler B, Kemming G, Habler O, et al. Inhaled prostacyclin (PGI_2) versus inhaled nitric oxide in adult respiratory distress syndrome. *Am J Respir Crit Care Med* 1996;**154**:1671–7.

88 Walmroth D, Schneider T, Shermuly R, Olschewski H, Grimminger F, Seeger W. Direct comparison of inhaled nitric oxide and aerosolized prostacyclin in acute respiratory distress syndrome. *Am J Respir Crit Care Med* 1996;**153**:991–6.

89 Olschewski H, Walmroth D, Shermuly R, Ghofrani A, Grimminger F, Seeger W. Aerosolized prostacyclin and iloprost in severe pulmonary hypertension. *Ann Intern Med* 1996;**124**:820–4.

90 Sinclair SE, Albert RK. Altering ventilation–perfusion relationships in ventilated patients with acute lung injury. *Intensive Care Med* 1997;**23**:942–50.

91 Staub NA. Pathophysiology of pulmonary edema. In: Staub NA, Taylor AE, eds, *Edema*. New York: Raven Press, 1984.

92 Wallin CJ, Rundgren M, Hjelmqvist H, Eriksson S, Leksell LG. Effects of rapid colloid expansion on pulmonary microvascular pressure and lung water in the conscious sheep. *Respir Physiol* 1997;**108**:225–31.

93 Dreyfuss D, Saumon G. Ventilator-induced lung injury: lessons from experimental studies (state of the art). *Am J Respir Crit Care Med* 1998;**157**:1–30.

94 Pinsky MR. The hemodynamic consequences of mechanical ventilation: an evolving story. *Intensive Care Med* 1997;**23**:493–503.

95 Sanchez de Léon R, Paterson JL, Sykes MK. Changes in colloid osmotic pressure and plasma albumin concentration associated with extracorporeal circulation. *Br J Anaesth* 1982;**54**:465–73.

96 Wallin CJ, Rosblad PG, Leksell LG. Quantitative estimation of errors in the indicator dilution measurement of extravascular lung water. *Intensive Care Med* 1997;**23**:469–75.

97 Velasquez M, Haller J, Amundsen T, Schuster JP. Regional lung water measurements with PET: accuracy, reproducibility, and linearity. *J Nucl Med* 1991;**32**:719–25.

98 Mayo JR, MacKay AL, Whittall KP, Baile EM, Pare PD. Measurement of lung water content and pleural pressure gradient with magnetic resonance imaging. *J Thorac Imaging* 1995;**10**:73–81.

99 Desai SR, Hansell DM. Lung imaging in the adult respiratory distress syndrome: current practice and new insights. *Intensive Care Med* 1997;**23**:7–15.

6: Regulation of the cardiovascular system

NIRAJ NIJHAWAN, DAVID C WARLTIER

Regulation of the cardiovascular system has two major homoeostatic goals: to maintain arterial pressure relatively constant and to provide sufficient perfusion to tissues to meet regional metabolic demands. When the requirements of an entire organism for blood flow are altered, the compensatory cardiovascular response involves changing the arterial perfusion pressure. On the other hand, when the perfusion to a particular organ system is altered, cardiovascular compensation occurs by adjusting the calibre of specific blood vessels. The most important variable that is controlled in the regulation of the circulation is arterial blood pressure. Arterial pressure has often been related to Ohm's law in physics. This implies that blood pressure (analogous to voltage) is directly proportional to the product of cardiac output (current) and peripheral vascular resistance (resistance). Neural and humoral control of arterial pressure are mediated through alterations of both cardiac output and/or peripheral resistance.

The physical characteristics of the vascular system are dynamic and more complex than previously realised. Age and certain pathophysiological conditions, such as hypertension, diabetes, and atherosclerosis, result in a progressive stiffening of the conduit (large artery) vessels related to intimal and smooth muscle changes. Vascular smooth muscle hypertrophy as a primary or a secondary phenomenon results in a hypersensitivity to control mechanisms. In any discussion pertaining to cardiovascular regulatory mechanisms, pathophysiological changes must be considered. Interestingly, ventricular hypertrophy may proceed with elevated or normal blood pressure. This appears to be related to the very important pulsatile component of ventricular load, which is not necessarily captured by measurements of blood pressure.[1] An understanding of the differential impact of conduit and resistance vessels will expand future investigations into cardiovascular control mechanisms as well as pharmocotherapy.

Acute mechanisms for regulation of arterial pressure are coordinated in the cardiovascular control centres of the brain stem. These centres regulate both cardiac output and peripheral resistance and, therefore, are able to

213

exert powerful control of arterial pressure. The brain stem cardiovascular centres are in turn influenced by impulses from other neural centres, as well as by numerous sensors within and external to the circulation.

Further regulation of the circulation is mediated by endogenous chemical substances, which are released into the circulation and have a direct effect on the heart and/or vasculature in both physiological and pathophysiological states. Many tissues have the ability to regulate blood flow by local mechanisms, preferentially altering regional perfusion without changes in cardiac output and systemic vascular resistance. Finally, the kidneys are the long term regulators of the entire circulation by manipulating the overall fluid status of an organism. This chapter addresses these different mechanisms individually, but ultimately all are closely integrated and function in unison to regulate the circulation.

Neural control of the heart and vasculature

Central nervous system cardiovascular centres

The critical central nervous system (CNS) cardiovascular control centres are located in the medulla oblongata and lower pons.[2] The centres for circulatory control are in close proximity to those regulating respiration, and together both comprise the CNS areas crucial for survival of the organism.

The centres for circulatory control have two major divisions, the vasomotor and the cardiac regions, which supply nervous innervation to the peripheral vasculature and heart, respectively.[3 4] The two divisions are neither anatomically nor functionally distinct, as significant overlap in both of these properties exists. Further subdivisions with more specialised functions have also been demonstrated in animal experiments utilising precise microelectrode stimulation, electrical ablation, and surgical transsection techniques. These subdivisions function in a highly integrated and coordinated manner to control arterial pressure.

The vasomotor centre is located bilaterally in the reticular substance of the medulla and lower third of the pons.[3] Although the exact organisation of the vasomotor centre has not been fully defined, experiments have identified certain areas that have specific functions. The vasoconstrictor area, also termed C-1, is located in the anterolateral portions of the upper medulla and contains a high concentration of neurons that secrete noradrenaline (norepinephrine). The C-1 area has been proposed to be one of the sites of action of α_2-adrenoceptor agonists such as clonidine and dexmedetomidine. C-1 neurons descend in the spinal cord and synapse with cells in the intermediolateral cell column. The neurons of the intermediolateral cell column are preganglionic neurons, which synapse further with adrenergic neurons. Adrenergic neurons send vasoconstrictor fibres to the periphery via the sympathetic nervous system (SNS).

A vasodilator region referred to as area A-1 is positioned bilaterally, but more medially, in the lower half of the medulla.[3] Neurons from this area project rostrally to and inhibit activity of the vasoconstrictor area (C-1), causing vasodilation. Finally, a sensory area, designated A-2, is located bilaterally in the tractus solitarius in the posterolateral portions of the medulla and lower pons. This region receives sensory neural input predominantly from the glossopharyngeal (cranial nerve IX) and vagus (cranial nerve X) nerves. Neurons arising from A-2 project to the vasoconstrictor and vasodilator areas modulating outputs from these regions. Thus, sensory area A-2 integrates reflex control for multiple circulatory functions. The baroreceptor reflex is a typical example.

The cardiac control centre can also be subdivided.[5] The cardioinhibitory area is well characterised and positioned in the nucleus ambiguous and the dorsal nucleus of the vagus nerve. Parasympathetic vagal efferents arising from this area send impulses to decrease heart rate and, to a lesser extent, reduce atrial contractility. Few parasympathetic fibres, however, innervate ventricular myocardium. The precise location of the cardiostimulatory area is less well defined, but appears to be present in the lateral medulla. Stimulation of this more diffuse region increases heart rate and myocardial contractility via activation of the SNS.

Both cardiostimulatory and cardioinhibitory areas, as well as the vasoconstrictor area, are tonically active, and these regions continuously emit low levels of efferent impulses at a rate of 0·5–2 impulses per second.[6] Activity of the vasoconstrictor area is responsible for a state of partial arteriolar contraction referred to as vasomotor tone. As the areas that control vasoconstriction and cardiac stimulation lie together laterally and superiorly in the cardiovascular control centre, these sites constitute the pressor area (Fig. 6.1).[4] Those areas that cause vasodilation and cardiac inhibition lie more medially, and form the depressor area (Fig. 6.1). Microelectrode stimulation of the pressor area increases heart rate, myocardiac contractility, and peripheral vascular resistance in experimental animals. Conversely, stimulation of the depressor area reduces heart rate and arterial pressure.

The cardiovascular control centres receive neural input from other regions within the brain.[7] The reticular substance of the pons, mesencephalon, and diencephalon send both excitatory and inhibitory impulses into the cardiovascular centres. The hypothalamus also has significant excitatory and inhibitory control, especially of the vasoconstrictor region. Finally, numerous areas of the cerebral cortex (for example, motor cortex, anterior temporal lobe, frontal cortex, anterior cingulate gyrus, amygdala, septum, and hippocampus) also project to the cardiovascular centres and elicit cardiovascular alterations associated with emotions.

Recently, imidazoline receptors have been found to have a distinct and important role in regulation of the cardiovascular system.[8] This receptor system, localised centrally, may be more specific for haemodynamic control than closely related α_2-adrenergic receptors. These receptors have traditionally been thought to be the key receptor system for central control of the sympathetic system. Although a specific endogenous imidazoline compound has not been isolated, the importance of the imidazoline receptors has been further highlighted by a correlation between mean arterial pressure and concentrations of "imidazoline like substances".[8] In the late

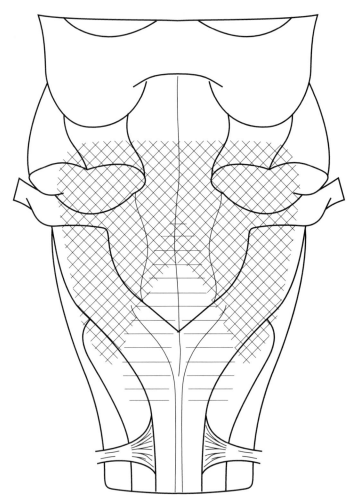

Fig 6.1 Schematic diagram of the brain stem of a cat demonstrating locations of the depressor (horizontal lines) and pressor (cross hatched) areas. (Reprinted with permission from Alexander.[4])

216

1980s, specific imidazoline binding sites, insensitive to catecholamines, were isolated. Imidazoline analogues cause a dose dependent reduction in arterial pressure when injected into the rostral ventrolateral medulla, whereas clonidine (an α_2 agonist known for reduction in centrally driven sympathetic tone) has minimal effect. Furthermore, research into imidazoline receptors has shown that the central sedative properties of α_2 agonists can be separated from their beneficial cardiovascular effects. This is an exciting area of investigation with the potential for revealing mechanisms of essential hypertension, as well as the development of novel specific antihypertensive drugs.

Autonomic nervous system

The cardiovascular control centres of the brain stem ultimately activate/deactivate the autonomic nervous system (ANS) which provides innervation of cardiac and vascular smooth muscle. The ANS represents the efferent or motor component of cardiovascular control and consists of two complementary divisions: the sympathetic and parasympathetic nervous systems (SNS and PNS, respectively). The SNS and PNS are commonly considered physiologically to be antagonistic, producing opposite effects on innervated tissues.

The SNS and PNS are bipolar, each consisting of two interconnected neurons.[9] The first, proximal neuron originates within the CNS, but does not make direct contact with the effector organ. This neuron is referred to as the preganglionic neuron and relays impulses from the CNS to the autonomic ganglion. Autonomic ganglia contain the cell bodies of the second, distal neuron (the postganglionic neuron), which innervates the effector organ. Both sympathetic and parasympathetic divisions have preganglionic neurons that are myelinated, slow conducting type B fibres with diameters of less than 3 μm (Table 6.1). Impulses are conducted in these fibres at 3–15 m/s. Postganglionic neurons of both divisions are unmyelinated type C fibres with diameters of less than 2 μm and conduct impulses at 0.5–2 m/s (Table 6.1).

Sympathetic nervous system

Preganglionic neurons of the SNS arise from the thoracic and first two lumbar (T1–L2) segments of the spinal cord.[10] The cell bodies of the preganglionic neurons are located in the intermediolateral grey column of the 14 spinal cord segments and have fibres that leave the spinal cord in the ventral (anterior) motor nerve roots (Fig. 6.2). These fibres pass via white (myelinated) communicating rami into one of 22 pairs of ganglia which comprise the paravertebral sympathetic chain. Once in the ganglia of the paravertebral sympathetic chain, the preganglionic fibre may follow any one of three courses. First, the fibre may synapse with the cell bodies of the postganglionic neuron in the ganglion at the level of exit. Second, the fibre

Table 6.1 *Nerve fibre classification*

Fibre type	Diameter (μm)	Myelin	Conduction velocity (m/s)
Type A			
α	12–20	+	120
β	5–12	+	120
γ	3–6	+	5–40
δ	2–5	+	5–40
ε	2	+	5
Type B	<3	+	3–15
Type C	0·3–1·2	−	0·5–2

+, myelinated; −, unmyelinated.

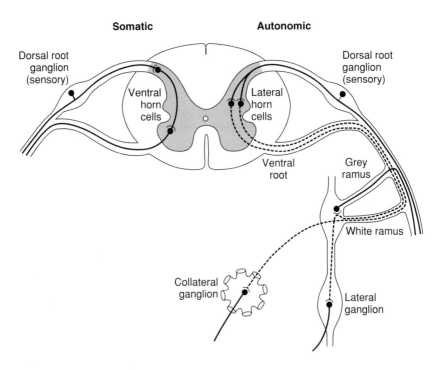

Fig 6.2 Schematic diagram of preganglionic fibres of the sympathetic nervous system. Preganglionic fibres exiting white rami can make synaptic connections in one of three ways: first, synapse can occur in paravertebral ganglia at the level of exit; second, preganglionic fibres can travel up or down the paravertebral sympathetic chain and synapse at other levels; third, fibres can exit the paravertebral chain without synapsing and travel to peripheral collateral ganglia. (Reprinted with permission from Lawson.[10])

may course upwards or downwards in the paravertebral sympathetic chain and synapse with postganglionic neurons at other levels. Finally, preganglionic fibres may travel for variable distances through the paravertebral chain and exit, without synapsing, to more peripheral, unpaired, collateral sympathetic ganglia where they synapse with postganglionic neurons (Fig. 6.2).[10] Thus, the cell bodies of postganglionic neurons are located either in the ganglia of the paired paravertebral sympathetic chains or in the more peripheral unpaired collateral ganglia. In contrast to the PNS, the SNS ganglia are almost always positioned closer to the spinal cord than the effector organs innervated. The coeliac and inferior mesenteric ganglia represent examples of unpaired peripheral collateral ganglia that are formed by the convergence of preganglionic neurons with numerous postganglionic cell bodies. Many fibres from postganglionic neurons pass back into spinal nerves via grey (unmyelinated) communicating rami. These neurons subsequently travel with the spinal nerves to innervate vascular smooth muscle.

The distribution of the SNS neurons to each organ is determined partly by the embryonic position from which the organ originates.[11] This is significant because the first five thoracic preganglionic neurons ascend into the neck to form three unique paired ganglia. These ganglia are the superior cervical, middle cervical, and stellate ganglia. The stellate ganglia are formed by fusion of the inferior cervical and first thoracic SNS ganglia. These three pairs of ganglia provide sympathetic innervation to the head, neck, upper extremities, heart, and lungs.

The distribution of the sympathetic system has considerable importance after intrathecal injection of local anaesthetics. As the level of the block rises above the T6 level, patients will have a greater degree of hypotension corresponding to the T6–9 sympathetic control of the mesenteric vessels. Anaesthetic blocks below T10 are associated with lesser degrees of hypotension, given the smaller number of veins available to sequester intravascular volume. Further cephalad spread of a spinal anaesthetic block reaching levels above T4 causes progressive interference with cardiac sympathetic function, resulting in even greater hypotension with a diminished compensatory reflex tachycardia contributed by T1–T4 fibres.

Parasympathetic nervous system

The cell bodies of the preganglionic neurons of the PNS are located in the brain stem and the sacral segments of the spinal cord. Cranial nerves III (oculomotor), VII (facial), IX (glossopharyngeal), and X (vagus) all contain preganglionic PNS neurons.[10] The preganglionic cell bodies of the second, third, and fourth sacral nerves are located in the intermediolateral grey column of the spinal cord. The paired vagus nerves contain about 75% of all fibres of the PNS, and have the most extensive distribution of any of the parasympathetic nerves, including innervation of the heart.

Preganglionic neurons of the PNS are quite different from the analogous preganglionic nerves in the SNS. PNS preganglionic fibres are longer and pass uninterrupted to ganglia near or in the innervated organ, which are generally not visible. As a consequence, the postganglionic neurons of the PNS are short because of the location of the corresponding ganglion. The proximity of the PNS ganglia to the effector organs limits the distribution of the postganglionic neurons, in contrast to postganglionic SNS fibres which are more widespread.

All preganglionic neurons of either division of the ANS release the neurotransmitter acetylcholine and are classified as cholinergic. The neurotransmitter released from postganglionic neurons in the PNS is acetylcholine. The neurotransmitter between postganglionic adrenergic neurons and effector organs in the SNS is noradrenaline (norepinephrine). Several types of non-adrenergic, non-cholinergic nerves have also been described in the past 20 years, revealing cardiovascular control mechanisms to have substantially greater levels of complexity.[12]

ANS effects on the circulation

The heart and peripheral vasculature are innervated by both the SNS and PNS. Alterations in heart rate (chronotropism), the strength of contraction (inotropism), and coronary blood flow are produced by both divisions of the ANS (Table 6.2). Cardiac vagal fibres are primarily distributed to the sinoatrial and atrioventricular nodes and to the atria, but are only minimally distributed to the ventricular myocardium. PNS stimulation leads to decreases in the rate of sinoatrial node discharge and reduces atrioventricular node excitability, causing slowing of impulse conduction to the ventricles via muscarinic receptors. Strong vagal discharge may cause complete sinoatrial node arrest or interrupt impulse conduction from the

Table 6.2 *Effects of adrenergic and cholinergic stimulation on the cardiovascular system*

	Adrenergic response	Cholinergic response
Heart		
Sinoatrial node	Tachycardia	Bradycardia
Atrioventricular node	Increased conduction	Decreased conduction
His–Purkinje system	Increased automaticity and conduction velocity	Minimal
Myocardium	Increased contractility	Minimal
Vasculature		
Skin and mucosa	Constriction	Dilatation
Skeletal muscle	Constriction (α) > dilatation (β_2)	Dilatation
Coronary	Constriction (α_1) and dilatation (β_2)	Dilatation (EDRF) and constriction
Pulmonary	Constriction	Dilatation (?)

EDRF, endothelium derived relaxing factor (NO).

atria to the ventricles. The PNS has little effect on myocardial contractility because of the lack of vagal efferent distribution to the ventricles. Any decrease in contractile force after PNS stimulation is most probably secondary to declines in heart rate. The human heart is tonically stimulated by both the PNS and SNS but vagal tone predominates. The degree of vagal tone is greatest in young individuals. Total pharmacological blockade of the ANS or cardiac denervation (for example, heart transplantation) results in higher resting heart rates by inhibition of this dominant vagal tone.

The SNS has the same supraventricular distribution as the PNS, but it also provides greater innervation of the ventricular myocardium.[13] Post-ganglionic fibres of the SNS arise in the paired stellate ganglia. The right stellate ganglion sends fibres primarily to the anterior epicardial surface and interventricular septum of the heart. Stimulation of these fibres leads to increases in heart rate via activation of β_1-adrenergic receptors. The left stellate ganglion distributes fibres to the lateral and posterior surfaces of both ventricles. Left stellate ganglion stimulation increases ventricular contractility while causing only minimal increases in heart rate. Experimental investigations have revealed that normal basal sympathetic tone maintains cardiac contractility at approximately 20% greater levels than the denervated heart.

SNS activation causes coronary arteriolar vasodilation indirectly through increases in myocardial oxygen consumption and coupling of myocardial metabolic requirements to blood flow.[14] Simultaneous α-adrenergic activation, however, causes large epicardial coronary artery vasoconstriction, limiting metabolically driven coronary vasodilation by about 30%. Parasympathetic activation causes coronary vasodilation in experimental animal models because of an acetylcholine mediated release of nitric oxide (endothelium derived relaxing factor). The direct stimulation of human coronary vascular smooth muscle by PNS, in the absence of a normally functioning vascular endothelium, may produce constriction leading to coronary spasm.

The peripheral vasculature is innervated by both divisions of the ANS, but the SNS has far greater importance in the regulation of vascular tone.[15] The distribution of parasympathetic nerves is relatively limited and PNS stimulation dilates vessels partially via endothelial mechanisms. The SNS causes vasoconstriction by stimulation of α-adrenergic receptors. The vasculature of the skin, kidneys, spleen, and mesentery has extensive sympathetic innervation. Vascular beds of the brain, heart, and muscle have significantly less innervation.

Vascular tone is the sum of the muscular forces intrinsic to the blood vessel wall, opposing an increase in vessel diameter.[6] The degree of tone is influenced by ANS activity, humoral and local metabolic substances, and autacoids with dilator or constrictor actions. Basal vasomotor tone results partially from low level, continuous impulses (0·5–2 impulses per second) from the lateral portion of the vasomotor centre in the medulla oblongata that pass via the SNS to maintain partial arteriolar and venular constriction. Circulating adrenaline from the adrenal medulla may add to regional constriction dependent on the relative concentration of α-constrictor versus β_2-vasodilator receptors. Increasingly, experimental evidence points to a larger role of chemical mediators in the control of basal vasomotor tone.

Basal vasomotor tone is normally maintained at approximately half-maximal constriction, enabling the arteriole to further constrict or dilate. Without basal vasomotor tone, the arteriole could only constrict during SNS stimulation. Thus, vasodilation can be produced by a reduction in the tonic sympathetic nerve activity without elicitation of "opposing" PNS. Basal vasomotor tone produces little resistance to flow in the venule compared with the arteriole. The importance of the degree of SNS stimulation on the venous circulation is, however, to increase or reduce venous capacitance. A small change in venous capacitance can produce large alterations in venous return and cardiac preload because up to 80% of the total blood volume can be stored in the veins.

Reflex control of the circulation

Intrinsic reflexes

Cardiovascular reflexes represent rapidly acting mechanisms to control the circulation using the central and autonomic nervous systems.[16] Reflex control of the circulation can be initiated either from within the cardiovascular system (intrinsic reflexes) or from other organs or systems (extrinsic reflexes). Intrinsic reflexes are the most important short term regulators of arterial pressure. These reflexes are produced by changes in arterial pressure or special chemical stimuli. Alterations in blood pressure are sensed by stretch receptors, pressoreceptors, baroreceptors, or mechanoreceptors. Chemoreceptors are sensitive to chemical stimuli, regulate respiration, and, secondarily, also influence the circulation.

Arterial baroreceptor reflexes – Arterial baroreceptors are specialised, pressure sensitive, nerve endings in walls of the aortic arch and internal carotid arteries just above the carotid bifurcation (carotid sinus) (Fig. 6.3). Afferent fibres from the baroreceptors travel in the aortic and carotid sinus nerves, which join the vagus and glossopharyngeal nerves, respectively, and connect with the cardiovascular centres in the medulla, commonly in the nucleus tractus solitarius. Cells from the nucleus tractus solitarius project to the C-1 area and inhibit this region by secretion of γ-aminobutyric acid (GABA). There is a small tonic discharge from baroreceptor afferents at a normal arterial pressure. When the baroreceptor endings are stretched, action potentials are generated and propagated at a frequency that is approximately proportional to the pressure change in the artery. Hence, increased arterial pressure sensed by the baroreceptors will increase the frequency of impulses travelling to the CNS. Afferent input produces greater activity in the medullary depressor area and inhibits the pressor and cardiac areas, causing decreases in myocardial contractility and heart rate, and reducing vasoconstrictor tone of both arterioles and veins. Therefore, increased blood pressure leads to reflex activity aimed at reducing the pressure back to a normal set point (the depressor reflex). The opposite effect for declines in blood pressure is also true (the pressor reflex). The arterial baroreceptor reflex provides a negative feedback mechanism for homoeostasis of arterial pressure.[16]

The baroreceptor reflex plays an important role in rapid control of arterial pressure, for example when rising from a recumbent position. The baroreceptor response can be experimentally elicited during sudden decreases or increases in arterial pressure produced by intravenous administration of sodium nitroprusside or phenylephrine, respectively (Smyth's procedure) (Fig. 6.4). The slope of the plot of heart rate (or R–R interval) versus systolic pressure during rapid changes in pressure obtained

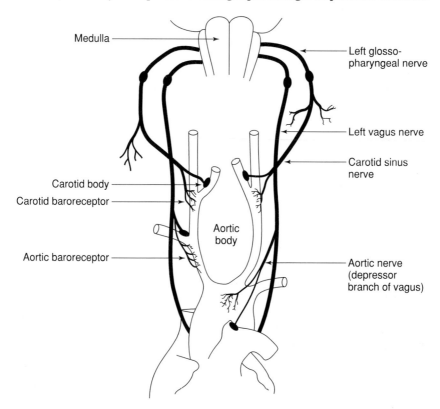

Fig 6.3 Diagram of the central connections of the aortic and carotid sinus baroreceptors. (Reprinted with permission from Smith and Kampine.[7])

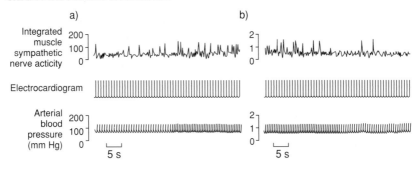

Fig 6.4 Baroreceptor reflex in a human subject: (a) A recording of the baroreceptor response after intravenous infusion of sodium nitroprusside. Note the increase in heart rate and sympathetic nerve activity in response to the decline in blood pressure. (b) The baroreceptor mediated decrease in heart rate and sympathetic nerve activity after an intravenous infusion of phenylephrine. (Reprinted with permission from Ebert.[17])

by this technique is a measure of the "sensitivity" of the baroreflex.[17] It has been proposed that such sensitivity may be reduced in patients prone to sudden death. Clamping of the common carotid artery or damage to the carotid sinus nerve during carotid endarterectomy surgery may elicit dramatic haemodynamic changes through alterations in the arterial baroreflex.

Arterial baroreceptors respond most effectively to the rate of change of arterial pressure. The response is greatest to changes of arterial pressure in the physiological range (80–150 mm Hg). Several subcategories of baro-receptors exist that respond to different pressure ranges. Arterial baro-receptors respond more actively to declines in arterial pressure than increases. Evidence suggests that the carotid baroreceptors are more sensitive to pressure changes than the aortic baroreceptors and operate at lower ranges of arterial pressure. Experimental investigations have deter-mined that arterial baroreceptors primarily influence reflex control of cardiac rate and contractility. Control of systemic vascular resistance is of secondary importance. The vessels most influenced by arterial baro-receptors are splanchnic arterioles and venules, with the venules being important in increasing venous return to the heart during the pressor reflex. Evidence also suggests that the arterial baroreceptors participate in stimulating the renin–angiotensin system via an increase in sympathetic tone.[18] Decreased baroreceptor responsiveness occurs with advancing age, hypertension, and coronary artery disease.

An important property of arterial baroreceptors is the ability to adapt to prolonged changes in arterial pressure. Arterial baroreceptors continue to function in hypertensive individuals or even during acute hypertensive episodes or exercise, but reset at a higher blood pressure range.[19] The higher pressure ultimately forms a new baseline range, but can be reversed if the increase in pressure is relieved. This resetting of the baroreceptor range demonstrates that these reflexes probably have no role in long term blood pressure regulation but, instead, respond only to acute changes in arterial pressure. In fact, resetting can be demonstrated within minutes to hours. The efferent portion of the baroreceptor reflex arc is blocked by many drugs used for the treatment of hypertension. As a result, orthostatic hypotension commonly occurs and, if severe, may lead to syncope. This condition may also be present secondary to pathological processes such as diabetes. Such "autonomic insufficiency" can lead to haemodynamic instability especially during anaesthesia.

Atrial and vena caval low pressure baroreceptors – The right and left atria and inferior and superior vena cava near the junction with the right atrium also contain specialised low pressure mechanoreceptors that respond to increases in central venous pressure.[7] These baroreceptors respond to pressure change but in a much lower range that arterial baroreceptors. The low pressure baroreceptors send impulses via large myelinated fibres in the vagus nerves to the CNS when the atria or vena cava are distended. The efferent portion of the reflex consists of SNS fibres to the sinoatrial node and subsequently causes tachycardia. This increase in heart rate caused by atrial stretch is known as the Bainbridge reflex and is abolished by vagotomy. Although the Bainbridge reflex has been observed in numerous species, the heart rate response to atrial filling in humans is complicated by numerous other factors, including the dominant arterial baroreflex, so this reflex probably plays only a secondary role.

Other baroreceptors have been isolated that are also stimulated by filling and distension of the atria but send impulses via unmyelinated vagal fibres to the CNS.[11] The reflex heart rate response is the opposite of that which occurs in the Bainbridge reflex, and the overall response is analogous to that of the arterial baroreceptors. An increase in venous return increases and positive pressure ventilation reduces discharge from the receptors. Arterial distension results in decreases in SNS activity, causing a decline in vasoconstriction of skeletal muscle, renal, and mesenteric arterioles, an increase in splanchnic venous capacitance, and a reduction in heart rate. The decrease in SNS activity is accompanied by a decline in renin secretion. Reduced circulating angiotension and aldosterone also decrease arteriolar vasoconstriction and lead to a diminution in plasma volume.

As with arterial baroreceptors, atrial baroreceptors adapt to a continuous increase in pressure by resetting.[7] This has been demonstrated in experimental animals where congestive heart failure leads to prolonged atrial distension, increased atrial pressure and attenuation of this reflex. This adaptation is reversed if the heart failure is relieved. It is also important to note that these atrial baroreceptors are stimulated not only by stretch but also by atrial muscle contraction. Hence, it is believed that the diuresis observed in certain clinical and experimental pathological conditions, such as paroxysmal atrial tachycardia and atrial fibrillation, may be the result of the unusual contractile activity in the atrial wall. Atrial natriuretic peptide may also play an important role. The low pressure baroreceptors are significant in the control of extracellular fluid volume. When volume is reduced, these receptors cause a reflex release of vasopressin and enhanced sympathetic tone, which activates the renin–angiotensin–aldosterone axis. In addition, SNS reflex constriction of the afferent arterioles occurs to conserve intravascular volume.[15] These actions increase volume and homoeostasis is maintained.

Ventricular reflexes – The ventricles contain receptors that are also stimulated by stretch or by strong ventricular contraction.[7] These receptors provide afferent input to the medulla via unmyelinated vagal fibres. The medulla responds by decreasing sympathetic tone and causing bradycardia and vasodilation. A very similar reflex response (that is, bradycardia and vasodilation accompanied by apnoea) can be elicited by injecting the drug, veratridine, into the heart or coronary circulation (especially the left circumflex perfusion territory in canine experiments). The unusual coronary chemoreceptor response is referred to as the Bezold–Jarisch reflex. Investigation suggests that this reflex may also be triggered by intracoronary injections of other pharmacological agents, including serotonin, capsaicin, nicotine, bradykinin, histamine and digitalis. A similar reflex has been noted after injection of contrast media during coronary angiography and in certain pathological conditions when specific metabolites accumulate in the coronary circulation, for example, in myocardial necrosis. It has been proposed that the coronary chemoreceptor reflex may be elicited during inferior wall myocardial infarction.

Arterial chemoreceptors – There are also arterial chemoreceptors located in the carotid and aortic bodies, small masses of tissue lying in close proximity to the carotid sinus and the aortic arch receptors (see Fig. 6.3), which have prominent effects on respiration and the circulation. The carotid body is the major chemoreceptor. The special nerve endings respond to decreases in the arterial partial pressure of oxygen (Pao_2), increases in the arterial partial pressure carbon dioxide ($Paco_2$), and increases in arterial hydrogen ion concentration. The afferent pathway is located in the same nerves as the adjacent baroreceptors. Arterial chemoreceptors serve primarily to cause an increase in respiratory minute volume, but secondarily these receptors produce sympathetic vasoconstriction during hypotension. This response is additive to that produced by arterial baroreceptors. The "secondary" circulatory reflex actions improve oxygen delivery to heart and brain through generalised peripheral vasoconstriction and increased arterial pressure. The increased arterial pressure occurs during hypotension secondary to severe depletion of intravascular volume and subsequent reduction in blood flow and ischaemia of the carotid and aortic bodies. The chemoreceptor response also contributes to formation of Mayer waves during recording of arterial pressure. Decreases in perfusion of the chemoreceptors during hypotension causes activation of the reflex and results in increases in arterial pressure. Increases in flow then deactivate the chemoreceptors and declines in arterial pressure occur. The repetitive cyclisation leads to large swings in pressure (Mayer waves) at a frequency of 2–3 cycles/min.

Extrinsic reflexes

Receptors of the afferent limbs of extrinsic reflex arcs are external to the circulatory system. These reflexes are less consistent than intrinsic reflexes and, in normal circumstances, play only a minor role in circulatory control. On the other hand, extrinsic reflexes are important and protective during certain types of environmental stresses and pathophysiological circulatory states. Afferent impulses enter the CNS via somatic nerves but the central processing of these reflexes is still uncertain. Examples of extrinsic reflexes include pain and cold, oculocardiac, CNS ischaemic, and Cushing reflexes.

Pain reflex – Pain, depending on severity, produces variable haemo-dynamic responses. Mild to moderate pain results in tachycardia and increases in arterial pressure mediated by the somatosympathetic reflex. This is a common finding in the postoperative period if analgesia is inadequate. Severe pain, as experienced by deep bone trauma or stretching of abdominal or perineal viscera, may elicit bradycardia, hypotension, and, at times, circulatory collapse and syncope.

Cold reflex – Cutaneous thermosensitive nerve endings respond to cold temperature and send impulses through somatic afferent fibres to the hypothalamus. This results in cutaneous vasoconstriction and piloerection. An example of this reflex is the cold pressor test in which application of intense local cold, such as immersion of a hand in ice water, leads to stimulation of both pain and cold receptors with a subsequent increase in arterial pressure. In certain patients with coronary artery disease, the cold pressor test can produce angina by either reflex coronary vasoconstriction or abruptly increased left ventricular afterload.

Oculocardiac reflex – Receptors stimulated by pressure or stretch in the extraocular muscles, conjunctiva, and globe send impulses through the ophthalmic division of the trigeminal nerve (cranial nerve V) to the CNS.[20] This leads to bradycardia and hypertension and possibly to more severe cardiac arrhythmias including asystole. This reflex does have a tendency to fatigue with repeated stimulation, most probably at the level of the cardioinhibitory centre.

CNS ischaemic reflex – The CNS ischaemic response occurs when severe hypotension (as in circulatory shock) reduces perfusion and causes hypoxia of the medullary vasomotor centre.[21] Chemoreceptors in the vasomotor centre sense local increases in P_{CO_2} and decreases in pH. As a result, there is an intense increase in SNS activity leading to a profound and generalised vasoconstriction. Simultaneously, an increase in PNS activity reduces heart rate. This reflex does not become active until mean arterial pressure decreases below 50 mm Hg (6·7 kPa) and is maximal at mean pressures of 15–20 mm Hg (2·0–2·7 kPa). The CNS ischaemic response does not participate in regulation of normal arterial pressure but is an emergency control system to restore cerebral blood flow when it is dangerously reduced.

The Cushing reflex – The Cushing reflex is another reflex that has an origin directly in the CNS. When intracranial pressure is acutely elevated, cerebral vessels are compressed. The decrease in cerebral perfusion pressure causes a reduction in arterial blood flow, and the CNS ischaemic response occurs. The decrease in blood flow to the vasomotor area results in an increase in SNS activity. This leads to progressive elevations in arterial pressure in an effort to exceed intracranial pressure and maintain adequate cerebral perfusion. Simultaneously, decreases in heart rate are observed which are mediated by the baroreceptor reflex.

Spinal shock and autonomic hyperreflexia

When the spinal cord is acutely trans-sected, all cord functions, including reflexes mediated through the CNS, are interrupted below the level of injury.[20] Vasoconstrictor tone regulated by the ANS is disrupted below the cord lesion and, if the spinal cord injury occurs at a high level (that is, C6–C7), spinal shock may result. Spinal shock is characterised by a fall in blood pressure as a result of lack of arteriolar and venular constriction as well as a loss of skeletal muscle pump action. The efferent limb of cardiovascular reflexes cannot compensate for the reduction in arterial pressure. This condition is analogous to the loss of control of blood pressure during spinal anaesthesia. Spinal shock typically lasts from one to three weeks.

After this period, local reflexes in the spinal cord below the level of disruption gradually return and a chronic stage, characterised by SNS overactivity or autonomic hyperreflexia, begins. Hyperreflexia occurs in response to cutaneous or visceral stimulation below the level of cord lesion in 85% of patients with spinal cord injury at or above the T6 level. The stimulus sends afferent impulses into the spinal cord, causing local activation of preganglionic sympathetic nerves and subsequent vasoconstriction. This reflex is normally modulated by inhibitory impulses from higher centres, but as a result of the trans-section, such impulses are blocked. The vasoconstriction causes hypertension and elicits the baroreceptor depressor reflex. The reflex mediated decline in SNS activity and increase in PNS activity occur only above the level of the cord trans-section, whereas vasoconstriction continues below this level. With high levels of trans-section, circulatory reflexes are insufficient to offset the effects of vasoconstriction, leading to persistent and sometimes severe hypertension.

Humoral control of the circulation

Catecholamines

The adrenal medulla is unique in that this gland is innervated by preganglionic SNS fibres which pass directly to it from the spinal cord.[10 22] Embryologically, cells of the adrenal medulla are derived from neural tissue and are analogous to postganglionic neurons. The adrenal medulla secretes primarily adrenaline (epinephrine) (80%) and also noradrenaline (norepinephrine) in response to SNS stimulation. As adrenaline and noradrenaline are released into the blood and exert functions at distal sites, these catecholamines function as hormones.

The release of catecholamines by the adrenal medulla occurs after acetylcholine is secreted by preganglionic SNS fibres. The cardiovascular response to the secreted adrenaline and noradrenaline is similar to direct stimulation by the SNS. The effects of those hormones are, however, significantly prolonged (10–30 seconds) compared with the duration of action of noradrenaline as a neurotransmitter. Adrenal medullary secretion may be considered to be additive to that of SNS stimulation in that some vessels that are poorly innervated are also constricted by circulating catecholamines.

Renin–angiotensin system

The renin–angiotensin system is another important humoral regulator of the cardiovascular system, particularly under conditions of stress.[18 23] The enzyme renin is synthesised in and released from juxtaglomerular cells of the renal cortex. Juxtaglomerular cells are modified vascular smooth muscle cells located in the tunica media of the afferent arteriole immediately proximal to the glomerulus. Renin is secreted into the blood in response to a decrease in renal artery pressure, reduced sodium delivery to the distal tubule (sensed by osmoreceptors of the macula densa region) and SNS stimulation via activation of β_1-adrenergic receptors. Renin cleaves the hepatically synthesised α_2-globulin, angiotensinogen, to form the decapeptide, angiotensin I. Angiotensin I is physiologically inactive but is rapidly hydrolysed to form the octapeptide angiotensin II by angiotensin converting enzyme which is found in high concentrations in the vascular endothelium of the lungs.

Angiotensin II produces vasoconstriction of arterioles in most vascular beds. It also stimulates SNS ganglion cells and facilitates impulse transmission in the SNS. Activation of presynaptic angiotensin receptors increases noradrenaline (norepinephrine) release. Angiotensin II directly stimulates the adrenal cortex to synthesise and secrete aldosterone. Aldosterone causes salt and water retention leading to expansion of plasma volume which further increases arterial pressure. Decreases in blood pressure or declines in sodium delivery to the macula densa (for example, haemorrhage, dehydration) lead to formation of angiotensin II. Angiotensin II increases arterial pressure by elevating the peripheral vascular resistance and by causing aldosterone secretion with subsequent salt and water retention. The renin–angiotensin–aldosterone axis system is of major importance in maintaining blood pressure, especially during periods of hypovolaemia, sodium deprivation, or inadequate cardiac output. Also, this system has been found to play a role in basal vascular tone as well as having an interplay with other regulatory systems such as the kinins.[24, 25]

Vasopressin

Vasopresson or antidiuretic hormone is a peptide synthesised in the supraoptic and paraventricular nuclei of the brain stem, which is transported to and released from the posterior pituitary gland.[26] Vasopressin secretion from the pituitary occurs in response to multiple physiological stimuli, including: an increase in plasma osmolality sensed by osmoreceptors located in the hypothalamus; a decrease in plasma volume detected by cardiopulmonary receptors, particularly in the left atrium; and increased plasma concentrations of angiotensin II. Vasopressin binds to specific receptors which cause the collecting ducts of the kidney to increase free water reabsorption (inhibit diuresis). An increase in plasma volume occurs, which has a negative feedback on further vasopressin release.

The vasoconstriction produced by vasopressin is generalised, affecting most regional circulations. Skin and gastrointestinal tract arteries are markedly constricted, whereas large epicardial coronary arteries and pulmonary arteries are constricted to a lesser extent. Severe and preferential constriction of small coronary collaterals can result in areas of regional myocardial ischaemia. Large quantities of vasopressin are released by the posterior pituitary gland during haemorrhage, and the constrictor action exerts an adjunctive pressor effect to that produced by baroreceptor reflexes.

Endothelium derived nitric oxide

Nitric oxide (NO) produced by vascular endothelium (formerly known as endothelium derived relaxing factor or EDRF) is a cell messenger that has important physiological and pathophysiological actions.[27 28] The primary effect of NO on the circulation is to relax vascular smooth muscle. A variety of endogenous mediators and pharmacological agents exerts haemodynamic effects by causing a release of NO from vascular endothelium. For example, acethylcholine will produce vasodilation in the presence of an intact endothelium in isolated vascular ring preparations. In contrast, acetylcholine causes vasoconstriction after endothelial denudation.

Nitric oxide is synthesised by at least two major NO synthase (NOS) isoforms. One is expressed constitutively in neurons and vasculature, and requires calcium and calmodulin binding for activation. This constitutive enzyme is involved in cell communication and is activated by an increase in intracellular calcium. The enzyme is in a soluble form in neural tissue, but it is membrane-bound in vascular endothelium. The other isoenzyme is expressed after induction by cytokines or endotoxin and participates in host defence. This inducible isoform has calmodulin bound as a subunit and produces NO continuously without requiring calcium. This isoenzyme may contribute to the pathophysiology associated with syndromes characterised by an overproduction of cytokines such as septic shock. It is present in macrophages, but is not normally found in endothelial cells or vascular smooth muscle unless induced by cytokines. The NOSs are mixed function mono-oxygenases which use NADPH. L-Arginine is oxidised in a stepwise manner to form NO and citrulline as primary products. NO synthases can be specifically and competitively inhibited by L-arginine analogues (for example, N^g-nitro-L-argenine methylester [L-NAME] and N^g-mono-methyl-L-arginine [L-NMMA]). The inhibitors have been used to elucidate the physiological and pathophysiological roles of NO. Administration of inhibitors of the synthesis of NO to experimental animals leads to considerable increases in arterial pressure, substantiating the premise that a basal release of NO normally occurs and that defects in NO synthesis may play a role in the aetiology of hypertension. The same inhibitors may also be useful in increasing arterial pressure in septic shock. The primary biological function of NO appears to be the activation of soluble guanylyl cyclase, which subsequently increases the cyclic guanosine $3':5'$-monophosphate (cGMP) content of several tissues including vascular smooth muscle. The cGMP may cause relaxation of vascular smooth muscle by several mechanisms, including the activation of cGMP dependent protein kinase, which in turn activates a calcium ATPase that causes extrusion of calcium from the cell or improves calcium uptake into the sarcoplasmic reticulum.

Nitric oxide plays an important and diverse role in cardiovascular regulation. Physiologically, it has significant roles in the maintenance of basal vascular tone and the modulation of platelet–vessel wall interactions. Conversely, an overproduction or underproduction of NO also has pathophysiological implications in hypotension associated within certain shock states, essential hypertension, and atherosclerosis. The release of NO may stem from stimuli such as intracellular calcium, changes in oxygen tension, vessel wall sheer stress, and other humoral mediators of vascular tone. NOS inhibitors may provide important avenues for the control of

231

certain hypotensive states, including septic shock where traditional therapies including administration of catecholamines have limited effectiveness. Furthermore, return of catecholamine sensitivity after the use of NOS inhibitors in patients with septic shock have been described. NO may also serve as the active moiety of certain antihypertensive agents that act to donate it.[29] L-Arginine may be another important agent that serves to control hypertension by being converted to NO via NOS.[30]

Atrial natriuretic peptide

Atrial natriuretic factor (ANP) is a peptide synthesised and stored in human atrial myocytes and secreted in response to distension of the atria (increased vascular volume or increased atrial pressure), adrenaline (epinephrine), vasopressin, or morphine.[31] Studies have determined that there is a larger amount of ANP synthesised and stored in the right than in the left atrium. ANP acts directly on the arterial and venous vasculature and kidneys to reduce arterial pressure and intravascular volume. It decreases blood pressure by relaxing vascular smooth muscle and sympathetic tone. ANP inhibits renin release and aldosterone secretion, thereby interfering with sodium retention and leading to natriuresis. Further renal effects include dilatation of afferent arterioles and possible constriction of efferent arterioles of the glomerulus, leading to increased filtration fraction and diuresis. Controversy exists about whether ANP inhibits sodium uptake in the inner medullary collecting ducts causing further natriuresis. ANP suppresses antidiuretic hormone secretion. No direct inotropic or chronotropic effects caused by this peptide have been observed, but some evidence indicates that at least a portion of the vasodilator action of ANP is mediated by NO.

Other humoral substances

There are several other endogenous substances that can be released into the circulation and affect the heart and vasculature. These include adenosine, histamine, the plasma kinins (kallidin and bradykinin), serotonin, and endothelins.

Adenosine is a ubiquitous endogenous nucleotide that stimulates A_1-, A_2-, and A_3-receptors to produce haemodynamic actions.[11] It has inhibitory effects on cardiac impulse conduction through the atrioventricular node (negative dromotropic effect). Adenosine is also a potent vasodilator. The local regulation of flow in the coronary circulation and other regions during an increase in oxygen demand is at least partially related to the release of adenosine.[22]

Histamine is one of several naturally occurring endogenous substances collectively referred to as autacoids.[7] Other autacoids include prostaglandins, angiotensin II, serotonin, and plasma kinins. Histamine is located in mass cells in the lungs, skin, and gastrointestinal tract and in basophils throughout the blood. The predominant circulatory effects of histamine are caused by dilatation of arterioles and capillaries. Histamine causes vasodilation by binding to H_1- and H_2-receptors directly on blood vessels. Histamine induced vasodilation leads to flushing, decreased systemic vascular resistance, reduced arterial pressure, and increased capillary permeability. This autacoid also has positive inotropic properties by directly stimulating cardiac H_2-receptors and indirectly by causing adrenaline (epinephrine) release from the adrenal medulla. Stimulation of cardiac H_2-receptors also causes positive chronotropic effects. Finally, coronary arteries have been shown to be vasoconstricted as a result of H_1-receptor stimulation and vasodilated after H_2-receptor stimulation.[32]

Plasma kinins are among the most potent endogenous vasodilators known.[33] Two examples of plasma kinins are kallidin and bradykinin, which are polypeptides formed by cleavage of α_2-globulin kininogens by kallikrein enzymes. Plasma kinins are approximately 10 times more potent as vasodilators than histamine. Kinins also cause increased capillary permeability and tissue oedema. vasodilation leads to a marked reduction in arterial pressure. In contrast, plasma kinins have been shown to constrict large veins, which subsequently elevates venous return. This increase in venous return increases stroke volume and cardiac output. Many of the actions of bradykinin are mediated by release of NO from vascular endothelium.

Kinins have been found to be increasingly important and may provide new pathways for understanding cardiovascular control mechanisms and therapies. These entities are clearly connected to the renin–angiotensin system. There is an inverse relationship between plasma kinin levels and angiotensin converting enzyme (ACE) and renin, respectively.[25] The renin–angiotensin system is linked to the kinins via ACE. This enzyme metabolises kinins to inactive products in addition to activating angiotensin II.

Serotonin (5-hydroxytryptamine) is also an endogenous vasoactive autacoid synthesised from tryptophan.[34] About 90% of endogenous serotonin exists in enterochromaffin cells of the gastrointestinal tract and the remainder in the CNS and platelets. The circulatory actions of serotonin are dependent on the specific vascular bed. It produces vasodilation in blood vessels in skeletal muscles and skin, while causing vasoconstriction particularly in splanchnic and renal vessels and, to a lesser extent, in cerebral and pulmonary vessels. It is also a potent venoconstrictor, but the resulting effects of increased venous return on cardiac output may be obscured by baroreceptor responses mediated by reflexes.

Within the past decade, a very important peptide system (endothelins) has been uncovered not only for its properties in the control of vascular tone but also for growth and development of the vascular system. Endothelins are possibly the most potent of all endogenous vasoconstrictors. These polypeptides may be involved in basal vascular tone and blood pressure in normal physiological states. Endothelins have a short half life and are therefore felt to have primarily a local action. The role of this system in human hypertension is unclear and difficult to ascertain given that plasma levels may not correlate accurately with their local effects. Finally, a number of endothelin antagonists are presently being developed as alternative antihypertensive agents or new drugs for the treatment of congestive heart failure.[35]

Local regulation of the circulation

Pressure autoregulation

Flow is locally controlled in certain vascular beds by a process termed "autoregulation"[36] (Fig. 6.5). By definition, autoregulation is the ability of an organ to maintain a relatively constant blood flow in the presence of changes in arterial perfusion pressure. The kidneys, brain, and heart are organs that exhibit autoregulation, whereas the skin and lungs are organs with minimal ability for autoregulation.

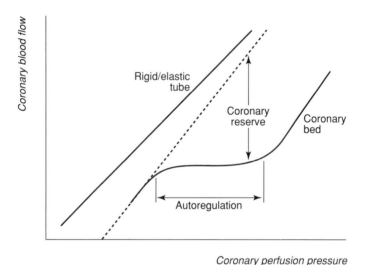

Fig 6.5 Pressure autoregulation in the normal coronary circulation. Note that during maximum vasodilation, autoregulation is abolished (dashed line) and pressure–flow relationships resemble those of a rigid/elastic tube. (Reprinted with permission from Goldberg and Warltier.[37])

A schematic diagram of the changes in blood flow to an organ over a wide range of perfusion pressures in the presence or absence of autoregulation is shown in Fig. 6.5. In the absence of autoregulation, pressure–flow relationships are linear, and increases in driving pressure lead to direct increases in perfusion. An autoregulatory curve is characterised by a large range of pressures during which flow remains relatively constant. vasodilation is achieved at lower perfusion pressures by relaxation of smooth muscle, and vascular smooth muscle constriction occurs at higher perfusion pressures to maintain constant flow. The ability to autoregulate assumes that a set point of basal vasomotor tone allows for this dilatation or constriction to occur. Flow varies directly with pressure when the limits of autoregulation are exceeded. In regional beds that are maximally vasodilated, for example by a drug such as dipyridamole, the process of autoregulation is eliminated and flow is directly dependent on driving pressure (Fig. 6.5).[37] Autoregulation of blood flow is affected to only a small extent by neural and humoral influences. Experimental investigations have demonstrated that the ability to autoregulate flow is largely an intrinsic property and even occurs in denervated tissues. As a result of this, autoregulation is considered to be a local phenomenon affected primarily by the active tone of arterioles.

Two major theories have been advanced to explain the mechanism of autoregulation.[36] The first of these is the myogenic theory which suggests that elevations in perfusion pressure lead to stretch and increases in tension of vascular smooth muscle cells. The distension of the smooth muscle directly causes vasoconstriction to maintain flow constant despite an increased driving pressure. Conversely, at low perfusion pressures, there is less muscle tension, vascular smooth muscle cells relax, and blood flow is maintained despite the decrease in pressure. Therefore, the degree of tension smooth muscle is exposed to is the stimulus for regulation, and subsequent constriction/dilatation serves as the mediator of this mechanism. Autoregulation is advantageous to vital organs such as the brain, heart, and kidneys because blood flow is optimised even during periods of hypo- and hypertension. It has also been proposed that the myogenic mechanism protects capillaries from excessively high blood pressures which could cause these fragile vessels to rupture.

The metabolic theory of autoregulation is based on the state of oxygenation in the surrounding tissues. A reduction in perfusion pressure leads to a decrease in blood flow and tissue Po_2 with concomitant increases in tissue Pco_2 and other metabolites related to normal cellular activity (for example, lactic acid, adenosine, K^+, and H^+). The reduced Po_2, increased Pco_2, and vasodilator substances directly cause arteriolar relaxation, and blood flow increases. High perfusion pressures supply ample O_2, remove CO_2, and wash out vasodilators leading to vasoconstriction and decreases in tissue blood flow. Regardless of the validity of either the myogenic or the metabolic theory, both are based on the premise that autoregulation of tissue flow is a negative feedback mechanism, maintaining constancy of arterial flow during large changes in perfusion pressure.

Matching of flow and metabolism

When tissues have greater metabolic activity, such as skeletal muscle during exercise or myocardium during increases in heart rate, arterioles in the tissue dilate and flow increases independently of changes in perfusion pressure. This process is referred to as active or functional hyperaemia.[19] The mechanism of functional hyperaemia is very similar to the metabolic theory of autoregulation. As the requirement of tissues for O_2 increases, there is a concomitant accumulation of byproducts of metabolism. For example, as more ATP is consumed during periods of increased metabolic activity, adenosine is released into the interstitium. The accumulation of this and other vasodilator substances leads to smooth muscle relaxation in arterioles with increases in tissue perfusion. This represents a powerful regulator of flow in which perfusion is closely coupled with metabolic demands. Investigations have demonstrated that, during intense exercise, active hyperaemia can increase skeletal muscle blood flow as much as 20-fold.

Reactive hyperaemia

When blood flow is interrupted by an arterial occlusion for a brief period and then suddenly restored, the resulting flow greatly exceeds previous levels for a short time before returning to the usual resting levels (Fig. 6.6). The increase in flow during early reperfusion is termed "reactive hyperaemia". Reactive hyperaemia is most probably related to the metabolic theory of tissue perfusion. Lack of perfusion causes a deprivation of oxygen and accumulation of vasodilating metabolites. The resulting degree and duration of the excess blood flow during the reactive hyperaemic response are proportional to the length of the blood flow interruption and severity of oxygen debt (Fig. 6.6).[38] This response emphasises a close connection between delivery of nutrients to tissues and the regulation of tissue perfusion. Reactive hyperaemia will occur after ischaemia (partial or total occlusion of arterial supply) or hypoxia (decreased Pao_2). The heart and brain have large, skeletal muscle intermediate, and liver, lung, and skin relatively small reactive hyperaemia responses.

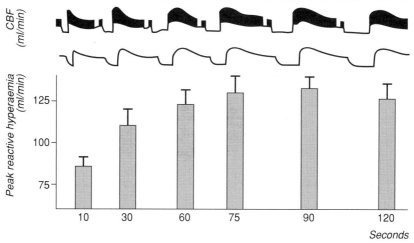

Fig 6.6 Average values (lower histogram) and chart recordings (top panel) of reactive hyperaemic responses of canine coronary blood flow (CBF) after 10, 30, 60, 75, 90, and 120 seconds of total coronary occlusion. Note that with increasing time of occlusion there is an increasing hyperaemic response. (Reprinted with permission from Warltier et al.[38])

Long term regulation of the circulation

Whereas circulatory reflexes provide acute and rapid control of the circulation, the concept of long term regulation is based upon the balance of blood volume and urinary output.[22] The kidneys provide the major long term control of the circulation. Reflex changes in haemodynamics, as mediated by baroreceptors, play no important role in long term adjustments because the receptors rapidly adapt to continued increases or decreases in pressure. Long term regulation follows a simple renal–body fluid mechanism: increases in arterial pressure produce increases in salt and water output through the kidneys, hence reducing extracellular fluid volume, blood volume, and venous return. Reduced venous return decreases cardiac output and arterial pressure. After several weeks, cardiac output returns to previous levels while reductions in systemic vascular resistance develop to maintain the lower arterial pressure. Conversely, a decline in blood pressure stimulates the kidneys to retain fluid which ultimately results in elevation of arterial pressure. Renal perfusion pressure and urinary output are directly related. This process occurs independently of any hormonal actions, but it is significantly amplified by the renin–angiotensin system.

The renal–body fluid mechanism is continuous and overriding, and undergoes no adaptation. It requires that small alterations in fluid volume lead to substantial changes in arterial pressure. It is also unique because it has the ability to return the blood pressure completely back to normal values. This is in contrast to short term regulating mechanisms, which cannot entirely re-establish normal arterial pressure. Overall, the renal–body fluid mechanism develops over hours to days and regulates the circulation over an infinite time span.

Conclusion

Several mechanisms involving the CNS, ANS, humoral and chemical substances, and circulatory reflexes act in combination to provide homoeostasis of the circulation. By functioning together to regulate cardiac output, peripheral vascular resistance, and venous capacitance, relatively constant arterial pressure and adequate tissue perfusion are maintained. The cardiovascular control mechanisms act in unison to provide important adaptive responses to stresses such as haemorrhage or exercise. Without such reflexes, even the simple act of assuming an upright position would be met with abrupt and large declines in cardiac output and arterial pressure threatening the status of the organism.

Acknowledgements

This work was supported by the Anesthesiology Research Training Grants GM 08377.

1 Mitchell GF, Pfeffer JM, Pfeffer MA. The heart and conduit vessels in hypertension. *Med Clin North Am* 1997;**81**:1247–71.
2 Dampney RA, Goodchild AK, Tan E. Identification of cardiovascular cell groups in the brain stem. *Clin Exp Hypertens [A]* 1984;**6**:205–20.
3 Hilton SM, Spyer KM. Central nervous regulation of vascular resistance. *Annu Rev Physiol* 1980;**42**:399–441.
4 Alexander RS. Tonic and reflex functions of medullary sympathetic cardiovascular centers. *J Neurophysiol* 1946;**9**:205–17.
5 Levy MN, Martin PJ, Stuesse SL. Neural regulation of the heart beat. *Annu Rev Physiol* 1981;**43**:443–53.
6 Calaresu FR, Yardley CP. Medullary basal sympathetic tone. *Annu Rev Physiol* 1988;**50**:511–24.
7 Smith JJ, Kampine JP. *Circulatory physiology: the essentials.* Baltimore, MD: Williams & Wilkins, 1990.
8 Dontenwill M, Tibirica E, Greney H, et al. Role of imidazoline receptors in cardiovascular regulation. *Am J Cardiol* 1994;**73**:3–6A.
9 Janig W. Pre- and postganglionic vasoconstrictor neurons: differentiation, types, and discharge properties. *Annu Rev Physiol* 1988;**50**:525–39.
10 Lawson NW. Autonomic nervous system physiology and pharmacology. In: Barash PG, Cullen BF, Stoelting RK, eds. *Clinical anesthesia.* Philadelphia: JB Lippincott, 1992:319–84.
11 Katz AM. *Physiology of the heart.* New York: Raven Press, 1992.

12 Ahluwalia A, Cellek S. Regulation of the cardiovascular system by non-adrenergic non-cholinergic nerves. *Curr Opin Nephrol Hypertens* 1997;**6**:74–9.

13 Hoffman BB, Lefkowitz RJ. Adrenergic receptors in the heart. *Annu Rev Physiol* 1982;**44**:475–84.

14 Feigl EO. Coronary physiology. *Physiol Rev* 1983;**63**:1–205.

15 Donald DE, Shepherd JT. Autonomic regulation of the peripheral circulation. *Annu Rev Physiol* 1980;**42**:429–39.

16 Shepherd JT, Mancia G. Reflex control of the human cardiovascular system. *Rev Physiol Biochem Pharmacol* 1986;**105**:1–99.

17 Ebert TJ. Autonomic balance and cardiac function. *Curr Opin Anaesthesiol* 1992;**5**:3–10.

18 Reid IA, Morris BJ, Ganong WF. The renin–angiotensin system. *Annu Rev Physiol* 1978;**40**:377–410.

19 Ludbrook J. Reflex control of blood pressure during exercise. *Annu Rev Physiol* 1983;**45**:155–68.

20 Stoelting RK, Dierdorf SF. *Anesthesia and co-existing disease.* New York: Churchill Livingstone, 1993.

21 Guyton AC. Acute hypertension in dogs with cerebral ischemia. *Am J Physiol* 1948;**154**:45–54.

22 Vatner SF, Cox DA. Circulatory function and control. *Textbook of internal medicine.* Philadelphia: JB Lippincott, 1992.

23 Mirenda JV, Grissom TE. Anesthetic implications of the renin–angiotensin system and angiotensin-converting enzyme inhibitors. *Anesth Analg* 1991;**72**:667–83.

24 Johnston CI. Franz Volhard Lecture. Renin–angiotensin system: a dual tissue and hormonal system for cardiovascular control. *J Hypertens* 1992;**10**:S13–26.

25 Scholkens BA. Kinins in the cardiovascular system. *Immunopharmacology* 1996; **33**:209–16.

26 Hays RM. Agents affecting the renal conservation of water. *Pharmacological basis of therapeutics.* New York: Macmillan, 1985.

27 Rich GF, Johns RA. Nitric oxide and the pulmonary circulation. *Adv Anesth* 1994;**11**:1–25.

28 Johns RA. Endothelium, anesthetics, and vascular control. *Anesthesiology* 1993; **79**:1381–91.

29 Welch G, Loscalzo J. Nitric oxide and the cardiovascular system. *J Cardiovasc Surg* 1994;**9**:361–71.

30 Maxwell AJ, Cooke JP. Cardiovascular effects of L-arginine. *Curr Opin Nephrol Hypertens* 1998;**7**:63–70.

31 Cogan MG. Renal effects of atrial natriuretic factor. *Annu Rev Physiol* 1990;**52**:699–708.

32 Ginsburg R, Bristow MR, Stinson EB, Harrison DC. Histamine receptors in the human heart. *Life Sci* 1980;**26**:2245–9.

33 Regoli D. Neurohumoral regulation of precapillary vessels: the kallikrein–kinin system. *J Cardiovasc Pharmacol* 1984;**6**(suppl 2):S401–12.

34 Marwood JF, Stokes GS. Serotonin (5HT) and its antagonists: involvement in the cardiovascular system. *Clin Exp Pharmacol Physiol* 1984;**11**:439–55.

35 Parris RJ, Webb DJ. The endothelin system in cardiovascular physiology and pathophysiology. *Vasc Med* 1997;**2**:31–43.

36 Olsson RA. Local factors regulating cardiac and skeletal muscle blood flow. *Annu Rev Physiol* 1981;**43**:385–95.

37 Goldberg AH, Warltier DC. The coronary circulation: Importance for anesthesiologists. *Semin Anesth* 1990;**9**:232–44.

38 Warltier DC, Gross GJ, Brooks HL. Pharmacologic- vs. ischemia-induced coronary artery vasodilation. *Am J Physiol* 1981;**240**:H767–74.

7: Cerebral circulation

DAVID K MENON

The brain receives 15% of the resting cardiac output (700 ml/min in the adult) and accounts for 20% of basal oxygen consumption. Mean resting cerebral blood flow (CBF) in young adults is about 50 ml/100 g brain per min. This mean value represents two very different categories of flow: 70 and 20 ml/100 g per min for grey and white matter, respectively. Regional CBF (rCBF) and glucose consumption decline with age, along with marked reductions in brain neurotransmitter content, and less consistent decreases in neurotransmitter binding.[1]

Functional anatomy of the cerebral circulation

Arterial supply

Blood supply to the brain is provided by the two internal carotid arteries and the basilar artery, which divides into the two posterior cerebral arteries. The anastomoses between these two sets of vessels gives rise to the circle of Willis (Fig. 7.1a). Functionally significant hypoplasia of the anterior and posterior communicating arteries is, however, common, and a classic "normal" polygonal anastomotic ring is found in less than 50% of brains.[2] Despite the anatomical variations described, certain patterns of regional blood supply from individual arteries are generally recognised (Fig. 7.1b). Cerebral ischaemia associated with systemic hypotension classically produces maximal lesions in areas where the zones of blood supply from two vessels meet, resulting in "watershed" infarctions. The presence of anatomical variants may, however, substantially modify patterns of infarction following large vessel occlusion. For example, in some individuals, the proximal part of one anterior cerebral artery is hypoplastic, and flow to the ipsilateral frontal lobe is largely provided by the contralateral anterior cerebral artery, via the anterior communicating artery. Occlusion of the single dominant anterior cerebral artery in such a patient may result in massive infarction of both frontal lobes: the unpaired anterior cerebral artery syndrome.

240

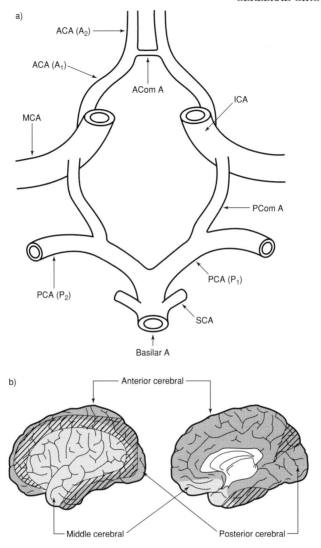

Fig 7.1 (a) Classic anatomy of the circle of Willis. ICA, internal carotid artery; AComA, anterior communicating artery; ACA, anterior cerebral artery (A_1, precommunicating segment of ACA; A_2, postcommunicating segment of ACA); MCA, middle cerebral artery; PComA, posterior communicating artery; PCA, posterior cerebral artery (P_1, precommunicating segment of PCA; P_2, post-communicating segment of PCA). (b) Classic patterns of blood flow distribution in the brain, showing contributions for the main components of the circle of Willis. Areas of the brain that are at the junction of two arterial territories are most at risk of hypoperfusion during global ischaemic insults, and may suffer *watershed* infarction.

241

Microcirculation

The cerebral circulation is protected from systemic blood pressure surges by a specially designed branching system and two resistance elements: the first of these lies in the large cerebral arteries and the second in vessels with a diameter of less than 100 μm. The architecture of the cerebral microvasculature is highly organised and follows the columnar arrangement seen with neuronal groups and physiological functional units.[3] Pial vessels on the surface of the brain give rise to arterioles that penetrate the brain at right angles to the surface and also to capillaries at all laminar levels. Each of these arterioles supplies a hexagonal column of cortical tissue, with intervening boundary zones, an arrangement that is responsible for columnar patterns of local blood flow, redox state,[4] and glucose metabolism seen in the cortex during hypoxia or ischaemia.[5] Capillary density in the cortex is one third of adult levels at birth, doubles in the first year, and reaches adult levels at four years. In the adult animal capillary density is related to the number of synapses, rather than the number of neurons or mass of cell bodies in a given region,[6] and can be closely correlated with the regional level of oxidative metabolism.[7, 8] Conventionally, functional activation of the brain is thought to result in "capillary recruitment", implying that some parts of the capillary network are non-functional during rest. Recent evidence suggests, however, that all capillaries may be persistently open,[8] and "recruitment" involves changes in capillary flow rates with homogenisation of the perfusion rate in a network.[9]

Venous drainage

The brain is drained by a system of infra- and extracerebral venous sinuses, which are endothelialised channels in folds of dura mater (Fig. 7.2). These sinuses drain into the internal jugular veins, which, at their origin receive minimal contributions from extra cerebral tissues. Measurement of oxygen saturation in the jugular bulb ($SJvo_2$) thus provides a useful measure of cerebral oxygenation. It has been suggested that the supratentorial compartment is preferentially drained by the right internal jugular vein, whereas the infratentorial compartment is preferentially drained by the left internal jugular vein. More recent data suggest, however, considerable interindividual variation in cerebral venous drainage.[10]

Cerebral blood volume: physiology and potential for therapeutic intervention

Most of the intracranial blood volume of about 200 ml is contained in these venous sinuses and pial veins, which constitute the capacitance vessels of the cerebral circulation; reduction in this volume can buffer rises in the volume of other intracranial contents (the brain and CSF). Conversely,

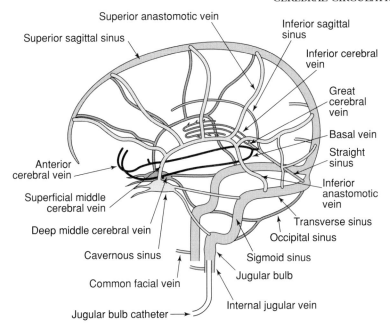

Fig 7.2 Venous sinuses of the brain, showing drainage of the superior sagittal sinus into the right jugular vein via the transverse and sigmoid sinus. Note that the first extracranial tributary of the internal jugular vein (the common facial vein or CFV) enters it below the lower level of the body of the second cervical vertebra. Consequently, a retrograde jugular catheter with its tip above this level samples blood that drains exclusively from intracranial contents.

when compensatory mechanisms to control intracranial pressure (ICP) have been exhausted, even small increases in cerebral blood volume (CBV) can result in steep rises in ICP (Fig. 7.3).

The position of the system on this curve can be expressed in terms of the pressure volume index (PVI), which is defined as the change in intracranial volume that produces a tenfold increase in ICP. This is normally about 26 ml,[11] but may be markedly lower in patients with intracranial hypertension, who are on the steep part of the intracranial pressure–volume curve (see effects of arterial carbon dioxide tension, $Pa\text{CO}_2$ on CBV).

With the exception of oedema reduction by mannitol, the only intracranial constituent whose volume can be readily modified by the anaesthetist via physiological or pharmacological interventions is the CBV. Although the CBV forms only a small part of the intracranial volume, and such interventions only produce small absolute changes (typically about 10 ml or less), they may result in marked reductions in ICP in the presence of intracranial hypertension. Conversely, inappropriate anaesthetic management may cause the CBV to increase. Again, although the absolute

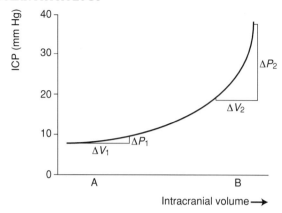

Fig 7.3 Intracranial pressure–volume curve. The pressure volume index (PVI), defined as the change in intracranial volume required to cause a tenfold increase in ICP, increases non-linearly, from approximately 25 ml in normals (A on the curve), to as little as 5 ml in patients with raised ICP (B on the curve).

magnitude of such an increase may be small, it may result in steep rises in ICP in the presence of intracranial hypertension.

The appreciation that pharmacological and physiological modulators may have independent effects on CBV and CBF is an important one for two reasons. First, interventions aimed at reducing CBV in patients with intracranial hypertension may have prominent effects on CBF and result in cerebral ischaemia[12] (Fig. 7.4). Conversely, drugs that produce divergent effects on CBF may have similar effects on CBV, and using CBF measurement to infer effects on CBV and hence ICP may result in erroneous conclusions.[13]

Determinants of cerebral perfusion

The inflow pressure to the brain is equal to the mean arterial pressure (MAP) measured at the level of the brain. The outflow pressure from the intracranial cavity depends on the ICP, because collapse of intracerebral veins is prevented by the maintenance of an intraluminal pressure 2–5 mm Hg above ICP. The difference between the MAP and the ICP thus provides an estimate of the effective cerebral perfusion pressure (CPP):

$$CPP = MAP - ICP.$$

Microcirculatory transport and the blood–brain barrier

Endothelial cells in cerebral capillaries contain few pinocytic vesicles, and are sealed with tight junctions, with no anatomical gap. Consequently,

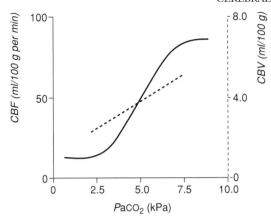

Fig 7.4 Relative effects of Pa_{CO_2} on cerebral blood flow (CBF) and voume (CBV). Hyperventilation is aimed at reducing CBV in patients with intracranial hypertension, but may be detrimental because of its effects on CBF. Note that the slope of CBF reactivity to Pa_{CO_2} is steeper than that for CBV (about 25% per kPa Pa_{CO_2} vs 20% per kPa Pa_{CO_2}, respectively).

unlike other capillary beds, the endothelial barrier of cerebral capillaries presents a high electrical resistance and is remarkably non-leaky, even to small molecules such as mannitol (molecular weight, M_w, 180 daltons). This property of the cerebral vasculature is termed the "blood–brain barrier" (BBB); it resides in three cellular components (the endothelial cell, astrocyte, and pericyte), and one non-cellular structure (the endothelial basement membrane) (Fig. 7.5). A fundamental difference between brain endothelial cells and the systemic circulation is the presence of inter-endothelial tight junctions termed the "zona occludens". The BBB is a function of the cerebral microenvironment rather than an intrinsic property of the vessels themselves, and leaky capillaries from other vascular beds develop a BBB if they are transplanted to the brain or exposed to astrocytes in culture.[14] Passage through the BBB is not simply a function of molecular weight; lipophilic substances traverse the barrier relatively easily, and several hydrophilic molecules (including glucose) cross the BBB via active transport systems to enter the brain interstitial space.[15] (Fig. 7.6). In addition, the BBB maintains a tight control of relative ionic distribution in the brain extracellular fluid. These activities are energy requiring and account for the fact that the mitochondrial density is exceptionally high in these endothelial cells, accounting for 10% of cytoplasmic volume.[16] Although the BBB is disrupted by ischaemia, this process takes hours or days rather than minutes, and much of the cerebral oedema seen in the initial period after ischaemic insults is cytotoxic rather than vasogenic.

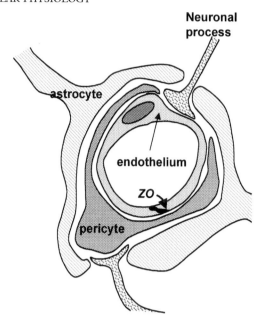

Fig 7.5 The components of the blood–brain barrier (see text).

Consequently, mannitol retains its ability to reduce cerebral oedema in the early phases of acute brain injury.

Measurement of rCBF

All clinical and many laboratory methods of measuring CBF or rCBF are indirect and may not produce directly comparable measurements. It is also important to treat results from any one method with caution, and attribute any observed phenomena to physiological effects only when demonstrated by two or more independent techniques. Methods of measuring CBF may be regional or global, and applicable either to humans or primarily to experimental animals. All of these methods have advantages and disadvantages (Table 7.1). All methods that provide absolute estimates of rCBF use one of two principles: either they measure the distribution of a tracer or they estimate rCBF from the wash-in or wash-out curve of an indicator. Other techniques do not directly estimate rCBF, but can be used either to measure a related flow variable (such as arterial flow velocity) or to infer changes in flow from changes in metabolic parameters. Some techniques that have been used for the measurement of CBF are described briefly.

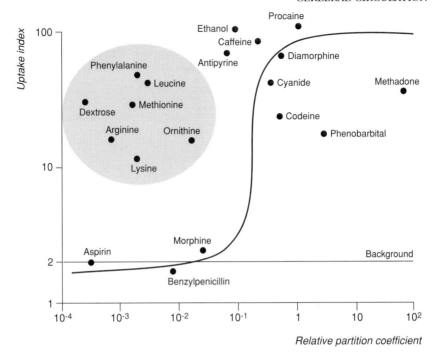

Fig 7.6 Correlation between brain uptake index and oil/water partition coefficients for different substrates. Although blood–brain barrier (BBB) permeability, in general, increases with lipid solubility, note that several substances, including glucose and amino acids, show high penetration as a result of active transport or facilitated diffusion. (After Oldendorf.[15])

The Kety–Schmidt technique[17]

The Kety–Schmidt technique involves the insertion of catheters into a peripheral artery and the jugular bulb. A diffusible tracer such as 10–15% inhaled nitrous oxide (N_2O) is administered, and paired arterial and jugular venous samples of blood are obtained at rapid intervals for measurement of N_2O levels. The resultant plot of concentration versus time produces an arterial and a venous curve (Fig. 7.7). The jugular venous level of N_2O rises more slowly than the arterial levels, because N_2O is being taken up by the brain as it is delivered. The rate of equilibration of the two curves measures the rate at which N_2O is being delivered to the brain, and thus provides a means of measuring global CBF.

Xenon-133 wash-out

An array of collimated scintillation counters is positioned over the head to plot the regional decay in radioactivity after the intracarotid[18] or intra-

Table 7.1 Methods of measuring cerebral blood flow

Technique	Global/regional	Comments
Human and laboratory methods		
Kety–Schmidt[17]	Global	Uses rate of uptake of N_2O to measure global CBF. Requires jugular bulb and arterial catheters. Repeated measures possible.
^{133}Xe wash-out[18 20]	Regional	Classic method uses wash-out curve of radioactive xenon after intracarotid injection to estimate CBF. Summated curves show fast and slow wash-out components (? grey and white matter). Primarily looks at cortex, poor resolution. Modifications include intravenous/inhalational/intra-aortic administration of xenon. Repeated measures possible.
Dynamic x ray CT	Regional	Looks at wash-out of stable xenon[138]/i.v. contrast[139] after inhalation. Repeated measures possible, but not at rapid intervals.
PET (H_2^{15}O)[140]	Regional	Uses distribution of radiolabelled markers to estimate rCBF. Repeated measures possible. Expensive equipment. Good resolution.
SPECT[141]	Regional	Uses distribution of radiolabelled tracer to estimate rCBF. Cheaper than PET, but resolution poorer. Repeated measurements difficult. Only measures relative CBF.
NIROS ($+O_2$ wash-in)[142]	?Regional	Detects rate of change of cerebral oxygenation state after step change in F_{IO_2}. Poorly defined volume and resolution. ?Accurate.

Continued/

Table 7.1 Continued

Technique	Global/regional	Comments
Laboratory methods		
H₂ clearance[143]	Regional	Measures wash-out of H_2 after inhalational administration. Very localised measurement (1–2 mm^3) with hydrogen electrode. Requires craniotomy. Repeated measures possible.
Autoradiography[144]	Regional	Uses distribution of radiolabelled tracer ([14C]-iodoantipyrine) to estimate rCBF. Excellent resolution. Single measurement only.
Radiolabelled microspheres[145]	Regional	Uses distribution of radiolabelled microspheres (15 μm diameter) to estimate rCBF; Resolution not as good as autoradiography. Repeated measurements with different radiolabels possible. Radiolabel injection in left atrium or aorta.
Indirect or non-quantitative measures		
MRI[146]	Regional	Utilises change in regional oxygenation during functional activation to show changes in rCBF. Superb resolution, absolute measures not possible. Excellent resolution, repeated measures easy. Modification with external label may permit quantitation, but repeated measures more restricted.
Doppler ultrasonography[147]	(Regional)	Measures flow velocity in middle cerebral artery using Doppler ultrasonography. Indirect measure of CBF.
NIROS[26]	(Regional)	Measures regional haemoglobin oxygenation and cytochrome redox state in restricted and poorly defined volume.
MRS[148]	Regional	Provides information regarding intracellular pH and tissue levels of ATP and lactate. Poor resolution. Repeatable.

Abbreviations: PET, positron emission tomography; SPECT, single photon emission tomography; NIROS, near infrared optical spectroscopy; MRI, magnetic resonance imaging; MRS, magnetic resonance spectroscopy; F_{IO_2}, fraction of inspired O_2.

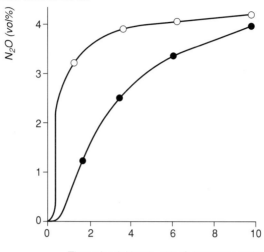

Fig 7.7 The Kety–Schmidt method of measuring global cerebral blood flow (CBF). The rate of increase in arterial (–○–) and jugular venous (–●–) concentrations of a diffusible tracer gas (N_2O in this instance) are compared. A rapid equilibration implies high CBF, whereas a slow equilibration is evidence of low CBF.

aortic[19] injection of ^{133}Xe. The wash-out curve for radioactivity is biexponential, and may be resolved into two monoexponential components, which represent a fast wash-out and a slow wash-out component. Although these are often referred to as grey matter and white matter components, it must be emphasised that there is no basis to support such an anatomical distinction, because the two curves represent pharmacokinetic compartments rather than specific neuroanatomical structures. The technique does provide two dimensional information regarding rCBF, but is invasive and primarily looks at superficial cortical blood flow. Further, intracarotid injection permits the assessment of only a single cerebral hemisphere at a time. One modification involves the inhalational[20] or intravenous administration of ^{133}Xe; although this makes the technique less invasive, problems arise because of recirculation and contamination by extracranial tissues. The simultaneous presence of activity in both cerebral hemispheres also leads to the "look-through" phenomenon, where rCBF reductions on one side may be missed because of activity sensed in deeper or contralateral tissues.

Tomographic rCBF measurement: dynamic CT, SPECT, PET, and fMRI

Tomographic information regarding rCBF may be obtained by quantifying the wash-out of a radiodense contrast agent, using rapid sequential *x* ray computed tomographic imaging (dynamic CT scanning). In the past, inhaled stable xenon has most often been used as the contrast agent. More recent studies have been performed using standard radioiodinated intravenous contrast agents.

Single photon emission tomography (SPECT) and positron emission tomography (PET) use γ emitting and positron emitting isotopes, respectively, to produce tomographic images of rCBF. PET, in addition to imaging cerebral blood flow (Fig. 7.8), can provide quantitative tomographic information on cerebral blood volume, oxygen metabolism, and oxygen extraction fraction (OEF). Functional magnetic resonance imaging (fMRI) produces tomographic images of rCBF in one of two ways. One technique uses an intravenous MR contrast agent (for example, gadopentate dimeglumine, Magnevist) in much the same way as the previous techniques in this section use other agents. MRI can also produce, without the use of external contrast agents, tomographic images of *changes* in rCBF *after* functional activation by imaging the increases in MR signal intensity produced by the decreases in regional deoxyhaemoglobin levels, which occur during flow metabolism coupling.

Detailed discussion of these techniques is beyond the scope of this chapter, and the interested reader is referred to the references in Table 7.1 for details.

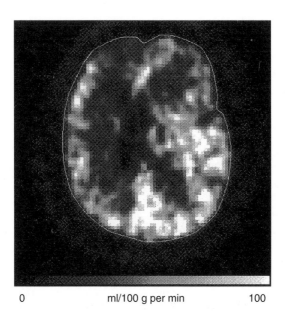

0   ml/100 g per min   100

Fig 7.8 PET images of cerebral blood flow (CBF) in a patient with a left temporoparietal contusion after a head injury. Note the marked heterogeneity in CBF values in the region of the contusion.

251

Continuous clinical monitoring of the adequacy of cerebral perfusion, in general, tends to use techniques other than those outlined in Table 7.1[21] (Fig. 7.9). The parameter most commonly monitored in head injured

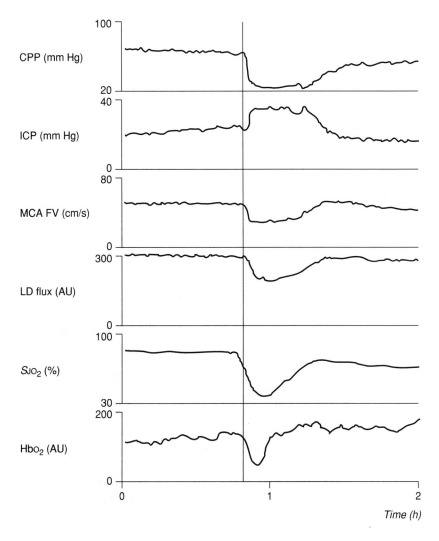

Fig 7.9 Continuous record of multimodality monitoring in a patient with acute head injury during a plateau wave in the intracranial pressure (ICP). Note the fall in the cerebral perfusion pressure (CPP) and reduction in the middle cerebral artery flow velocity (FV) measured using transcranial Doppler and reduction in laser Doppler signal intensity (FLUX), suggesting reduced capillary flow. The ischaemia associated with the reduction in CPP produces jugular venous desaturation (SjO_2 catheter) and a fall in oxyhaemoglobin signal (NIRS). (Recording courtsey of Dr Marek Czosnyka.)

patients is the cerebral perfusion pressure, although many centres are increasingly using fibreoptic jugular venous oximetry[22] and transcranial Doppler measurement of middle cerebral artery flow velocity.[23] Monitoring of the processed EEG[24] or evoked potentials[25] provides information regarding the consequences of reduced CBF, and this technique has been used in the context of cardiopulmonary bypass and carotid endarterectomy. Near infrared optical spectroscopy[26] and laser Doppler flowmetry[27] are investigational techniques whose roles have not been clearly defined.

Transcranial Doppler ultrasonography

Transcranial Doppler ultrasonography (TCD) measures the velocity of red blood cells (RBCs) flowing through the large vessels at the base of the brain using the Doppler shift principle. As the diameter of these basal vessels is not affected by common physiological variables, such as MAP and Pa_{CO_2}, flow velocity (FV) in these vessels provides an index of flow. Although many of the intracranial arteries may be studied, the middle cerebral artery is most commonly insonated (Fig. 7.10) because it is easy to detect, receives a substantial proportion of the blood flow from the internal

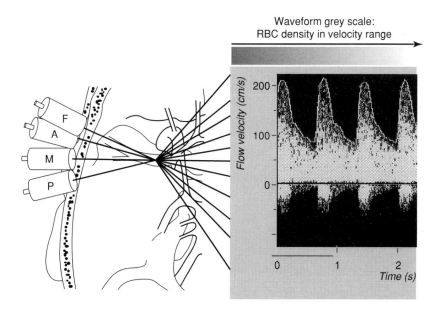

Fig 7.10 Transcranial Doppler ultrasonography (TCD) waveform from the left middle cerebral artery. Note the three axes on the TCD waveform, which include time on the x axis and red blood cells (RBCs) flow velocity on the y axis. The grey scale of the waveform is the third axis, and represents the population density of RBCs at any given velocity.

253

carotid artery, and allows easy probe fixation. Provided that the angle of insonation and the diameter of the vessel insonated remain constant, relative changes in CBF velocity correlate closely with changes in CBF.[28–30] Changes in TCD velocities and waveform patterns can be used to detect cerebral ischaemia, hyperaemia, and vasospasm.[31] In addition, the characteristics of the TCD waveform may be used to provide a non-invasive estimate of cerebral perfusion pressure (CPP).[32]

Jugular venous oximetry

Cerebral oxygenation has conventionally been assessed by jugular bulb oximetry. Conventionally, the superior saggital sinus is thought to drain primarily into the right internal jugular vein, and it is common practice to place jugular bulb catheters on this side in order to monitor the oxygenation in the supratentorial compartment. More recent data suggest that supratentorial venous drainage is less lateralised, and a case has been made for bilateral jugular bulb catheterisation.[33] Normal jugular bulb oxygen saturations (S_Jvo_2) tend to run at 65–70%. Reductions in S_Jvo_2 or increases in arteriojugular differences in oxygen content (Da_Jo_2) to greater than 9 ml/dl provide useful markers of inadequate CBF[33] (Fig. 7.11) and can guide therapy,[34] and S_Jvo_2 values below 50% have been shown to be associated with a worse outcome in head injury.[35] Conversely, marked elevations in S_Jvo_2 may provide evidence of cerebral hyperaemia.

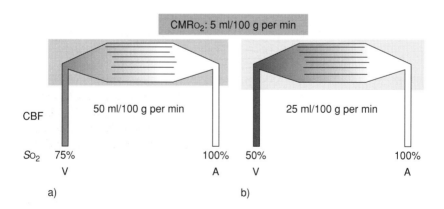

Fig 7.11 Use of jugular bulb oximetry to assess the adequacy of cerebral blood flow (CBF). Reductions in CBF force an increase in oxygen extraction by the brain if cerebral metabolic requirements for O_2 (CMR_{O2}) requirements are to be met. This is reflected by a fall in jugular venous oxygen saturation (S_Jvo_2); (a) normal and (b) reduced CBF.

Physiological determinants of regional cerebral blood flow and volume

Flow–metabolism coupling

Increases in local neuronal activity are accompanied by increases in regional cerebral metabolic rate (rCMR). Until recently, the increases in rCBF and oxygen consumption produced during such functional activation were thought to be closely coupled to the cerebral metabolic rate of utilisation of O_2 (CMRo$_2$) and glucose (CMRglu). However, it has now been clearly shown that increases in rCBF during functional activation tend to track glucose utilisation, but may be far in excess of the increase in oxygen consumption.[36] This results in regional *anaerobic* glucose utilisation, and a consequent local decrease in oxygen extraction ratio and an increase in local haemoglobin saturation. The resulting local decrease in deoxy-haemoglobin levels is used by functional MRI techniques to image the changes in rCBF produced by functional activation. Despite this revision of the proportionality between increased rCBF and CMRo$_2$ during functional activation in the brain, the relationship between rCBF and CMRglu is still accepted as linear.

The cellular mechanisms underlying these observations are elucidated by recent publications, which have highlighted the role played by astrocytes in the regulation of cerebral metabolism.[37] These data suggest that astrocytes utilise glucose glycolytically and produce lactate, which is transferred to neurons where it serves as a fuel in the citric acid cycle.[38] Astrocytic glucose utilisation and lactate production appear to be, in large part, coupled by the astrocytic reuptake of glutamate released at excitatory synapses (Fig. 7.12).

The regulatory changes involved in flow–metabolism coupling have a short latency (about 1 s) and may be mediated by either metabolic or neurogenic pathways. The former category includes the increases in perivascular K^+ or adenosine concentrations that follow neuronal depolarisation. The cerebral vessels are richly supplied by nerve fibres, and the mediators thought to play an important part in neurogenic flow metabolism coupling are acetylcholine[39] and nitric oxide,[40] although roles have also been proposed for 5-hydroxytryptamine, substance P, and neuropeptide Y.

Autoregulation

Autoregulation refers to the ability of the cerebral circulation to maintain CBF at a relatively constant level in the face of changes in CPP by altering cerebrovascular resistance (CVR) (Fig. 7.13). Although autoregulation is maintained irrespective of whether changes in CPP arise from alterations in MAP or ICP, autoregulation tends to be preserved at lower levels when falls in CPP are the result of increases in ICP rather than decreases in MAP

255

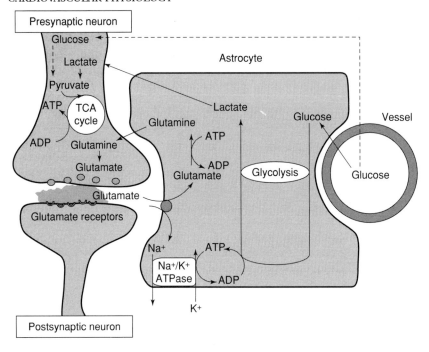

Fig 7.12 Relationship of astrocytes to oxygen and energy metabolism in the brain. Glucose taken up by astrocytes undergoes glycolysis for generation of ATP to meet astrocytic energy requirements (for glutamate reuptake, predominantly). The lactate that this process generates is shuttled to neurons, which utilise it aerobically in the citric acid cycle.

caused by hypovolaemia.[41][42] One possible reason for this may be the cerebral vasoconstrictive effects of the massive levels of catecholamines secreted in haemorrhagic hypotension, because lower MAP levels are tolerated in hypotension if the fall in blood pressure is induced by sympatholytic agents,[43][44] or occurs in the setting of autonomic failure.[45] Autoregulatory changes in CVR probably arise from myogenic reflexes in the resistance vessels, but these may be modulated by activity of the sympathetic system or the presence of chronic systemic hypertension.[46] Thus, sympathetic blockade or cervical sympathectomy shifts the autoregulatory curve to the left, whereas chronic hypertension or sympathetic activation shifts it to the right. These modulatory effects may arise from angiotensin-mediated mechanisms. Primate studies suggest that nitric oxide is unlikely to be important in pressure autoregulation.[47]

In reality, the clear cut autoregulatory thresholds seen with varying CPP in Fig. 7.13a are not observed; the autoregulatory "knees" tend to be more gradual, and there may be wide variations in rCBF at a given value of CPP in experimental animals and even in neurologically normal individuals.[48] It

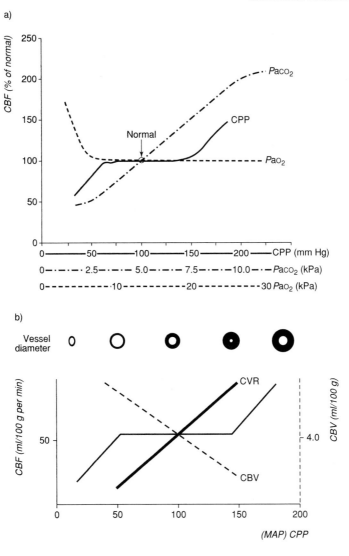

Fig 7.13 Effect of changes in cerebral perfusion pressure (CPP), Pa_{CO_2}, and Pa_{O_2} on cerebral blood flow (CBF). (a) Note the increase in slope of the CBF/Pa_{CO_2} curve as basal CBF increases from 20 ml/100 g per min (white matter) to 50–70 ml/100 g per min (grey matter). (b) Note that maintenance of CBF with reductions in CPP is achieved by cerebral vasodilation, which results in reductions in cerebrovascular resistance. This results in an increase in cerebral blood volume (CBV), which has no detrimental effects in healthy subjects. These CBV increases may, however, result in critical increases in intracranial pressure (ICP) in patients with intracranial hypertension, who operate on the steep part of the intracranial pressure–volume curve.

257

has been demonstrated that symptoms of cerebral ischaemia appear when the MAP falls below 60% of an individual's lower autoregulatory threshold.[49] Generalised extrapolation from such individualised research data to the production of "safe" lower limits of MAP for general clinical practice is, however, hazardous for several reasons:

1 There may be wide individual scatter in rCBF autoregulatory efficiency, even in normal subjects.
2 The coexistence of fixed vascular obstruction (for example, carotid atheroma or vascular spasm) may vary the MAP level at which rCBF reaches critical levels in relevant territories.
3 The autoregulatory curve may be substantially modulated by the mechanisms used to produce hypotension. Earlier discussion made the distinction between reductions in CPP produced by haemorrhagic hypotension, intracranial hypertension, and pharmacological hypotension. The effects on autoregulation may also vary with the pharmacological agent used to produce hypotension. Thus, neuronal function is better preserved at similar levels of hypotension produced by halothane, nitroprusside, or isoflurane in comparison to trimethephan.[50]
4 Autoregulatory responses are not immediate: estimates of the latency for compensatory changes in rCVR range from 10 to 60 s.[51]

Some recent studies suggest that, especially in patients with impaired autoregulation, the cardiac output and pulsatility of large vessel flow may be more important determinants of rCBF than CPP itself.[52]

Arterial carbon dioxide tension

Cerebral blood flow is proportional to $Paco_2$, subject to a lower limit below which vasoconstriction results in tissue hypoxia and reflex vasodilatation, and an upper limit of maximal vasodilatation (Fig. 7.13a). On average, in the middle of the physiological range, each kiloPascal change in $Paco_2$ produces a change of about 15 ml/100 g per min in CBF. The slope of the $Paco_2$/CBF relationship depends, however, on the baseline normocapnic rCBF value, being maximal in areas where it is high (for example, grey matter; cerebrum) and least in areas where it is low, (for example white matter; cerebellum, and spinal cord). Moderate hypocapnia ($Paco_2$ of about 3·5 kPa) has long been used to reduce CBV in intracranial hypertension, but this practice is under review for two reasons:

1 The CO_2 response is directly related to the change in perivascular pH; consequently, the effect of a change in $Paco_2$ tends to be attenuated over time (hours) as brain extracellular fluid (ECF) bicarbonate levels fall to normalise interstitial pH.[53]
2 It has now been shown that "acceptable" levels of hypocapnia in head injured patients can result in dangerously low rCBF levels.[12 54]

Prostaglandins may mediate the vasodilation produced by CO_2;[55] more recent work suggests that nitric oxide may also be involved,[56] perhaps in a permissive capacity.[57]

Effects on CBV and ICP

Grubb et al[58] studied the CBF/$Paco_2$ response curve in primates and demonstrated that the CBF changed by approximately 1.8 ml/100 g per min for each change in $Paco_2$ of 1 mm Hg (133 Pa). In the same experiment, however, the CBV/$Paco_2$ curve was much flatter (about 0·4 ml/100 g per mm Hg [0·3 ml/100 g per kPa] change in $Paco_2$). It follows from these figures that, although a reduction in $Paco_2$ from 40 to 30 mm Hg (5·3 to 4 kPa) would result in about a 40% reduction in CBF (from a baseline of about 50 ml/100 g per min), it would only result in a 0·4% reduction in intracranial volume. This may seem trivial, but, in the presence of intracranial hypertension, the resultant 5 ml decrease in intracranial volume in an adult brain could result in a halving of ICP because the system operates on the steep part of the intracranial compliance curve.[59]

Arterial oxygen pressure and content

Classic teaching is that CBF is unchanged until $Paco_2$ levels fall below approximately 7 kPa, but rises sharply with further reductions[60] (see Fig. 7.13a). Recent TCD data from humans, however, suggest cerebral thresholds for cerebral vasodilatation as high as 8·5 kPa (about 89–90% arterial O_2 saturation or Sao_2).[61] This non-linear behaviour is because tissue oxygen delivery governs CBF; the sigmoid shape of the haemoglobin–O_2 dissociation curve means that the relationship between Cao_2 (arterial O_2 content) and CBF is inversely linear. These vasodilator responses to hypoxaemia appear to show little adaptation with time,[62] but may be substantially modulated by $Paco_2$ levels.[63 64] Nitric oxide does not appear to play a role in the vasodilatory response to hypoxia.[56]

Some studies suggest that hyperoxia may produce cerebral vasoconstriction, with a 10–14% reduction on CBF with inhalation of 85–100% O_2, and a 20% reduction in CBF with 100% O_2 at 3·5 atmospheres.[65] There are no human data to suggest that this effect is *clinically* significant.

Haematocrit

As in other organs, optimal O_2 delivery in the brain depends on a compromise between the oxygen carrying capacity and the flow characteristics of blood; previous experimental work suggests that this may be best achieved at a haemotocrit of about 40%. Some recent studies in the setting of vasospasm after subarachnoid haemorrhage have suggested that modest haemodilution to a haematocrit of 30–35% may improve neurological outcome by improving rheological characteristics[66] and increasing rCBF.

259

This may, however, result in a reduction in O_2 delivery if maximal vasodilatation is already present and, as clinical results in the setting of acute ischaemia have not been uniformly successful, this approach must be viewed with caution.

Autonomic nervous system

The autonomic nervous system mainly affects the larger cerebral vessels, up to and including the proximal parts of the anterior, middle, and posterior cerebral arteries. β_1-Adrenergic stimulation results in vasodilatation whereas α_2-adrenergic stimulation vasoconstricts these vessels. The effect of systemically administered α or β agonists is less significant. Significant vasoconstriction can, however, be produced by extremely high concentrations of catecholamines (for example, in haemorrhage) or centrally acting α_2 agonists (for example, dexmedetomidine).

Pharmacological modulation of CBF

Inhaled anaesthetics

All the potent fluorinated agents have significant effects on CBF and CMR. The initial popularity of halothane as a neurosurgical anaesthetic agent was reversed by the discovery that it was a potent cerebral vasodilator, producing decreases of 20–40% in cerebrovascular resistance in normocapnic individuals at 1·2–1·5 MAC (MAC = minimum alveolar concentration).[67 68] In another study, 1% halothane was shown to result in clinically significant elevations in ICP in patients with intracranial space occupying lesions.[69] Preliminary studies with enflurane and isoflurane suggested that these agents might produce smaller increases in cerebrovascular resistance (CVR) at equivalent doses.[70] As enflurane may produce epileptogenic activity, its use in the context of neuroanaesthesia decreased. Several studies, however, compared the effects of isoflurane and halothane on CBF, with conflicting results. Although some studies showed that halothane produced larger decreases in CVR, others found no difference. Examination of the patterns of rCBF produced by these two agents provides some clues to the origin of this discrepancy. Halothane selectively increases cortical rCBF, while markedly decreasing subcortical rCBF, whereas isoflurane produces a more generalised reduction in rCBF.[71 72] A review of published comparisons of the CBF effects of the two agents suggests that studies that estimated CBF using techniques that preferentially looked at the cortex (for example, ^{133}Xe wash-out) tended to show that halothane was a more potent vasodilator, whereas most studies that have used more global measures of hemispheric CBF (for example, the Kety–Schmidt technique) have found little difference between the two agents at levels of around 1 MAC (Fig. 7.14).

Both agents tend to reduce global CMR, but the regional pattern of such an effect may vary, with isoflurane producing greater cortical metabolic suppression[73] (reflected by its ability to produce EEG burst suppression at higher doses). Both the rCBF and rCMR effects of the two anaesthetics are markedly modified by baseline physiology and other pharmacological agents. Thus, CBF increases produced by both agents are attenuated by hypocapnia (more so with isoflurane[74 75]), and thiopental attenuates the relative preservation of cortical rCBF seen with halothane. It is difficult to predict accurately what the effect of either agent would be on CBF in a given clinical situation, but this would be a balance of its suppressant effects on rCMR (with autoregulatory vasoconstriction) and its direct vasodilator effect (which is partially mediated via both endothelial and neuronal nitric oxide).[56 76]

Although initial reports suggests that halothane could "uncouple" flow and metabolism,[76] more recent studies clearly show that at concentrations commonly in use for neuroanaesthesia (0·5–1 MAC) neither halothane[77] nor isoflurane[77 78] completely disrupts flow–metabolism coupling, although

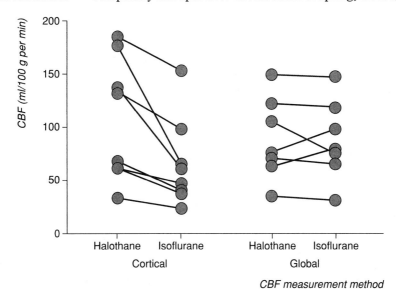

CBF measurement method

Fig 7.14 Comparison of mean ±SD CBF in animals anaesthetised with 0·5–1·5 MAC isoflurane or halothane, either in the same study or in comparable studies from a single research group with identical methodology within a single publication.[149–160] In studies shown on the left, CBF was estimated using techniques likely to be biased towards cortical flow (for example, ^{133}Xe wash-out) and shows that halothane produces greater increases in CBF. In studies on the right, CBF was estimated using techniques that measured global CBF (for example, the Kety–Schmidt method); the difference in effects on CBF between the two agents is much less prominent.

their vasodilator effects may alter the slope of this relationship. These vasodilator effects may become more prominent at higher concentrations.

In equi-MAC doses, nitrous oxide is probably a *more* powerful vasodilator than either halothane or isoflurane;[79 80] this fact, coupled with its lack of CMR depression,[81] produces a particularly unfavourable pharmaco-dynamic profile in patients with raised ICP.[82 83] Further, the vasodilatation produced by nitrous oxide is not decreased by hypocapnia,[84] although the resulting increases in ICP can be attenuated by the administration of other CMR depressants such as the barbiturates.[85]

Although initial studies suggested that desflurane[86] and sevoflurane[87] had effects on the cerebral vasculature that appear very similar to isoflurane, more recent studies have shown distinct differences between these agents.

Although high dose desflurane, like isoflurane, can produce EEG burst suppression, this effect may be attenuated over time.[88] It is not known whether this adaptation represents a pharmacokinetic or a pharmaco-dynamic effect. Initial clinical reports suggest that desflurane may cause a clinically significant rise in ICP in patients with supratentorial lesions,[89] despite its proven ability to reduce $CMRo_2$ as documented by EEG burst suppression.[88 90] These increases in ICP, which are presumably related to cerebral vasodilatation, appear to be independent of changes in systemic haemodynamics.[91]

In humans, sevoflurane produces some increase in TCD flow velocities at high doses (≥ 1.5 MAC), but these appear to be less marked than desflurane, and were reported to be unassociated with increases in ICP in patients with supratentorial space occupying lesions.[92] In other studies, 1.5 MAC sevoflurane caused no increase in middle cerebral artery flow velocities,[93] and did not affect CO_2 reactivity or pressure autoregulation.[94]

Intravenous anaesthetics

Thiopentone,[95] etomidate,[96] and propofol[97 98] all reduce global CMR to a minimum of approximately 50% of baseline, with a coupled reduction in CBF, although animal studies suggest small differences in the distribution of rCBF changes with individual agents. Decreases in CBV have been demonstrated with barbiturates[99] and probably occur with propofol and etomidate as well. Maximal reductions in CMR are reflected in an isoelectric EEG, although burst suppression is associated with only slightly less CMR depression.[95] Initial doubts that CBF reductions produced by propofol were secondary to falls in MAP have proved to be unfounded.[97 98]

Even high doses of thiopental or propofol[100] do not appear to affect autoregulation, CO_2 responsiveness, or flow–metabolism coupling.

Opioids

Although high doses (3 mg/kg) of morphine and moderate doses of fentanyl (15 μg/kg) have little effect on CBF and CMR, high doses of fentanyl (50–100 μg/kg)[101] and sufentanil[102] depress CMR and CBF. Results with alfentanil, in doses of 0·32 mg/kg, show no reduction in rCBF.[103] These effects are variable and may be prominent only in the presence of N_2O, where CMR may be reduced by 40% from baseline.[104] Bolus administration of large doses of fentanyl or alfentanil may be associated with increases in ICP in patients with intracranial hypertension,[105] probably as a result of reflex increases in CBF that follow an initial decrease in CBF (caused by reductions in MAP and cardiac output produced by large bolus doses of these agents). These effects are unlikely to be clinically significant if detrimental haemodynamic and blood gas changes can be avoided.

Other drugs

Ketamine can produce increases in global CBF and ICP,[106] with specific increases in rCMR and rCBF in limbic structures.[107] These changes may be partially attenuated by hypocapnia, benzodiazepines, or halothane.[108] Sedative doses of benzodiazepines tend to produce small decreases in CMR and CBF;[109] however, there is a ceiling effect and increasing doses do not produce greater reductions in these variables.[110] α_2 Agonists such as dexmedetomidine reduce CBF in humans.[111] There are good data, in animal models at least[112] to show that CBF reductions produced by intraventricular dexmedetomidine are probably direct vascular effects of the agent, and *not* exclusively the consequence of either systemic hypotension or coupled falls in rCBF arising from reductions in neuronal metabolism.

Most non-depolarising neuromuscular blockers have little effect on CBF or CMR, although large doses of *d*-tubocurarine may increase CBV and ICP secondary to histamine release and vasodilatation. In contrast, suxamethonium (succinylcholine) can produce increases in ICP, probably secondary to increases in CBF mediated via muscle spindle activation. These effects, however, are transient and mild[113 114] and can be blocked by prior precurarisation[115] if necessary; they provide no basis for avoiding suxamethonium in patients with raised ICP when its rapid onset of action is desirable for clinical reasons.

CBF in disease

Ischaemia

Graded reductions in CBF are associated with specific electrophysiological and metabolic consequences (Table 7.2). Some of these thresholds for metabolic events are well recognised, but others, such as the

263

Table 7.2 Electrophysiological and metabolic consequences of graded reductions in cerebral blood flow (CBF)

CBF (ml/100 g per min)	Electrophysiological/metabolic consequence
>50	Normal neuronal function
?	Immediate early gene activation
?	Cessation of protein synthesis
?	Cellular acidosis
20–23	Reduction in electrical activity
12–18	Cessation of electrical activity
8–10	ATP rundown, loss of ionic homoeostasis
<8	Cell death (also depends on other modifiers: duration, CMR, etc)

CMR, cerebral metabolic rate.

development of acidosis, cessation of protein synthesis, and the failure of osmotic regulation, have only recently received attention.[116] Ischaemia is thus a continuum between normal cellular function and cell death; cell death, however, is not merely a function of the severity of ischaemia, but is also dependent on its duration and several other circumstances that modify its effects. Thus, the effects of ischaemia may be ameliorated by the CMR depression produced by hypothermia or drugs, exacerbated by increased metabolic demand associated with excitatory neurotransmitter release, or compounded by other mechanisms of secondary neural injury (such as cellular calcium overload or reperfusion injury) (Fig. 7.15).

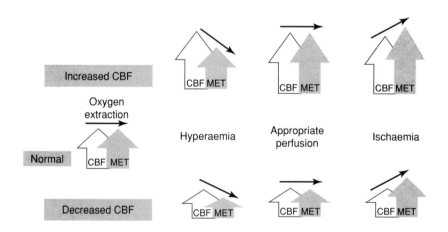

Fig 7.15 Relationship of cerebral blood flow (CBF) to the presence of ischaemia under conditions of varying metabolism. Changes in CBF levels compared with physiological levels may be misleading, because a diagnosis of ischaemia or hyperaemia demands that CBF levels be assessed in the context of metabolic requirements.

Head injury

Severe head injury is accompanied by both direct and indirect effects on CBF and metabolism, which show both temporal and spatial variations. CBF may be high, normal, or low soon after the ictus, but is typically reduced.[117] Of patients undergoing CBF studies within 6–8 hours of a head injury, 30% have significant cerebral ischaemia.[118] Global hypoperfusion in these studies was associated with a 100% mortality rate at 48 hours, and regional ischaemia with significant deficits. CBF patterns also vary with relation to the time after injury[116] (Fig. 7.16). Initial reductions are replaced, especially in patients who achieve good outcomes, by a period of relative increase in CBF, which towards the end of the first week post ictus may be replaced by reductions in CBF that are the consequence of vasospasm associated with subarachnoid haemorrhage.[120] CBF changes are non-uniform in the injured brain. Blood flow tends to be reduced in the immediate vicinity of intracranial contusions,[121] [122] and cerebral ischaemia associated with hyperventilation may be extremely regional and not reflected in global monitors of cerebrovascular adequacy[123] (Fig. 7.17).

Elevations in ICP result in reductions in CPP and cerebral ischaemia, which lead to secondary neuronal injury. There is strong evidence that maintenance of a CPP above 60 mm Hg improves outcome in patients with head injury and raised ICP.[124] Traditionally, patients with intracranial hypertension have been nursed head-up in an effort to reduce ICP. It is important to realise, however, that such manoeuvres will also reduce the effective MAP at the level of the head and run the risk of reducing CPP. Feldmann et al[125] suggest that a 30° head-up elevation may provide the optimal balance by reducing ICP without decreasing CPP.

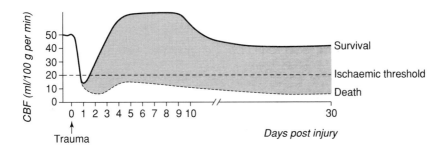

Fig 7.16 Spectrum of cerebral blood flow (CBF) patterns after severe head injury. Following an initial period of ischaemia lasting less than 24 hours, CBF begins to rise and may exceed normal values on days 2 to 4. CBF may fall to subnormal levels at later time points, chiefly as a result of the presence of vasospasm secondary to traumatic subarachnoid haemorrhage. CBF levels may never rise in some patients, especially those who have a poor outcome.

265

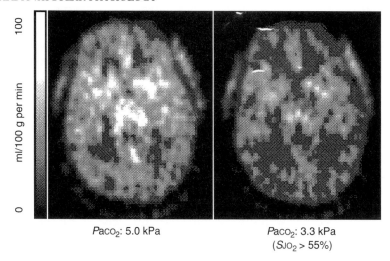

Pa_{CO_2}: 5.0 kPa Pa_{CO_2}: 3.3 kPa
($SJ_{O_2} > 55\%$)

Fig 7.17 PET image of cerebral blood flow (CBF) showing the effect of hyperventilation within the first 24 hours after head injury. Despite the maintenance of SJ_{O_2} values at acceptable levels, hyperventilation results in increases in the volume of brain tissue where CBF falls below recognised thresholds of ischaemia.

Hypertensive encephalopathy

Current concepts of the causation of hypertensive encephalopathy are based on the forced vasodilatation hypothesis.[126] Severe acute or sustained elevations in MAP overcome autoregulatory vasoconstriction in the resistance vessels and result in forced vasodilatation. These vasodilated vessels, exposed to high intraluminal pressures, leak fluid and protein and result in cerebral oedema, which is multifocal and later diffuse.

Subarachnoid haemorrhage

Cerebral autoregulation and CO_2 responsiveness are grossly distorted after subarachnoid haemorrhage (SAH), more so in patients in worse clinical grades[127] (Fig. 7.18). Such patients may be unable to compensate for reductions in MAP produced by anaesthetic agents and develop clinically significant deficits.[128] Clinically significant vasospasm after SAH occurs in up to 30–40%[129] of patients, typically several days after the initial bleed and may be caused by one or more of several mechanisms. NO may be taken up by haemoglobin in the extravasated blood or be inactivated to peroxynitrite ($ONOO^-$) by superoxide radicals (O^-) produced during ischaemia and reperfusion. Alternatively, spasm may be secondary to lipid peroxidation of the vessel wall by various oxidant species, including superoxide and peroxynitrite. Other authors have proposed a role for endothelin.[130 131] Vasospasm tends to be worst in patients with the largest

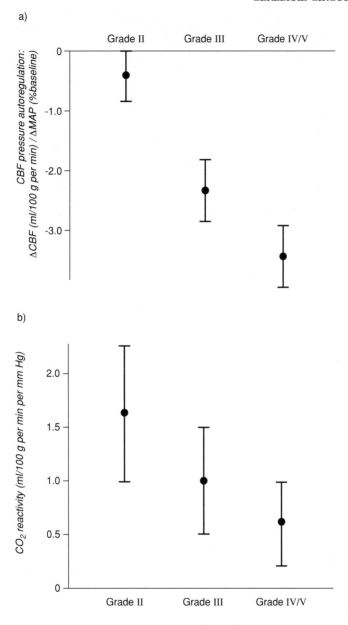

Fig 7.18 Effect of Hunt and Hess grade of aneurysmal subarachnoid haemorrhage on (a) pressure autoregulation and (b) cerebral blood flow (CBF) reactivity to changes in Pa_{CO_2}.

amounts of subarachnoid blood,[132] suggesting that the blood itself contributes to the phenomenon. Vasospasm is associated with parallel reductions in rCBF and $CMRo_2$ in the regions affected.

The clinical impact of late vasospasm has been substantially modified by the routine use of Ca^{2+} channel blockers such as nimodipine[133] and by the routine use of hypertensive hypervolaemic haemodilution[134] (triple H therapy). Triple H (3H) therapy involves the use of colloid administration (with venesection if needed) to increase filling pressures and reduce haematocrit to 30–35%. If moderate hypertension is not achieved with volume loading, vasopressors and inotropes are used to maintain mean blood pressures as high as 120–140 mm Hg. The hypertensive element of this therapy protects non-autoregulating portions of the cerebral vasculature from hypoperfusion, whereas the haemodilution improves rheological characteristics of blood and facilitates flow through vessels whose calibre is reduced by spasm. Such interventions have been shown to produce clinically useful improvements in rCBF in regions of ischaemia.[135]

Mechanisms in rCBF control

Some of the mechanisms involved in cerebrovascular control are shown in Fig. 7.19. Several of these have been referred to earlier. In addition, the level of free Ca^{2+} is important in determining vascular tone, and arachidonate metabolism can produce prostanoids that are either vasodilators (for example, prostacyclin, PGI_2) or vasoconstrictive (for example, thromboxane, TxA_2). Endothelin (ET), produced by endothelin converting enzyme (ECE) in endothelial cells, balances the vasodilator effects of nitric oxide in a tonic matter by exerting its influences at ET_A receptors in the vascular smooth muscle.

Nitric oxide in the regulation of cerebral haemodynamics[56]

Recent interest has focused on the role of NO in the control of cerebral haemodynamics. NO is synthesised in the brain from the amino acid L-arginine by the constitutive form of the enzyme nitric oxide synthase (NOS). This form of the enzyme is calmodulin-dependent and requires Ca^{2+} and tetrahydrobiopterin for its activity; it differs from the inducible form of the enzyme, which is present in mononuclear blood cells and is activated by cytokines. Under basal conditions, endothelial cells synthesise NO which diffuses into the muscular layer and, via a cGMP-mediated mechanism, produces relaxation of vessels. There is strong evidence to suggest that NO exerts a tonic dilatory influence on cerebral vessels. It is important to emphasise that data on NO obtained from peripheral vessels cannot always be translated to the cerebral vasculature; for example, some of the endothelium derived relaxant factor (EDRF) activity in cerebral vessels may be caused by compounds other than NO. There is growing evidence that carbon monoxide (CO), produced by haem oxygenase, may be responsible for significant cerebral vasodilatation, especially when NO production is reduced.[136]

Nitric oxide plays an important role in cerebrovascular responses to functional activation, excitatory amino acids, hypercapnia, ischaemia, and SAH. Further, NO may play an important part in mediating the vasodilatation produced by volatile anaesthetic agents,[56] although other mechanisms, including a direct effect on the vessel wall, cannot be excluded.

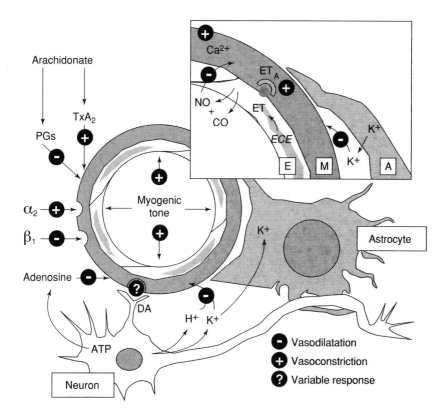

Fig 7.19 Mechanisms involved in the regulation of regional cerebral blood flow (rCBF) in health and disease. The diagram shows a resistance vessel in the brain in the vicinity of a neuron (N) and an astrocyte (A). Other abbreviations: E, endothelium; M, muscular layer; PGs = prostaglandins; TxA_2, thromboxane A_2; ET, endothelin; ECE, endothelin converting enzyme; ET_A, ET_A receptor; NO, nitric oxide; CO, carbon monoxide; DA, dopamine. The inset box shows the detail of the vessel wall and adjacent glial cell process. See text for details.

CARDIOVASCULAR PHYSIOLOGY

Neurogenic flow–metabolism coupling

Although the last 10 years have focused on flow–metabolism coupling being effected by a diffusable extracellular mediator, there is now accumulating evidence to suggest that dopaminergic neurons may play a major part in such events, and in addition may control blood–brain barrier permeability.[137]

1 Edvinsson L, Mackenzie ET, McCulloch J. The aged brain. In: *Cerebral blood flow and metabolism*. New York: Raven Press, 1993:647–60.
2 Alpers BJ, Berry RG, Paddison RM. Anatomical studies in the circle of Willis in normal brains. *Arch Neurol Psychiatry* 1959;**81**:409–18.
3 Collins RC. Intracortical localization of 2-deoxyglucose metabolism on-off metabolic columns. In: Passonneau JV, Hawkins RA, Lust WD, Welsh FA, eds, *Cerebral metabolism and neural function*. Baltimore: Williams & Wilkins, 1980:338–51.
4 Welsh FA. Regional evaluation of ischaemic metabolic alterations. *J Cereb Blood Flow Metab* 1984;**4**:309–16.
5 Pulsinelli WA, Duffy TE. Local cerebral glucose metabolism during controlled hypoxaemia in rats. *Science* 1979;**204**:626–9.
6 Duning HS, Wolff HG. The relative vascularity of various parts of the central and peripheral nervous system in the cat and its relation to function. *J Comp Neurol* 1937;**67**:433–50.
7 Sokoloff L, Reivich M, Kennedy C, et al. The [^{14}C]-deoxyglucose method for measurement of local cerebral glucose utilization: Theory, procedure, and normal values in the conscious and anesthetized albino rat. *J Neurochem* 1977;**28**:897–916.
8 Göbel U, Theilen H, Kuschinsky W. Congruence of total and perfused capillary network in rat brains. *Circ Res* 1990;**66**:271–81.
9 Kuschinsky W, Paulson OB. Capillary circulation in the brain. [Review]. *Cerebrovasc Brain Metabol Rev* 1992;**4**:261–86.
10 Beards SC, Yule S, Kassner A, Jackson A. Anatomical variation of cerebral venous drainage: the theoretical effect on jugular bulb blood samples. *Anaesthesia* 1998;**53**:627–33.
11 Shapiro K, Marmarou A, Shulman K. Characterization of clinical CSF dynamics and neural axis compliance using the pressure-volume index. I. The normal pressure–volume index. *Ann Neurol* 1980;**7**:508–13.
12 Chesnut RM. Hyperventilation in traumatic brain injury: Friend or foe? *Crit Care Med* 1997;**25**:1275–8.
13 Todd MM, Weeks J. Comparative effect of propofol, pentobarbital and isoflurane on cerebral blood flow and volume. *J Neurosurg Anesthesiol* 1996;**8**:296–303.
14 Janzer RC, Raff MC. Astrocytes induce blood–brain barrier properties in endothelial cells. *Nature* 1987;**325**:253–7.
15 Oldendorf WH. Lipid solubility and drug penetration of the blood brain barrier. *Proc Soc Exp Biol Med* 1974;**147**:813–16.
16 Oldendorf WH, Cornford ME, Brown WJ. The large apparent work capability of the blood brain barrier. A study of the mitochondrial content of capillary endothelial cells in brain and other tissues of the rat. *Ann Neurol* 1977;**1**:409–17.
17 Kety SS and Schmidt CF. The determination of cerebral blood flow in man by use of nitrous oxide in low concentrations. *Am J Physiol* 1945;**143**:53–66.
18 Ingvar DH, Lassen NA. Quantitative determination of regional cerebral blood flow in man. *Lancet* 1961;**ii**:806–7.
19 Prough DS, Stump DA, Roy RC, et al. Response of cerebral blood flow to changes in carbon dioxide tension during hypothermic cardiopulmonary bypass. *Anesthesiology* 1986;**64**:576–81.

20 Mallett BL, Veall N. Investigation of cerebral blood flow in hypertension, using radioactive xenon inhalation and extracranial recording. *Lancet* 1963;**i**:1081–2.

21 Cruz J, Raps EC, Hoffstad OJ, Jaggi JL, Gennarelli TA. Cerebral oxygenation monitoring [Review]. *Crit Care Med* 1993;**21**:1242–6.

22 Bodenham A, Webster NR. New practical beside procedures on the intensive care unit. *Ballière's Clin Anesthesiol* 1992;**6**:425–41.

23 Mayberg TS, Lam AM. Management of central nervous system trauma. *Curr Opin Anaesthesiol* 1993;**6**:764–71.

24 Faught E. Current role of electroencephalography in cerebral ischaemia [Review]. *Stroke* 1993;**24**:609–13.

25 Zentner J, Schramm J. Monitoring the central nervous system. *Curr Opin Anaesthesiol* 1993; **6**:784–90.

26 Wyatt JS. Noninvasive assessment of cerebral oxidative metabolism in the human newborn [Review]. *J R Coll Phys Lond* 1994;**28**:126–32.

27 Bolognese P, Miller JI, Heger IM, Milhorat TH. Laser-Doppler flowmetry in neuro-surgery [Review]. *J Neurosurg Anesthesiol* 1993;**5**:151–8.

28 Bishop CCR, Powell S, Rutt D, et al. Transcranial Doppler measurement of the middle cerebral flow velocity: A validation study. *Stroke* 1986; **17**:913–15.

29 Dahl A, Russell D, Nyberg-Hanson R, et al. A comparison of regional cerebral blood flow and middle cerebral artery flow velocities:simultaneous measurements in healthy subjects. *J Cereb Blood Flow Metab* 1992;**12**:1049–54.

30 Matta BBF, Lam AM. Isoflurane and desflurane do not dilate the middle cerebral artery appreciably (Abstract). *Br J Anaesth* 1995;**74**:486–7P.

31 Menon DK. Monitoring the central nervous system. *Curr Anaesth Crit Care* 1997;**6**:254–63.

32 Czosnyka M, Matta BF, Smielewski P, et al. Cerebral perfusion pressure in head-injured patients: a noninvasive assessment using transcranial Doppler ultrasonography. *J Neurosurg* 1998;**88**:802–8.

33 Metz C, Holzschuh M, Bein T, et al. Monitoring of cerebral oxygen metabolism in the jugular bulb: Reliability of unilateral measurements in severe head injury. *J Cereb Blood Flow Metab* 1998;**18**:332–43.

34 Cruz J. The first decade of continuous monitoring of jugular bulb oxyhemoglobin saturation: management strategies and clinical outcome. *Crit Care Med* 1998;**26**344–51.

35 Shienberg M, Kanter MJ, Robertson CS, et al. Continuous monitoring of jugular venous oxygen saturation in head-injured patients. *J Neurosurg* 1992;**76**:212–17.

36 Fox PT, Raichle ME, Mintun MA, Dence C. Nonoxidative glucose consumption during focal physiologic neural activity. *Science* 1988;**241**:462–4.

37 Tsacopoulos M, Magistretti PJ. Metabolic coupling between glia and neurons. *J Neurosci* 1996;**16**:877–85.

38 Pellerin L, Magistretti PJ. Glutamate uptake into astrocytes stimulates anaerobic glycolysis: a mechanism coupling neuronal activity to glucose utilization. *Proc Natl Acad Sci USA* 1994;**91**:10625–9.

39 Edvinsson L, Mackenzie ET, McCulloch J. Perivascular nerve fibres in brain vessels. In: *Cerebral blood flow and metabolism.* New York: Raven Press, 1993:57–91.

40 Kontos HA. Nitric oxide and nitrosothiols in cerebrovascular and neuronal regulation [Review]. *Stroke* 1993;**24**:1155–8.

41 Miller JD, Stanek A, Langfitt TW. Concepts of cerebral perfusion pressure and vascular compression during intracranial hypertension. *Prog Brain Res* 1972;**35**:411–32.

42 Miller JD, Stanek AE, Langfitt TW. Cerebral blood flow regulation during experimental brain compression. *J Neurosurg* 1973;**39**:186–96.

43 Fitch W, MacKenzie ET, Harper AM. Effects of decreasing arterial blood pressure on cerebral blood flow in the baboon: Influence of the sympathetic nervous system. *Circ Res* 1975;**37**:550–7.

44 Heistad DD, Marcus ML, Sandberg S, Abboud FM. Effect of sympathetic nerve stimulation on cerebral blood flow and on large cerebral arteries of dogs. *Circ Res* 1977;**41**:342–50.

45 Thomas D, Bannister RG. Preservation of autoregulation of cerebral blood flow in autonomic failure. *J Neurol Sci* 1980;**44**:205–12.

271

46 Strandgaard S, Olesen J, Skinhoj E, Jassen NA. Autoregulation of brain circulation in severe arterial hypertension. *BMJ* 1973;**1**:507–10.

47 Thompson BG, Pluta RM, Girton ME, Oldfield EH. Nitric oxide mediation of chemoregulation but not autoregulation of cerebral blood flow in primates. *J Neurosurg* 1996;**84**:71–8.

48 Bentsen N, Larsen B, Lassen NA. Chronically impaired autoregulation of cerebral blood flow in long-term diabetes. *Stroke* 1975;**6**:497–502.

49 Strandgaard S. Autoregulation of CBF in hypertensives. The modifying influence of prolonged antihypertensive treatment on the tolerance to acute, drug induced hypotension. *Circulation* 1976;**53**:720–7.

50 Michenfelder JD, Theye RA. Canine systemic and cerebral effects of hypotension induced by hemorrhage, trimethaphan, halothane, or nitroprusside. *Anesthesiology* 1977; **46**:188–95.

51 Aaslid R, Lindegaard K-F, Sorteberg W, Nornes H. Cerebral autoregulation dynamics in humans. *Stroke* 1989;**20**:45–52.

52 Davis DH, Sundt TM Jr. Relationship of cerebral blood flow to cardiac output, mean arterial pressure, blood volume, and alpha and beta blockade in cats. *J Neurosurg* 1980;**52**:745–54.

53 Koehler RC, Traystman RJ. Bicarbonate ion modulation of cerebral blood flow during hypoxia and hypercapnia. *Am J Physiol* 1982;**243**:H33–40.

54 Stringer WA, Hasso AN, Thompson JR, Hinshaw DB, Jordan KG. Hyperventilation-induced cerebral ischaemia in patients with acute brain lesions: demonstration by Xenon-enhanced CT. *Am J Neuroradiol* 1993;**14**:465–84.

55 Pickard JD, MacKenzie ET. Inhibition of prostaglandin synthesis and the response of baboon cerebral circulation to carbon dioxide. *Nature (New Biol)* 1973;**245**:187–8.

56 Maktabi MA. Role of nitric oxide in regulation of cerebral circulation in health and disease. *Curr Opinion Anaesthesiol* 1993;**6**:799–83.

57 Okamoto H, Hudetz AG, Roman RJ, et al. JP Neuronal NOS-derived NO plays permissive role in cerebral blood flow response to hypercapnia. *Am J Physiol* 1997;**272**:H559–66.

58 Grubb RL Jr, Raichle ME, Eichling JO, Ter-Pogossian MM. The effects of changes in $PaCO_2$ on cerebral blood volume, blood flow and vascular mean transit time. *Stroke* 1974;**5**:630–9.

59 Kosteljanetz M. Acute head injury: pressure-volume relations and cerebrospinal fluid dynamics. *Neurosurgery* 1986;**18**:17–24.

60 McDowall DG. Interrelationships between blood oxygen tension and cerebral blood flow. In: Payne JP, Hill DW, eds, *Oxygen measurements in blood and tissues*. London: Churchill, 1966:205–14.

61 Gupta AK, Menon DK, Czosnyka M, et al. Thresholds for hypoxic cerebral vasodilatation in volunteers. *Anesth Analg* 1997;**85**:817–20.

62 Krasney JA, Jensen JB, Lassen NA. Cerebral blood flow does not adapt to sustained hypoxia. *J Cereb Blood Flow Metab* 1990;**10**:759–64.

63 Krasney JA, McDonald B, Matalon S. Regional circulatory responses to 96 hours of hypoxia in conscious sheep. *Respir Physiol* 1984;**57**:73–88.

64 Krasney JA, Hajduczok G, Miki K, Matalon S. Peripheral circulatory responses to 96 hours of eucapnic hypoxia in conscious sheep. *Respir Physiol* 1985;**59**:197–211.

65 Purves MJ. *The physiology of the cerebral circulation*. Cambridge: Cambridge University Press, 1972.

66 Adams HP. Prevention of brain ischaemia after aneurysmal subarachnoid haemorrhage. *Neurol Clin* 1992;**10**:251–68.

67 Christensen MS, Hoedt-Rasmussen K, Lassen NA. Cerebral vasodilatation by halothane anesthesia in man and its potentiation by hypotension and hypercapnia. *Br J Anaesth* 1967;**39**:927–31.

68 Wollman H, Alexander SC, Cohen PJ, Chase PE, Melman E, Behar MG. Cerebral circulation of man during halothane anesthesia. Effects of hypocarbia and of d-tubocurarine. *Anesthesiology* 1964;**25**:180–4.

69 Jennett WB, Barker J, Fitch W, McDowall DG. Effects of anaesthesia on intracranial pressure in patients with space-occupying lesions. *Lancet* 1969;**i**:61–4.

70 Murphy FL, Kennell EM, Johnstone RE. The effects of enflurane, isoflurane, and halothane on cerebral blood flow and metabolism in man. Abstracts of the Meeting of The American Society of Anesthesiologists 1974:61–2.

71 Hansen TD, Warner DS, Todd MM, Vust LJ, Trawick DC. Distribution of cerebral blood flow during halothane versus isoflurane anesthesia in rats. *Anesthesiology* 1988;**69**:332–7.

72 Hansen TD, Warner DS, Todd MM, Vust LJ. Effects of nitrous oxide and volatile anaesthetics on cerebral blood flow. *Br J Anaesth* 1989;**63**:290–5.

73 Scheller MS, Todd MM, Drummond JC. Isoflurane, halothane and regional cerebral blood flow at various levels of $PaCO_2$ in rabbits. *Anesthesiology* 1986;**64**:598–604.

74 Drummond JC, Todd MM. The response of the feline cerebral circulation to $PaCO_2$ during anesthesia with isoflurane and halothane and during sedation with nitrous oxide. *Anesthesiology* 1985;**62**:268–73.

75 Okamoto H, Meng W, Ma J et al. Isoflurane-induced cerebral hyperaemia in neuronal nitric oxide synthase gene deficient mice. *Anesthesiology* 1997;**86**:875–84.

76 Kuramoto T, Oshita S, Takeshita H, Ishikawa T. Modification of the relationship between cerebral metabolism, blood flow, and the EEG by stimulation during anesthesia in the dog. *Anesthesiology* 1979;**51**:211–17.

77 Hansen TD, Warner DS, Todd MM, Vust LJ. The role of cerebral metabolism in determining the local cerebral blood flow effects of volatile anaesthetics: evidence for persistent flow–metabolism coupling. *J Cereb Blood Flow Metab* 1989;**9**:323–8.

78 Maekawa T, Tommasino C, Shapiro HM, Kiefer-Goodman J, Kohlenberger RW. Local cerebral blood flow and glucose utilisation during isoflurane anesthesia in the rat. *Anesthesiology* 1986;**65**:144–51.

79 Sakabe T, Kuramoto T, Kumagae S, Takeshita H. Cerebral responses to the addition of nitrous oxide to halothane in man. *Br J Anaesth* 1976;**48**:957–62.

80 Lam AM, Mayberg TS, Eng CC, Cooper JO, Bachenberg LK, Mathisen TL. Nitrous oxide-isoflurane anesthesia causes more cerebral vasodilation than an equipotent dose of isoflurane in humans. *Anesth Analg* 1994;**78**:462–8.

81 Reasoner D, Warner DS, Todd MM, McAllister A. Effects of nitrous oxide on cerebral metabolic rate in rats anaesthetized with isoflurane. *Br J Anaesth* 1990;**65**:210–15.

82 Henriksen HT, Jorgensen PB. The effect of nitrous oxide on intracranial pressure in patients with intracranial disorders. *Br J Anaesth* 1973;**45**:486–92.

83 Moss E, McDowall DG. ICP increases with 50% nitrous oxide in oxygen in severe head injuries with controlled ventilation. *Br J Anaesth* 1979;**51**:757–61.

84 Kaieda R, Todd MM, Warner DS. The effects of anaesthetics and $PaCO_2$ on the cerebrovascular, metabolic, and electroencephalographic responses to nitrous oxide in the rabbit. *Anesth Analg* 1989;**68**:135–43.

85 Phirman JR, Shapiro HM. Modification of nitrous oxide induced intracranial hypertension by prior induction of anaesthesia. *Anesthesiology* 1977;**46**:150–1.

86 Young WL. Effects of desflurane on the central nervous system. *Anesth Analg* 1992;**75**(suppl 4):32–7.

87 Scheller MS, Tateishi A, Drummond JC, Zornow MH. The effects of sevoflurane on cerebral blood flow, cerebral metabolic rate for oxygen, intracranial pressure and the electroencephalogram are similar to those of isoflurane in the rabbit. *Anesthesiology* 1988;**68**:548–51.

88 Lutz LJ, Milde JH, Milde LN. The cerebral functional, metabolic, and hemodynamic effects of desflurane in dogs. *Anesthesiology* 1990;**73**:125–31.

89 Muzzi DA, Losasso TJ, Dietz NM, Faust RJ, Cucchiara RF, Milde LN. The effect of desflurane and isoflurane on cerebrospinal fluid pressure in humans with supratentorial mass lesions. *Anesthesiology* 1992;**76**:720–4.

90 Rampil IJ, Lockhart SH, Eger EI, Weiskopf RB. Human EEG dose response to desflurane. *Anesthesiology* 1990;**73**:A1218.

91 Tonner PH, Scholz J, Krause T, Paris A, von Knobelsdroff G, Schulte an Esch J. Administration of sufentanil and nitrous oxide blunts cardiovascular responses to desflurane but does not prevent an increase in middle cerebral artery flow velocity. *Eur J Anaesthesiol* 1997;**14**:389–96.

92 Bundgaard H, von Oettingen G, Larsen KM, et al. Effects of sevoflurane on intracranial pressure, cerebral blood flow and cerebral metabolism. A dose–response study in patients subjected to craniotomy for cerebral tumours. *Acta Anaesthesiol Scand* 1998;**42**:621–7.

93 Heath KJ, Gupta S, Matta BF. The effects of sevoflurane on cerebral heamodynamics during propofol anesthesia. *Anesth Analg* 1997;**85**:1284–7.

94 Gupta S, Heath K, Matta BF. Effect of incremental doses of sevoflurane on cerebral pressure autoregulation in humans. *Br J Anaesth* 1997;**79**:469–72.

95 Kassel NF, Hitchon PW, Gerk MK, Sokoll MD, Hill TR. Alterations in cerebral blood flow, oxygen metabolism, and electrical activity produced by high dose sodium thiopental. *Neurosurgery* 1980;**7**:598–603.

96 Milde LN, Milde JH, Michenfelder JD. Cerebral functional, metabolic, and haemodynamic effects of etomidate in dogs. *Anesthesiology* 1985;**63**:371–7.

97 Ramani R, Todd MM, Warner DS. The cerebrovascular, metabolic and electroencephalographic effects of propofol in the rabbit – a dose response study. *J Neurosurg Anesth* 1992;**4**:110–19.

98 Van Hemelrijck J, Van Aken H, Plets C, Goffin J, Vermaut G. The effects of propofol on intracranial pressure and cerebral perfusion pressure in patients with brain tumours. *Acta Anaesthesiol Belg* 1989;**40**:95–100.

99 Weeks J, Todd MM, Warner DS, Katz J. The influence of halothane, isoflurane, and pentobarbital on cerebral plasma volume in hypocapnic and normocapnic rats. *Anesthesiology* 1990;**73**:461–6.

100 Fox J, Gelb AW, Enns J, Murkin JM, Farrar JK, Manninen PH. The responsiveness of cerebral blood flow to changes in arterial carbon dioxide is maintained during propofol–nitrous oxide anesthesia in humans. *Anesthesiology* 1992;**77**:453–6.

101 Carlsson C, Smith DS, Keykhah MM, Englebach I, Harp JR. The effects of high dose fentanyl on cerebral circulation and metabolism in rats. *Anesthesiology* 1982;**57**:375–80.

102 Keykhah MM, Smith DS, Carlsson C, Safo Y, Englebach I, Harp JR. Influence on sufentanil on cerebral metabolism and circulation in the rat. *Anesthesiology* 1985;**63**:274–80.

103 McPherson RW, Krempasanka E, Eimerl D, Traystman RJ. Effects of alfentanil on cerebral vascular reactivity in dogs. *Br J Anaesth* 1985;**57**:1232–8.

104 Murkin JM, Ferrar JK, Tweed WA, McKenzie FN, Guiraudon G. Cerebral autoregulation and flow/metabolism coupling during cardiopulmonary bypass: the influence of $PaCO_2$. *Anesth Analg* 1987;**66**:825–32.

105 Sperry RJ, Bailey PL, Reichman MV, Peterson PB, Pace NL. Fentanyl and sufentanil increase intracranial pressure in head trauma patients. *Anesthesiology* 1992;**77**:416–20.

106 Åkeson J, Böjrkman S, Messeter K, Rosén I, Helfer M. Cerebral pharmacodynamics of anaesthetic and subanaesthetic doses of ketamine in the normoventilated pig. *Acta Anaesthesiol Scand* 1993;**37**:211–18.

107 Davis DW, Mans AM, Biebuyck JF, Hawkins RA. The influence of ketamine on regional brain glucose use. *Anesthesiology* 1988;**69**:199–205.

108 Menon DK, Burdett NG, Carpenter TA, Hall LD. Functional MRI of ketamine-induced changes in rCBF: An effect at the NMDA receptor? [Abstract]. *Br J Anaesth* 1993;**7**:767.

109 Forster A, Juge O, Morel D. Effects of midazolam on cerebral blood flow in human volunteers. *Anesthesiology* 1982;**56**:453–5.

110 Fleischer JE, Milde JH, Moyer TP, Michenfelder JD. Cerebral effects of high-dose midazolam and subsequent reversal with RO 15–1788 in dogs. *Anesthesiology* 1988;**68**:234–42.

111 Zornow MH, Fleischer JE, Scheller MS et al. Dexmedetomidine and alpha 2-adrenergic agonist, decreases cerebral blood flow in the isoflurane anesthetised dog. *Anesth Analg* 1990; **70**:624–30.

112 McPherson RW, Koehler RC, Kirsch JR, Traystman RJ. Intraventricular dexmedetomidine decreases cerebral blood flow during normoxia and hypoxia in dogs. *Anesth Analg* 1997;**84**:139–47.

113 Ducey JP, Deppe AS, Foley FT. A comparison of the effects of suxamethonium, atracurium and vecuronium on intracranial haemodynamics in swine. *Anaesth Intensive Care* 1989;**17**:448–55.

114 Kovarik WD, Lam AM, Slee TA, Mathisen TL. The effect of succinylcholine on intracranial pressure, cerebral blood flow velocity and electroencephalogram in patients with neurologic disorders [Abstract]. *Anesthesiology* 1991;**75**:207.

115 Stirt AJ, Grosslight KR, Bedford RF, Vollmer D. "Defasciculation" with metocurine prevents succinylcholine-induced increases in intracranial pressure. *Anesthesiology* 1987;**67**:50–3.

116 Siesjo BK. Pathophysiology and treatment of focal cerebral ischaemia. Part I: Pathophysiology. *J Neurosurg* 1992;**77**:169–84.

117 Robertson CS, Contant CF, Gokaslan ZL, Narayan RK, Grossman RG. Cerebral blood flow, arteriovenous oxygen difference, and outcome in head injured patients. *J Neurol Neurosurg Psychiatry* 1992; **55**:594–603.

118 Bouma GJ, Muizelaar JP, Stringer WA, Choi SC, Fatouros P, Young HF. Ultra early evaluation of regional cerebral blood flow in severely head-injured patients using Xenon-enhanced computerized tomography. *J Neurosurg* 1992;**77**:360–9.

119 Martin NA, Patwardhan RV, Alexander MJ, et al. Characterization of cerebral hemodynamic phases following severe head trauma: hypoperfusion, hyperaemia and vasospasm. *J Neurosurg* 1997;**87**:9–19.

120 Martin NA, Doberstein C, Zane C, Caron MJ, Thomas K, Becker DP. Posttraumatic cerebral arterial spasm: transcranial Doppler ultrasound, cerebral blood flow and angiographic findings. *J Neurosurg* 1992;**77**:575–83.

121 Marion DW, Darby J, Yonas H. Acute regional cerebral blood flow changes caused by severe head injuries. *J Neurosurg* 1991;**74**:407–14.

122 McLaughlin MR, Marion DW. Cerebral blood flow within and around cerebral contusions. *J Neurosurg* 1996;**85**:871–6.

123 Menon DK, Minhas P, Herrod NJ, et al. Cerebral ischaemia associated with hyperventilation: a PET study. *Anesthesiology* 1997;**87**:A176.

124 Chan KH, Dearden NM, Miller JD, Andrews PJ, Midgley S. Multimodality monitoring as a guide to treatment of intracranial hypertension after severe brain injury. *Neurosurgery* 1993;**32**:547–52.

125 Feldman Z, Kanter MJ, Robertson CS, et al. Effect of head elevation on intracranial pressure, cerebral perfusion pressure and cerebral blood flow in head injured patients. *J Neurosurg* 1992;**76**:207–11.

126 Lassen NA, Agnoli A. The upper limit of autoregulation of cerebral blood flow on the pathogenesis of hypertensive encephalopathy. *Scand J Clin Lab Invest* 1973;**30**:113–16.

127 Voldby B, Enevoldsen EM, Jensen FT. Cerebrovascular reactivity in patients with ruptured intracranial aneurysm. *J Neurosurg* 1985;**62**:59–67.

128 Pickard JD, Matheson M, Patterson J, Wyper D. Prediction of late ischemic complications after cerebral aneurysm surgery by the intraoperative measurement of cerebral blood flow. *J Neurosurg* 1980;**53**:305–8.

129 Kassell NF, Peerless SJ, Durward QJ, Beck DW, Drake CG, Adams HP. Treatment of ischaemic deficits from vasospasm with intravascular volume expansion and induced arterial hypertension. *Neurosurgery* 1982;**11**:337–43.

130 Yamaura I, Tani E, Maeda Y, Minami N, Shindo H. Endothelin-1 of canine basilar artery in vasospasm. *J Neurosurg* 1992;**76**:99–105.

131 Clozel M, Watanabe H. BQ-123, a peptidic endothelin ET_A receptor antagonist, prevents the early cerebral vasospasm following subarachnoid hemorrhage after intracisternal but not intravenous injection. *Life Sci* 1993;**52**:825–34.

132 Jakobsen M, Skjødt T, Enevoldsen E. Cerebral blood flow and metabolism following subarachnoid hemorrhage: effect of subarachnoid blood. *Acta Neurol Scand* 1991;**8**:226–33.

133 Pickard JD, Murray GD, Illingworth R, et al. Effect of oral nimodipine on cerebral infarction and outcome after subarachnoid hemorrhage: British aneurysm nimodipine trial. *BMJ* 1989;**298**:636–42.

134 Origitano TC, Wascher TM, Reichman OH, Anderson DE. Sustained increased cerebral blood flow with prophylactic hypervolemic haemodilution ("Triple-H" Therapy) after subarachnoid haemorrhage. *Neurosurgery* 1990;**27**:729–38.

135 Darby JM, Yonas H, Marks EC, Durham S, Snyder RW, Nemoto EM. Acute cerebral blood flow response to dopamine-induced hypertension after subarachnoid hemorrhage. *J Neurosurg* 1994;**80**:857–64.

136 Zakhary R, Gaine SP, Dinennan JL, et al. Heme oxygenase 2: Endothelial and neuronal localisation and role in endothelial-dependent relaxation. *Proc Natl Acad Sci USA* 1996;**93**:795–8.

137 Iadecola C. Neurogenic control of the cerebral microcirculation: is dopamine minding the store? *Nature Neurosci* 1998;**1**:363–4.

138 Yonas H, Gur D, Latchaw RE, Wolfson SK. Xenon computed tomographic blood flow mapping. In: Wood JH, ed, *Cerebral blood flow. Physiologic and clinical aspects.* New York: McGraw-Hill, 1987:220–42.

139 Miles KA, Hayball M, Dixon AK. Colour perfusion imaging: a new application of computed tomography. *Lancet* 1991;**337**:643–5.

140 Herscovitch MD, Powers WJ. measurement of regional cerebral blood flow by positron emission tomography. In: Wood JH, ed, *Cerebral blood flow. Physiologic and clinical aspects.* New York: McGraw Hill, 1987:257–71.

141 Holman BL, Hill TC. Perfusion imaging with single-photon emission computed tomography. In: Wood JH, ed, *Cerebral blood flow. Physiologic and clinical aspects.* New York: McGraw-Hill, 1987:243–56.

142 Elwell CE, Owen-Reece H, Cope M, et al. Measurement of adult cerebral haemodynamics using near infrared spectroscopy. *Acta Neurochir* 1993;suppl 59:74–80.

143 Farrar JK. Hydrogen clearance technique. In: Wood JH, ed, *Cerebral blood flow. Physiologic and clinical aspects.* New York: McGraw-Hill, 1987:275–87.

144 Ginsburg MD. Autoradiographic measurement of local cerebral blood flow. In: Wood JH, ed, *Cerebral blood flow. Physiologic and clinical aspects.* New York: McGraw-Hill, 1987:299–308.

145 Warner DS, Kassell NF, Boarini DJ. Microsphere cerebral blood flow determination. In: Wood JH, ed, *Cerebral blood flow. Physiologic and clinical aspects.* New York: McGraw-Hill, 1987:288–98.

146 Pritchard JW, Rosen BR. Functional study of the brain by NMR. *J Cereb Blood Flow Metab* 1994;**14**:365–72.

147 Newell DW, Aaslid R, eds, *Transcranial Doppler.* New York: Raven Press, 1992.

148 Menon DK, Peden CJ, Hall AS, Sargentoni J, Whitwam JG. Magnetic resonsance for the anaesthetist: Part I: Principles, applications, safety aspects. *Anaesthesia* 1992;**47**:240–55.

149 Madsen JB, Cold GE, Eriksen HO, Eskesen V, Blatt-Lyon B. CBF and CMRo$_2$ during craniotomy for small supratentorial cerebral tumours in enflurane anaesthesia. A dose–response study. *Acta Anaesthesiol Scand* 1986;**30**:633–6.

150 Madsen JB, Cold GE, Hansen ES, Bardrum B. Cerebral blood flow, cerebral metabolic rate of oxygen and relative CO_2-reactivity during craniotomy for supratentorial cerebral tumours in halothane anaesthesia. A dose–response study. *Acta Anaesthesiol Scand* 1987;**31**:454–7.

151 Madsen JB, Cold GE, Hansen ES, Bardrum B. The effect of isoflurane on cerebral blood flow and metabolism in humans during craniotomy for small supratentorial cerebral tumours. *Anesthesiology* 1987;**66**:332–6.

152 Kaieda R, Todd MM, Warner DS. The effects of anaesthetics and $PaCO_2$ on the cerobrovascular, metabolic, and electroencephalographic responses to nitrous oxide in the rabbit. *Anesth Analg* 1989;**68**:135–43.

153 Todd MM, Drummond JC. A comparison of the cerebrovascular and metabolic effects of halothane and isoflurane in the cat. *Anesthesiology* 1984;**60**:276–82.

154 Eintrei C, Lesezniewski W, Carlsson C. Local application of [133]Xenon for measurement of regional cerebral blood flow (rCBF) during halothane, enflurane and isoflurane anesthesia in humans. *Anesthesiology* 1985;**63**:391–4.

155 Scheller MS, Todd MM, Drummond JC. Isoflurane, halothane and regional cerebral blood flow at various levels of $PaCO_2$ in rabbits. *Anesthesiology* 1986;**64**:598–604.

156 Michenfelder JD, Sundt TM, Fode N, Sharborough FW. Isoflurane when compared to enflurane and halothane decreases the frequency of cerebral ischemia during carotid endarterectomy. *Anesthesiology* 1987;**67**:336–40.

How to search the catalogue

...ave logged in, you can carry out a simple or advanced
...e catalogue for books or journals by entering keywords,

How to reserve an item

...of the search will be displayed. Click on the title to see if
...available in your library, if not then click on place hold
...u will be contacted when the item is ready for collection

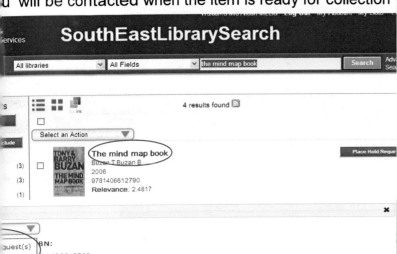

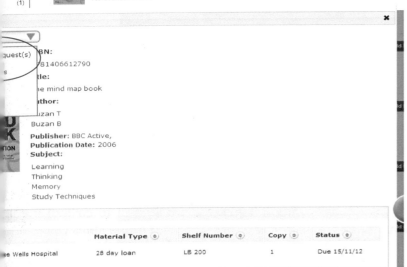

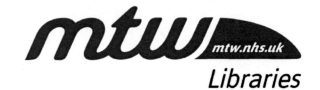

Libraries

Quick guide
How to Manage your Library Account online using the Library Catalogue

www.southeastlibrarysearch.nhs.uk

Library ID: MTW_____

Library PIN: _____

Need more help?

For training on the Library Catalogue and other courses:

contact: Alison Millis (Training & Outreach Manager)
email: alison.millis@nhs.net
Phone: 01892 635994 or 07500 814120
                    or contact the library
email: mtw-tr.library@nhs.net
Phone :   Maidstone Hospital: 01622 224647
              Tunbridge Wells Hospital: 01892 635884 or 635489

How to manage your library account online

How to log in

From the home page of www.southeastlibrarysearch.nhs.uk click on My Library account (see below)

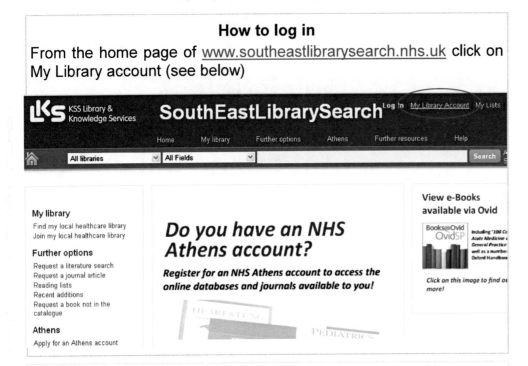

Enter your Library ID (include the prefix MTW) and PIN (4 digits). Contact Library staff if you do not know your Library PIN or have problems logging in

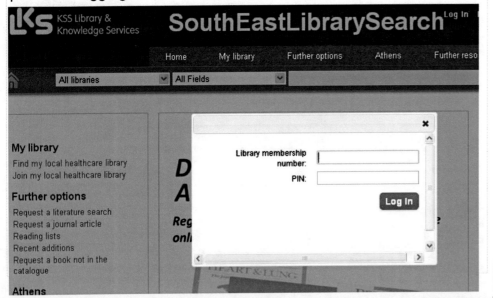

How to renew your

To renew your books click on 'My Librar[...] page & select 'Checkouts' tab (see belo[...]

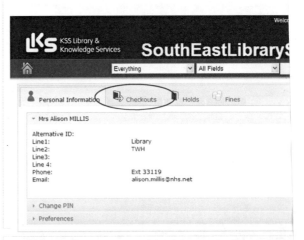

Either select all or select individual items [...]

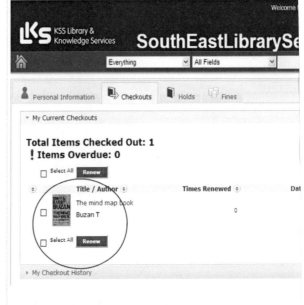

* If you have overdue items – you will need [...] can renew them, or if you have renewed thes[...] then we will need to see the items before we [...]

Once you h[...] search of th[...]

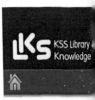

The results [...] the item is [...] request. Y[...]

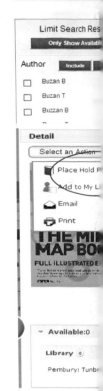

157 Gelman S, Fowler KC, Smith LR. Regional blood flow during isoflurane and halothane anaesthesia. *Anesth Analg* 1984;**63**:557–65.

158 Stullken EH Jr, Milde JH, Michelfelder JD, Tinker JH. The nonlinear responses of cerebral metabolism to low concentrations of halothane, enflurane, isoflurane and thiopental. *Anesthesiology* 1977;**46**:28–34.

159 Hansen TD, Warner DS, Todd MM, Vust LJ, Trawick DC. Distribution of cerebral blood flow during halothane versus isoflurane anesthesia in rats. *Anesthesiology* 1988;**69**:332–7.

160 Boarini DJ, Kassell NJ, Coesler HC, Butler M, Sokoll MD. Comparison of systemic and cerbrovascular effects of isoflurane and halothane. *Neurosurgery* 1984;**15**:400–9.

8: Renal, splanchnic, skin, and muscle circulations

NGUYEN D KIEN, JOHN A REITAN

Renal circulation

The major functions of the kidneys include:

1 Excretion of the end products of systemic metabolism while retaining essential nutrients.
2 Regulation of the volume and composition of body fluids.
3 Production of endocrine substances, including renin, prostaglandins, and kinins, which are important for the control of the pressure, volume, and flow of blood.

Anatomy

The kidneys are bilateral, bean shaped organs, which lie in a retroperitoneal position on either side of the vertebral column beneath the diaphragm. An adult human kidney weighs between 115 and 170 g with the upper and lower borders situated between the twelfth thoracic and third lumbar vertebrae. The right kidney is slightly more caudal in position because of the liver. Located on the concave border facing the vertebral column is an indentation called the hilus through which the ureter, blood and lymph vessels, and a nerve plexus pass into the renal sinus. The cut surface of a bisected kidney reveals an outer region called the cortex and an inner region called the medulla. The cortex is divided into the outer cortical layer and the inner juxtamedullary layer. The medulla is made up of 4–18 conical pyramids. The base of each pyramid faces the cortex and the apex (called the papilla) extends into the renal sinus and is covered by a funnel shaped calyx. It is through these calyces that the urine is drained from the kidney into the pelvis and the ureter.

The kidney is innervated by the renal plexus of the sympathetic division of the autonomic nervous system. The nerve fibres enter the kidney alongside the arterial vessels. Their branches supply the renal vasculature throughout the cortex and the outer region of the medulla.

The functional unit of the kidney is the nephron. There are approximately 10^6 nephrons in each kidney. Each nephron consists of a glomerulus, a capillary network through which plasma is filtered, and the uriniferous tubule, a long and cylindrical tube where filtered plasma is modified into urine.

Glomerulus

The glomerulus is composed of a capillary network that invaginates into the dilated blind end of the nephron called Bowman's capsule.[1] The glomerulus is the filtration barrier between blood and urine that is responsible for the production of an ultrafiltrate of plasma. The glomerular capillaries are covered by a thin fenestrated endothelium. The endothelial cells form an initial barrier to the passage of blood constituents from the capillary to Bowman's capsule. Beneath the endothelium is the basement membrane of the glomerulus. This extracellular membrane, consisting of fibrils in a glycoprotein matrix, serves as a retaining wall of large sized proteins. The largest cells of the glomerulus are the visceral epithelial cells, which are partially responsible for the synthesis and maintenance of the glomerular basement membrane. The mesangial cells are similar to the visceral epithelial cells. These cells contain filaments and are capable of phagocytosis. They produce prostaglandins and appear to have a role in the counter regulation of the effect of vasoconstrictors.

Juxtaglomerular apparatus

The juxtaglomerular apparatus is an area of the nephron where the distal tubal comes into contact with the arterioles.[2] It is composed of:

- juxtaglomerular granular cells
- extraglomerular mesangium
- the macula densa.

The juxtaglomerular granular cells are modified smooth muscle cells which produce, store, and release renin. The extraglomerular mesangium is connected with the intraglomerular mesangium, and is composed of cells that are similar to the mesangial cells. The extraglomerular mesangium has been suggested as a functional link of the mesangium, glomerular arterioles, and macula densa.

The juxtaglomerular apparatus is a major structural component of the renin–angiotensin system. It is involved in the autoregulation of renal blood flow and glomerular filtration rate. Changes in sodium or chloride concentration at the macula densa, or alterations in the volume and stretch of the afferent arteriole, are thought to affect the control of renin release.

279

Renal tubule

The renal tubule consists of the proximal tubule, the loop of Henle, and the distal tubule. Bowman's capsule opens into the first section of the renal tubule, called the proximal tubule, which lies within the cortex. The proximal tubule contains a large number of lysosomes that are responsible for the normal turnover of intracellular constituents by autophagocytosis. Proteins are absorbed from the tubule lumen by endocytosis or pinocytosis. The proximal tubule is lined with cuboidal epithelium with microvilli that increase the surface area for reabsorption and secretion. The proximal tubule plays a major role in the reabsorption of various ions, water, and organic solutes such as glucose and amino acids. Approximately half of the filtrate is reabsorbed in the proximal tubule.

The transition from the proximal tubule to the loop of Henle occurs abruptly at the outer layer of the medulla. The loop of Henle consists of a straight segment of the proximal tubule, the descending thin limb, and the thick ascending limb. The descending thin limb has permeability properties that are important for maintaining medullary hypertoxicity and the delivery of a dilute fluid to the distal tubule.

The distal tubule begins close to the macula densa and extends into the cortex where two or more nephrons combine to form a cortical collecting duct. The distal tubule is involved in the active transport of sodium chloride. Its function is regulated by various hormones including vaso-pressin, parathyroid hormone, and calcitonin, which exert their effects by activating the adenylate cyclase system. The cells of the distal tubule are similar to those of the proximal tubule, except they have fewer microvilli. The distal tubule connects to the collecting duct via the connecting tubule which plays an important role in potassium secretion.

The collecting duct extends from the cortical region through the medulla to the tip of the papilla. It collects fluid from several nephrons, travels along the conical pyramid, and terminates at the minor calyx. The collecting duct is also involved in potassium secretion and urine acidification.

There are two types of nephrons separated by their locations in the kidney. About 85% of nephrons are located in the cortex and are called cortical nephrons. The remaining 15% are found close to the medulla and are called the juxtamedullary nephrons. The nephrons filter approximately 180 litres of plasma each day through the glomerular component. Only 1% is excreted as urine, the remaining plasma fluid being reabsorbed into the circulation through the tubules.

Vascular supply

The renal vasculature is characterised by two capillary networks surrounding the glomerulus and the tubule.[3] The renal artery usually divides into the anterior and posterior main branches before entering the renal parenchyma. These main branches divide further into segmental

280

arteries which give rise to the interlobar arteries in the renal sinus. These vessels advance to the junction of the cortex and medulla where they divide and form arcuate arteries. Their divisions tend to lie in a plane parallel to the kidney surface at the corticomedullary junction. As the arcuate arteries advance towards the kidney surface and branch into the interlobular arteries (also known as cortical radial arteries), further divisions occur to form the afferent arterioles. The arterioles eventually divide into several branches which form the capillary network of the glomerulus. The wall structure of the intrarenal arteries and the afferent arterioles resembles that of vessels found in other organs, indicating that these vessels can regulate the glomerular capillary flow through their well developed smooth muscles.[4] Afferent arterioles are composed of one to three layers of smooth muscles. As the arterioles approach the glomerulus, the smooth muscle cells are replaced by granular cells of the juxtaglomerular apparatus.

The glomerular capillaries exit Bowman's capsule to form the efferent arterioles. The efferent arterioles are smaller in size than the afferent arterioles. This feature is a contributing factor in raising the glomerular pressure. The efferent arterioles supply the renal tubules in the form of a capillary network called the peritubular capillaries. Near the corticomedullary junction, the efferent arterioles become larger, longer, and more muscular than those in the outer cortex. The arteriolar smooth muscle is replaced by pericytes as the efferent arterioles extend into the medulla to form long loops of thin walled vessels called vasa recta. The peritubular capillaries eventually reunite to form interlobular veins which converge into the arcuate and interlobar veins. They run between the pyramids and give rise to several trunks that leave the kidney through a single renal vein at the hilus. Unlike the arterial system, which lacks collateral vessels, the venous network anastomoses at several levels. This allows normal drainage of blood even when a large venous branch is occluded.

Control of the renal circulation

The kidneys receive approximately 20% of cardiac output. They are capable of increasing flow even further, although they constitute less than 0·5% of the total body weight. This marked renal blood flow is well in excess of that required to provide renal tissue with sufficient oxygen and nutrients. Therefore, renal blood flow is regulated to maintain an optimum delivery of filtrate to the nephrons and adequate reabsorption of fluid back into the vascular system. The factors that control renal circulation are divided into intrinsic factors (autoregulation and renal nerves) and extrinsic factors (hormonal and other endogenous vasoactive agents).

Autoregulation
Regulation of the renal blood flow depends closely on changes of vascular resistance secondary to constriction or relaxation of vascular smooth

muscles. Autoregulation is the intrinsic ability of the kidney to maintain a relatively constant blood flow over a range of renal perfusion pressure from 75 to 180 mm Hg. Outside this pressure range, afferent arteriolar resistance is less responsive and flow becomes pressure dependent.[5] As this vascular reaction is demonstrable in isolated kidneys, autoregulation of renal blood flow is generally assumed to be mediated by factors intrinsic to the kidney. It is well accepted that blood flow to the renal cortex is autoregulated. Whether there is also blood flow autoregulation in the medulla remains controversial.

Currently, two theories are proposed to explain autoregulation. One is the myogenic theory first discussed by Bayliss in 1902.[6] It has been shown that a vasoconstrictor is released from renal vessels when the transmural pressure difference increases, supporting a relationship between the endothelium and the vascular smooth muscle, which mediates the autoregulation. The second theory postulates a tubuloglomerular feedback mechanism which enables autoregulation of both renal blood flow and glomerular filtration rate. Within the autoregulatory range, there is a coupling between renal blood flow and glomerular filtration rate, which supports the postulate that the principal autoregulatory actions on renal vascular resistance occur at preglomerular arterioles.[7] The tubuloglomerular feedback theory is based on a relationship between the distal tubular Na^+ delivery and the intrarenal release of renin.[8] Changes in distal tubular flow and/or solute can affect renal blood flow and thus modulate glomerular filtration rate. Recent data support a close interaction between the tubuloglomerular feedback and the myogenic mechanisms (Fig 8.1). Thus, the renal vascular bed is believed to consist of a rapid (myogenic

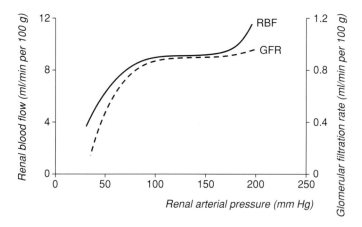

Fig 8.1 An example of autoregulation in the kidney that demonstrates the flow and filtration stability between 75 and 180 mm Hg blood pressure. ———— renal blood flow; – – – glomerular filtration rate.

response) and a slow (tubuloglomerular feedback mechanism) component of renal autoregulation.

Renal nerves

The renal nerves contain both afferent and efferent nerve fibres which release noradrenaline (norepinephrine).[9] Both noradrenaline and adrenaline (epinephrine) released from the adrenal medulla activate α_1-adrenoceptors and cause vasoconstriction, which decreases both renal blood flow and glomerular filtration rate. Renal nerves also release dopamine (DA) which activates specific dopamine receptors existing in abundance in the renal tissues. Activation of the DA_1-receptors causes significant increases in both cortical and medullary blood flows.[10] In addition, the release of neuropeptide Y and noradrenaline from sympathetic activation can stimulate Y-receptors and contribute to the modulation of renal vascular resistance.[11]

Renin-angiotensin system

Renin is a proteolytic enzyme that is synthesised in the epithelial cells of the juxtaglomerular apparatus and secreted into the surrounding interstitium. It cleaves angiotensin I from angiotensinogen. Angiotensin I is converted into angiotensin II which exerts both direct and indirect adrenergic actions on renal arterioles. Angiotensin II can also act as a circulating hormone. It is a potent vasoconstrictor; however, its most important action is to stimulate aldosterone production and secretion by the adrenal cortex. Thus, an increase in renin release from the kidney will lead to an increase in Na^+ reabsorption secondary to a higher blood level of aldosterone. The increased reabsorption of Na^+ will facilitate water movement from the interstitial space and increase plasma volume. The renin–angiotensin system shuts off once the volume deficit is corrected.[12] Although angiotensin II has potent vasoconstrictor effects on the afferent arterioles, its primary action appears to be on the efferent arterioles. Vasoconstriction of the efferent arterioles can contribute to the maintenance of the glomerular filtration, particularly when renal plasma flow is reduced. There are two main angiotensin II receptors: AT_1 and AT_2. Activation of these receptors increases the sensitivity of the tubuloglomerular feedback mechanisms and augments autoregulation. Blockade of the renin–angiotensin system, however, has no effect on autoregulation.[13]

Antidiuretic hormone

This hormone, also called vasopressin, is synthesised in the hypothalamus and released from the posterior pituitary gland. The release of antidiuretic hormone (ADH) can be stimulated by changes in the volume and osmolality of body fluids or by activation of the sympathetic nervous system. This hormone acts on the collecting tubules where it inhibits diuresis and increases water reabsorption leading to increased plasma volume. Thus, ADH modulates urinary concentration via an increase in osmotic water permeability and a decrease in medullary blood flow by constricting juxtamedullary arterioles.[13] Although ADH is involved in the maintenance of the volume and osmolality of plasma, the magnitude and direction of such involvement remain controversial. The conflicting results may result from different dosages of ADH, varying states of fluid balance, and the influence of other vasoactive agents.

Prostaglandins

Prostaglandin E_2 (PGE$_2$) and prostacyclin (PGI$_2$) are produced within the kidney during haemorrhagic hypovolaemia. The production of these substances is stimulated by sympathetic nerve activity and angiotensin II. During haemorrhage, prostaglandin synthesis occurs within the kidneys, which causes vasodilation in the afferent and efferent arterioles to prevent severe renal vasoconstriction and ischaemia. Therefore, prostaglandins appear to play a role in modulating the renal vascular effects of other vasoactive agents, including vasoconstrictor hormones and bradykinins. As prostaglandin inhibitors do not significantly alter renal blood flow autoregulation, the contribution of prostaglandins to the control of basal or resting renal blood flow is considered to be minimal.[14]

Atrial natriuretic peptide

Atrial natriuretic peptide (ANP) is a recently discovered peptide that appears to be involved in the regulation of renal function and Na^+ balance. ANP is released primarily from cardiac atria in response to atrial distension secondary to volume expansion. This peptide is a rapidly acting, potent natriuretic and diuretic substance, which can also exert direct vasodilator effects on the systemic vasculature. There are membrane receptors for ANP throughout the renal cortical and medullary vasculature, particularly at the glomerular capillaries. Infusion of ANP increases renal blood flow, glomerular filtration rate, papillary plasma flow, and sodium excretion caused by a direct vasodilator effect.[15] As ANP can inhibit renin secretion and aldosterone release, and increase urinary kallikrein excretion, part of the renal effects of ANP may be indirect. Nevertheless, ANP appears to have an important role in the control of Na^+ balance during conditions of altered plasma volume. The Na^+ excretion may be partially mediated by the vasodilator effect of ANP which increases the glomerular filtration rate.

Adenosine

It has been proposed that adenosine may play a role in the regulation of renal blood flow and glomerular filtration.[16] Administration of adenosine causes significant changes in renal vascular resistance, glomerular filtration rate, and renin release. Responses of renal vascular resistance to intrarenal infusion of adenosine include an initial transient vasoconstriction of the afferent arterioles, possibly by interaction with the renin–angiotensin system, and is followed by a dilatory phase that may be associated with a marked vasodilation caused by both direct and indirect mechanisms. The vasoconstriction of the afferent arterioles combined with the vasodilation of the efferent arterioles can result in sustained decreases in glomerular filtration pressure and rate. In addition, adenosine can exert a direct and powerful inhibition of renin release by the juxtaglomerular cells. In general, adenosine appears to be an important mediator in the control of renal blood flow. Further studies are, however, necessary to delineate the effects of adenosine on both the renal and the systemic vasculature.

Kinins

Administration of bradykinin released from plasma kallikrein causes marked renal vasodilation. Infusion of kinin antagonist decreases papillary blood flow by 20% without changing outer cortical blood flow, indicating that kinins exert a vasodilatory influence on the papillary vessels. The role of kinin in regulating medullary haemodynamics is not, however, clear because more than 90% of the renal kallikrein is found in the cortex and a very small fraction in the medulla and papilla.

Nitric oxide

The role of endothelium derived relaxing factor (EDRF) or nitric oxide (NO) is being extensively investigated. Recent data suggest that about 30% of renal vascular resistance may be controlled by NO. The collecting duct and vasa recta capillaries seem to be the major sites of NO synthesis.[17] NO inhibitor infused into the renal medulla decreases papillary blood flow without changes in cortical blood flow, renal blood flow, or mean arterial pressure.[18] Systemic inhibition of NO, however, significantly decreases renal blood flow without affecting the glomerular filtration rate.[19] During NO blockade, renal autoregulation remains intact. Apparently, NO blockade shifts the myogenic response to a lower renal arterial pressure and thus modulates autoregulation. It has been speculated that NO blockade inhibits the myogenic response, but autoregulation is sustained by a strong activation of the tubuloglomerular feedback mechanism.[7] In the presence of NO deficiency in the cells of the macula densa, the tubuloglomerular feedback mechanism becomes increasingly sensitive, which leads to elevated sodium and water retention and thereby hypertension. The release of NO in response to changes in vessel tension is postulated to be associated with the activation of membrane receptors or to involve a complex enzymatic pathway. Inflammation mediators such as tumour necrosis factor modify the release of NO from either endothelial or non-endothelial cells.[20]

285

Other vasoactive substances such as serotonin and histamine have been proposed as mediators involved in the control of renal haemodynamics. Current data, however, suggest that their role in regulating the renal circulation appears to be limited. Future studies should examine the possible role of endothelin in the local control of renal blood flow.

Fig 8.2 demonstrates the main contributors to renal circulatory control.

Effects of anaesthetic drugs on renal blood flow

Anaesthetic drugs are associated with significant sympathetic and endocrine changes, particularly those with sympathomimetic properties such as pentobarbital (pentobarbitone), and ketamine can stimulate the release of catecholamines. An increased blood level of adrenaline causes significant renal vasoconstriction and triggers renin release from the juxtamedullary nephrons. The formation of angiotensin II from renin leads to profound vasoconstriction of the renal vessels, and associated decreases in both the renal blood flow and glomerular filtration rate. Surgical stress may also induce further release of catecholamines, ADH, and aldosterone into the circulation. Opioids generally decrease regional vascular resistance by both local and systemically mediated mechanisms, but changes in perfusion pressure are moderated by reflex increases in sympathetic activity. They also appear to have no significant effect on renal blood flow. A low concentration of propofol has no effect on blood pressure, heart rate, or renal nerve activity. At moderate to high doses, renal nerve activity decreased by 22–50%, but the effect of propofol on renal blood flow still has to be elucidated.

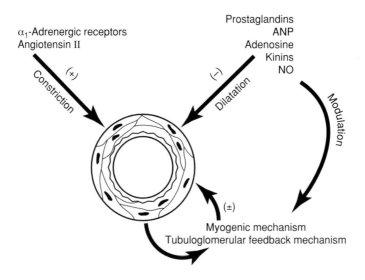

Fig 8.2 Factors controlling renal blood flow.

In healthy volunteers in the absence of surgical stimuli, as well as in patients undergoing surgery, inhalational anaesthetic drugs are associated with dose dependent decreases in renal blood flow, glomerular filtration rate, and urine production. These anaesthetic drugs have both direct and indirect effects on renal blood flow. The direct effects on the renal bed can be intensified in certain clinical conditions, including dehydration, pain, and loss of blood volume. They are accompanied by indirect factors such as depressed myocardial performance, altered vascular resistance, or decreased intravascular volume associated with most inhalational anaesthetic agents. Data from laboratory animals clearly demonstrate changes in active ion transport during anaesthesia. It has been suggested that an interaction with adrenaline is involved in the augmented Na^+ transport, whereas the inhibition of Na^+ transport is related to a direct effect of inhalational anaesthetic drugs. At concentrations of 3% or higher, halothane causes significant decreases in renal blood flow and oxygen consumption. The effects of enflurane and isoflurane on renal blood flow are considerably less than those of halothane. All inhalational anaesthetic drugs at high concentrations, however, possess potent vasodilator properties which may lead to loss of autoregulation.

Spinal or epidural anaesthesia may cause significant reductions in glomerular filtration rate and renal plasma flow when arterial blood pressure is markedly reduced. When the reduction of perfusion pressure is corrected, renal haemodynamics are normalised, suggesting that perfusion pressure is an important factor in sustaining normal circulation in the kidney. No change in plasma renin levels is observed with either spinal or epidural anaesthesia. Therefore, the decrease in renal blood flow during spinal or epidural anaesthesia is possibly caused by a reduction in venous return and decreased cardiac output.

In summary, anaesthetic drugs are associated with an increase in renal vascular resistance. It is still, however, controversial whether anaesthetic drugs alter renal autoregulation.

Splanchnic circulation

Anatomy

The splanchnic circulation is composed of gastric, small intestinal, colonic, pancreatic, hepatic, and splenic circulations.[21][22] They are arranged in parallel with one another and fed by three arteries:

1 The coeliac artery, which perfuses the hepatic artery, the stomach, the spleen, and part of the pancreas.
2 The superior mesenteric artery which supplies branches to the pancreas, small intestines, and part of the colon.

287

3 The inferior mesenteric artery which supplies the rest of the colon.

The stomach is composed of three histologically distinct layers: the mucosa, submucosa, and muscularis externa. The mucosa receives approximately three quarters of resting blood flow. Gastric arteries pierce the muscularis layer and form a network of branches into the submucosal area. This submucosal plexus gives rise to smaller branches that form a secondary arcade within the smooth muscles at the base of the mucosa. The venous system is parallel to the arterial vessels.

The mesenteric vasculature to the small and large intestine is composed of several circuits coupled both in series and in parallel. The three parallel circuits serve the muscularis, the submucosa, and the mucosa. Each of these circuits possesses a series coupled component consisting of resistance arterioles, precapillary sphincters, the capillaries themselves, postcapillary sphincters, and the venous capacitance vessels. The resistance arterioles are the primary determinants of vascular resistance and they regulate blood flow both to the splanchnic bed as a whole and through each of the parallel circuits. The mucosa has an enormous surface area for absorption created by villi and microvilli. The mucosa is the metabolically active area in the gut and receives well over half of the total resting organ blood flow. The small intestinal villi are oxygenated via a countercurrent circulation whereby a central, small artery diffuses oxygen across to the parallel submucosal veins. As a result of this anatomical configuration, the tips of the villi have the lowest tissue oxygen tension (Po_2), and ischaemia to this area may be induced by relatively small changes in blood flow.[23] The submucosa and mucosa both have a parallel capillary plexus. Venous drainage from the small intestinal veins joins with veins from the colon, which subsequently join with splenic veins to form the portal system.[24]

The pancreas receives its blood supply from several branches of the coeliac and superior mesenteric arteries. It also drains into the portal system.

The splenic circulation is unusual in that the internal red pulp has a complex mesh like structure which filters the blood passing through it. Blood flowing through the spleen may bypass the red pulp and constitutes a fast compartment, whereas blood perfusing the red pulp has a considerably increased transit time and may be considered to be the slow compartment. Splenic blood flow is approximately 250 ml/min. The oxygen content of splenic venous blood is quite high because of the fast compartment and adds significantly to the portal oxygen saturation.

The liver is unique in that it has both an arterial and a venous afferent blood supply. The hepatic artery provides approximately 30–40% of total hepatic blood flow, with the rest coming from the portal veins. In the normal resting adult, about 500 ml/min perfuse the liver via the hepatic artery whereas an additional 1300 ml/min flow via the portal system. The portal blood flows through hepatic sinusoids, which puts it in close contact with the metabolic cells of the liver parenchyma. Hepatic arterial blood flow also supplies nutrients to the connective tissue within the liver itself, especially the walls of the collecting ducts which form the intrahepatic biliary system. The hepatic sinuses are lined with endothelium similar to that found in capillaries, but the permeability of this endothelium is extreme and allows for rapid, easy diffusion of components within the blood into the hepatic parenchyma and back. The sinusoids drain into venules which form the hepatic veins; these, in turn, empty into the inferior vena cava. There is a well organised intrahepatic lymph system as well, which accounts for more than half of the total body lymph flow.

Overall, splanchnic blood flow requires about a quarter of the cardiac output in normal resting adults and, by coincidence, the splanchnic capacitance venous system serves as a large reservoir for almost a quarter of the total blood volume of the body.[25]

Control of the splanchnic circulation

The resistance arterioles are the primary determinant of vascular resistance in the splanchnic system, and therefore regulate blood flow through this bed as a whole and through each parallel circuit. In this sort of control system, the relationship between flow and resistance can be described by the haemodynamic version of Ohm's law:

$$\text{Resistance} = \frac{\text{Pressure}}{\text{Flow}}.$$

In the case of the mesenteric circulation, this would be the hydrostatic difference between the arterial and venous pressures divided by flow across the gut.

The control of splanchnic blood flow is by a combination of neuroreflex and hormonal factors.[23 26] Neural control of the mesenteric circulation is almost exclusively sympathetic in origin. The parasympathetic fibres originating from the vagi have little effect on splanchnic blood flow, although they are most important in the regulation of secretion and motility of the gut. The sympathetic postganglionic fibres act directly on the vascular smooth muscle of the arterioles. In this way increased sympathetic activity decreases blood flow to splanchnic organs. In addition, sympathetic outflow to the splanchnic bed contracts the venous smooth muscles of the capacitance veins in the splanchnic circulation, and may expel a large volume of pooled blood from the splanchnic reservoir into the systemic circulation. Most of these sympathetic ganglia arise from the coeliac plexus with lesser contributions from the superior and inferior mesenteric plexus. Through the sympathetic system, the mechanoreceptor reflexes – particularly the low pressure cardiopulmonary receptor systems – are closely involved in splanchnic arterial and venous vascular tone.[27] Interestingly, β_2-adrenoceptors are also present in the mesenteric circulation and activation of these receptors causes vasodilation.

Circulating substances that may alter vascular resistance in the splanchnic bed include adrenaline, noradrenaline, angiotensin II, vasopressin, and gastrointestinal peptides such as glucagon, vasoactive intestinal peptide (VIP), and cholecystokinin.[28] The role of adenosine in control of the splanchnic circulation is controversial, but research has shown: (1) its presence in normal gut, and (2) that blockade of its receptors alters mesenteric blood flow significantly.[29] Thus, adenosine probably plays an important local role in increasing regional blood flow. In fact, most of the gastrointestinal peptides are vasodilators; they rarely reach a concentration high enough to be vasoactive in the systemic circulation as a whole. The catecholamines, including angiotensin and vasopressin, probably achieve a concentration that is centrally vasoactive only under circumstances of significant shock.

In addition to the classic gastrointestinal hormones, various vasoactive substances, including histamine, serotonin, bradykinin, and prostaglandins, which are produced and stored in the splanchnic organs, have been shown to affect organ blood flow in this region.[30] Many of the changes observed with these substances are in patients or study models with compromised splanchnic function.[24] The action of these hormones may be independent or in combination with other regulatory mechanisms.

Regional production and circulatory effects from vasoactive substances have been shown in normal subjects.[32] The potent vasoconstrictor, endothelin-1 (ET-1) induces paracrine actions in the mesenteric vessels through its local production and breakdown. NO inhibits the formation of ET-1 in humans and thereby counteracts its constricting action on the gut's vasculature.[33] Apparently, this interactive relationship between ET-1 and NO is another step in the complex regulatory pathways for the splanchnic circulation.

Autoregulation in the splanchnic circulation is demonstrated by compensatory dilatation of the resistance arterioles in response to an acute reduction of perfusion pressure which serves to restore the decreased tissue perfusion partially. Splanchnic autoregulation is less pronounced than in the cerebral, cardiac, or renal circulation. The response is evident, however, as a mechanism whereby initial levels of hypoperfusion are rapidly ameliorated by marked arteriolar vasodilation which partially restores blood flow. This phenomenon is a variation of the postischaemic hyperperfusion mechanism seen in many areas of the body, and is the result of a direct myogenic response to the reduction in perfusion pressure and the accumulation of local ischaemic metabolites in the region, including adenosine, which may be the principal metabolic mediator of autoregulation. Interestingly, the oxygen consumption in the small intestine is even more rigorously autoregulated than blood flow, with the result that oxygen uptake in this organ remains constant when arterial perfusion pressures are varied fourfold.[34] The portal venous system does not autoregulate so that, as the portal venous pressure and flow are raised, resistance either remains constant or may decrease.

In addition to autoregulation of blood flow within the individual organ as a whole, the splanchnic circulation responds to reductions in perfusion pressures by redistributing blood flow to various levels within the individual organ. This redistribution is achieved by changes in the relative resistance of the arterioles and precapillary sphincters, gating the parallel vascular circuits in the various layers of the organ. In shock, for example, this response usually favours the mucosa at the expense of the muscularis layers. The gut is protected from ischaemic injury by its unique ability to increase oxygen extraction as much as sixfold, thereby maintaining oxygen consumption at near normal levels over a broad range of flows and avoiding the usual hypoxic sequelae, particularly in areas at risk such as the tips of the villi. This protective mechanism is the result not only of the "mass effect" of rapid diffusion of oxygen along a steeper concentration gradient, but also of the opening of hypoperfused capillary beds. The net result is an increase in perfused capillary density as flow is reduced within the mucosa of the gut. This provides an important defence against splanchnic ischaemia.

An illustrated overview of the central mechanisms for splanchnic blood flow is shown in Fig 8.3.

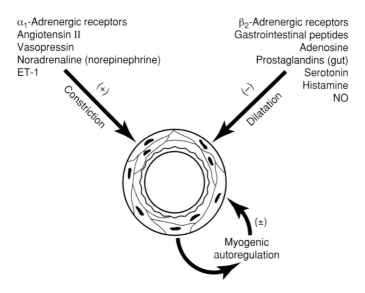

Fig 8.3 Factors influencing blood flow through the splanchnic circulation.

The effects of anaesthetic drugs on the splanchnic blood flow

Animal studies have shown that some intravenous anaesthetic drugs, particularly propofol, result in an increase in total liver blood flow with contributions from both the hepatic artery and portal systems. These data mark propofol as a vasodilator in this region. Human studies have, however, indicated an initial fall in hepatic flow followed by a return towards normal levels. Barbiturates also may cause a decrease in overall splanchnic blood flow, most pronounced in the portal system because of the relative venoplegia caused by higher doses of these drugs. Midazolam may also reduce splanchnic flow initially, with a rebound increase from the splanchnic reservoir shortly thereafter.

Opioids, in small doses, produce a central sympathetic withdrawal and relative increase in vascular capacitance in this circulation.[35]

The change in splanchnic blood flow after regional anaesthesia of the central neural axis is dictated by the level of block obtained. Spinal and epidural anaesthetic drugs at T10 and below have little effect upon splanchnic flow. Raising the block level to the T4 dermatome reduces total splanchnic blood flow by at least 25% in humans. Inclusion of the sympathetic outflow from the coeliac and mesenteric plexus produces the withdrawal of resting venous tone and the subsequent reduction in transhepatic flow.

With inhalational anaesthetic agents, there is most often a reduction in portal blood flow, particularly by halothane. Isoflurane and enflurane apparently increase hepatic arterial blood flow which facilitates an increase in oxygen delivery to the liver with these anaesthetic agents.[36] Moreover, noradrenaline spillover (a result of increased sympathetic nerve activity) was reduced in the mesenteric circulation of pigs during isoflurane anaesthesia, thus suggesting a relative vasodilation by the anaesthetic in that region.[37]

Of equal importance in the anaesthetised patient are the physiological consequences of ventilation. During inspiration with controlled ventilation, the diaphragm compresses the liver, which causes an increase in hepatic venous pressure and decreased transhepatic conductance. With expiration, there is a reversal of this and splanchnic flow increases dramatically. Positive end expiratory pressure will decrease mesenteric arterial flow, portal blood flow, and total splanchnic blood flow.[38] Interestingly, hypocapnia, which often accompanies controlled ventilation, reduces portal blood flow because of an increase in the resistance in mesenteric and splenic arteries and portal veins. On the other hand, hepatic arterial resistance is decreased and hepatic arterial blood flow thereby maintained. Increases in circulating carbon dioxide levels most commonly increase portal and total hepatic blood flows, probably mediated through carbon dioxide as a direct vasodilator and the increase in cardiac output resulting from stimulation of the central nervous system. Concurrently, there is an initial transient decrease in hepatic arterial flow followed by an increase towards the normocapnic control values. This phenomenon in the hepatic artery is compatible with a typical escape phenomenon of hepatic arterial vasculature from sudden sympathetic stimulation.

Cutaneous circulation

Anatomy

The largest organ in the body is the skin with a surface area of approximately 1.9 m^2 and a weight of about 2 kg in a 70 kg adult. The blood flow to the skin, including the microcirculation, is approximately 10 times greater than the metabolic needs of the cutaneous system. Under normothermic conditions, the venular plexus in the cutaneous circulation has the potential of being one of the larger reservoirs of blood volume in the body. The gross anatomy of the cutaneous circulation reflects the ability of the skin circulation to dissipate or preserve heat within the body as a whole and the anatomy reflects this functional need.[39][40]

The cutaneous vascular system is divided into three interconnected levels:

1 The deep subdermal or subcutaneous plexus
2 The middle or cutaneous plexus
3 The superficial or subpapillary plexus.

The subdermal plexus is the major vascular network of the overlying skin. Vessels of this plexus generally run in the subcutaneous fatty or areolar tissue. The arterial blood supply to the skin comes primarily from muscular cutaneous arteries which perforate the subcutaneous tissue from underlying muscle. These arteries and their concomitant veins ascend through the reticular dermis to the papillary dermis. Here the artery forms a superficial arteriolar plexus with terminal arterioles which project into capillary loops through the epidermis. The collecting venous system forms a double layered horizontal network at the subcutaneous dermal junction, and returns into the subcutaneous and muscular area via collecting venules. Total skin flow is made up of the blood perfusing through these vessels as well as bypasses (shunts) at deeper levels – primarily in the hands and feet – where the arteriovenous anastomoses are prominent in changing skin flow for thermal regulation.[41][42]

The skin is the primary site of exchange of body heat with the external environment.[43] Hence, changes in cutaneous blood flow in response to various metabolic states and environmental conditions provide the main mechanism by which temperature homoeostasis occurs. Skin blood flow is, under normal circumstances, about 5–6% of the resting cardiac output.

This can decrease markedly in a cold environment when heat retention is necessary. Alternatively, the skin vessels may dilate to increase flow up to seven times the normal state when heat loss is required by hypermetabolic states. Specialised areas of the skin, including the palm, fingers, sole, toes, and the face, possess the capability for remarkable vasodilation and constriction.[44] There may be as much as a 75-fold change in flow from cold to hot environments.

Control of the cutaneous circulation

The potential for skin vessels to generate great increases in vascular conductance makes this circulation an important regional flow area during changes in the environment and during anaesthesia.

Cutaneous resistance vessels and the venous plexus in the subcutaneous dermal junction are richly innervated with sympathetic vasoconstrictor nerves which maintain a relatively high degree of neurogenic activity and, hence, vascular tone. This predominant vasoconstrictor tone is mediated by hormonal action of circulating catecholamines at postjunctional α-adrenergic receptors. In addition, there is an active dilator system that is activated under thermal, physical, or emotional stress. The mechanism for this active dilatation is not clear and may involve the release of a yet-to-be-determined neurotransmitter on cutaneous blood vessels or, more probably, involves a release of a vasodilator substance from activated sweat glands.[45] The substance most commonly mentioned or identified is bradykinin. Recent studies have shown, however, that calcitonin gene related peptide (CGRP), a vasoactive polypeptide, can increase regional blood flow in the skin under resting conditions at the expense of other organ flow, primarily the splanchnic circulation. From this work it has been proposed that normal regional blood flow changes in the skin may be mediated to some extent by CGRP acting as a local vasodilator and produced by neuronal activity.[46]

In the context of total body circulatory control, investigators have shown that the sympathetic vasomotor fibres in the skin vasculature exert significant influence on overall homoeostasis. Such control is exerted from both the low pressure cardiopulmonary and the high pressure arterial baroreceptor areas. These conclusions deviate from the previous literature in which baroreflex sympathetic vasoconstriction in the human skin was proposed to be more or less selectively mediated from cardiopulmonary low pressure receptors.[47]

The afferent control of resistance vessels in the skin is interesting in that arterioles in non-peripheral areas are innervated by two distinct sympathetic nerve types:

1 Adrenergic vasoconstrictor nerves similar to those in all arterioles.
2 A specialized sympathetic active vasodilator nerve.

Arterioles in the peripheral skin seem to be innervated solely by sympathetic vasoconstrictor nerves. The remarkable dilatation that occurs in these areas under thermal stress is solely the result of withdrawal of sympathetic support.[48]

Temperature sensors lie predominantly in the preoptic area of the anterior hypothalamus, although they may be situated in the abdominal viscera and spinal cord as well. Increased heat to these areas causes vasodilation and cold elicits vasoconstriction. Such reflex activity is mediated through cardiovascular centres in the brain. Increased thermal content in the blood causes inhibition of normal sympathetic vasoconstriction at the preganglionic neuron level, which results in opening of arteriovenous anastomoses (shunts) in the extremities – the nose, ears, and mouth. Under normal sympathetic activity these shunts are closed, and withdrawal of sympathetic activity opens them for thermal regulation. Aortic and carotid chemoreceptor stimulation secondary to acidaemia, hypercapnia, or hypoxaemia may cause a decrease in sympathetic tone to the cutaneous arterioles with subsequent vasodilation. This effect is the opposite of that seen in the muscle, splanchnic, and renal circulations.[49]

Regional cutaneous blood flow control to non-peripheral areas includes a cholinergic pathway to eccrine sweat glands in the skin. Recent work has shown that some afferent sympathetic preganglionic and postganglionic fibres innervate and activate the glands as well. When the cholinergic and sympathetic pathways to the glands are activated, they trigger the release of bradykinin alone or other local vasodilator substances, possibly NO, serotonin (5-HT) or other peptides.[50 51]

The only parasympathetic innervation to affect skin blood vessels reaches the sweat glands via the sudomotor nerve. Activation of this system increases the output of the enzyme kallikrein. This substance, in turn, splits the polypeptide bradykinin from globulin in the perivascular interstitial tissues and induces a most potent vasodilatory effect.

Figure 8.4 illlustrates the control mechanisms for regulation of cutaneous blood flow.

Effects of anaesthetic drugs on the cutaneous blood flow

In humans, propofol administration causes an increase in flow, recorded by laser Doppler, which is probably the result of decreased sympathetic tone caused by the anaesthetic drug plus the direct vasodilating effect of propofol itself. A similar, though smaller, increase in skin blood flow may be observed with thiopental and other short acting barbiturates as well.

Opiate anaesthesia, in particular morphine anaesthesia, has been shown to increase forearm skin flow, and the neurocomponent is thought to be mediated centrally rather than by a local inhibition of adrenergic receptors. In addition, there is a centrally mediated effect upon the venous system, in that a significant venodilatation occurs approximately five minutes after delivery of centrally acting morphine. Most probably, in both cases, sympathetic mediated vasoconstriction is reduced and resultant vasodilation occurs.

With local anaesthetic drugs there is vasodilation of the arterioles and venules at high concentrations; however, small amounts of local anaesthetic drugs have a mild constrictive effect on the precapillary arteriolar vessels. Mepivacaine may also have a postcapillary constrictive effect in small concentrations. Overall, at concentrations used in clinical practice, the direct acting vasodilatory effects of the local anaesthetic drugs predominate.[52]

Most of the potent inhalational anaesthetic drugs cause some degree of sympathoplegia which results in opening of the arteriovenous anastomoses in the extremities – nose, ears, and mouth. These shunts, normally closed, are opened during anaesthesia and may lead to an accelerated body hypothermia. Indeed, the relative vasodilation in the cutaneous vessels may be one of the causes of dilated superficial veins whenever these agents are used.

Under regional anaesthesia, a relative sympathoplegia again occurs and conductance within the skin of the affected limb will increase, whereas blood flow through the cutaneous tissues in non-blocked limbs will decrease by reflex compensatory mechanisms. At least a T8 epidural sensory level is, however, necessary for a complete blockade of the distal intraneurally recorded skin sympathetic activity in the lower extremity.[53]

In summary, the cutaneous circulation is greatly influenced by anaesthesia and, although normally possessing thermoregulatory capacities, it may be significantly inhibited by anaesthetic drugs to mimic poikilothermic adaptation.

Muscle circulation

Anatomy

Skeletal muscle comprises approximately 40% of the total body mass. The density of the capillary networks varies greatly between the two basic muscle fibre types that are present in humans.[54] The slow twitch, or red, fibres are numerous in more slowly contracting muscles which help maintain posture and fulfil isometric functions. The fast twitch, or white, fibres are most numerous in the fast contracting muscles such as those used for running and quick movement. Numerous animal studies have demonstrated that resting blood flow and capillary density, as well as oxygen consumption, vary with the type of muscle that is being perfused. In general, the capillary density for slow twitch fibres is approximately two to three times that seen in fast twitch fibres in the same muscles. Other animal studies have shown that oxidative enzymes, as well as blood flow, are several times higher in the slow contracting muscles compared with the fast twitch muscles, which have a much higher activity of glycolytic enzymes and rely more on anaerobic metabolism. Apparently, slow twitch muscles respond better to prolonged activation and long term aerobic function.

In resting muscle, the precapillary arterioles exhibit intermittent asynchronous contractions and relaxations which, in effect, limit the number of capillary beds that are being perfused. This very action allows sudden recruitment and an increase in the number of nutrient capillary beds that perfuse the muscle when muscle activity begins. As a result of this, total blood flow through resting skeletal muscle varies between 2 and 5 ml/min per 100 g. With exercise, this can increase in trained athletes to more than 125 ml/min per 100 g.[55] Dynamic rhythmic exercise has a large, rapid effect on vascular contracture which is not explained by known neural, metabolic, myogenic, or hydrostatic influences.[56] The muscle relaxation between contractions draws blood from the arteries into the veins, and effectively reduces arterial driving pressure. During the subsequent contraction venous blood is pumped centrally raising the central venous pressure. The consequent increase in muscle blood flow, coupled with the decrease in arterial pressure and raised central venous pressure, markedly increases the calculated conductance. This rhythmic contraction and relaxation, in effect, pumps blood across the muscle bed.

The anatomical architecture of the muscle and the increase in intramuscular pressure causing hindrance to blood flow itself determine the increase in perfusion pressure observed during exercise. In the forearm, the circulation is initially arrested during voluntary isometric contraction of more than 70% maximal. In the calf, tensions of only 20–30% of maximal voluntary contraction are necessary to interrupt blood flow.[54] The increase in vascular resistance during strong muscle contraction occurs chiefly in the larger supply vessels – the branched arteries down into the muscle bed. The manner in which this vascular bed is occluded keeps red cells in the capillary and so provides a continuous, albeit dwindling, supply of nutrient oxygen during contraction.

Overall, the sequence of vascular segments in the muscle beds is similar to those seen in other parts of the bodies – that is, large arteries, small branched arteries, arterioles, precapillary arterioles, capillaries, then postcapillary venules, venules, and collecting veins which return blood to the central circulation. At the capillary level, only between 20% and 25% of the circuits are open in the resting muscle and these have decreased conductance from sympathetic tone and intramuscular pressure.

Control of the muscle circulation

Blood flow to skeletal muscle depends on the pressure gradient through the vessel complex and the calibre in the resistance vessels. Local modulation of vessel size is dependent on chemical and physical events near or within the environment of the resistance vessels, as a result of changes in nervous innervation of the vessels and circulating vasoactive agents.

The resting tone in the resistance arterioles is relatively high in the non-active muscle.[57] There is an intrinsic basal vascular resistance, or contractile property, in these small vessels and those of 50–100 μm in diameter tend to have more myogenic tone than the larger vessels up to 400 μm in diameter. In isolated muscle, the change from continuous to pulsatile perfusion causes a gradual increase in vascular resistance, presumably by the periodic stretch of the arterioles, which provides a continuing stimulus to the smooth muscle cells in the vessel walls.[58 59] This phenomenon was a concept initiated by Bayliss early in this century, who suggested that distension of the resistance blood vessels by intravascular pressure contributes to the basal vascular resistance through a direct action on the vascular smooth muscle. The phenomenon of autoregulation in the muscle vascular bed relies on this myogenic theory and resides primarily at the precapillary arterioles. Recent observations strongly suggest that myogenic regulatory mechanisms contribute directly or indirectly to circulatory homoeostasis in the following ways: intravenous pressure induces a tonic excitatory activation which initiates an intrinsic myogenic basal tone in the arterial microvessels. This, in turn, induces variable vascular resistance (total peripheral resistance) mainly from the myogenic tone, and basically serves to maintain normal arterial pressure at rest. Lastly, it produces an improved nutritional flow and exchange characterised by blood flow recruitment, capillary recruitment, and adjustments to the capillary perfusion/defusion ratio for optimum exchange of nutrients in a heterogeneous capillary network.[60] This myogenic control seems to initiate and maintain basal vascular tone. In synergism with metabolic vasodilators, it modifies the autoregulation of blood flow through the muscle itself. Both the humoral and neurogenic β-adrenergic effects depress myogenic reactivity and counter the α-adrenergic constriction.

Nervous control

The direct vasoconstricting activity of the sympathetic nervous system on the muscle blood flow is through the α-adrenergic receptor system. Vasoconstrictor fibres emerge from the ventral roots of the lower thoracic through upper lumbar segments with maximum outflow through L3. In addition, there is cholinergic innervation of the resistance vessels in the muscle bed. This is limited to cholinergic vasodilator fibres from the lumbar region for lower limb innervation. The sympathetic nerves follow the somatic nerves to the vessels innervated and continue along the adventitial surface of the vessels. Only the outer layers of smooth muscle cells within the vessels are in contact with noradrenergic vessels. These axons form varicosities which are demyelinated Schwann cells. Within these varicosities, the vesicles for storage of neurotransmitter substance are situated. At the neuroeffector junction, arterial baroreceptors and chemoreceptors, the cardiopulmonary low pressure mechanoreceptors, the receptors in the skeletal muscle, and those originating from centres in the brain signal alterations in the amount of noradrenaline delivered by the terminal nerves into the junctional clefts near the vascular smooth muscle cells. The actual release of noradrenaline is initiated by action potentials generated within the ganglionic cell body.

Both sympathetic nerve stimulation and exogenous noradrenaline cause vasoconstriction for skeletal muscle resistance vessels. Small amounts of noradrenaline metabolites appear in the venous drainage after nerve stimulation. This indicates that reuptake into the sympathetic nerve terminals must be the main route for terminating action of the released noradrenaline on the muscle vessels. In animal studies, complete ablation of sympathetic activity to a resting limb muscle results in less than a threefold increase in blood flow. Conversely, maximal stimulation of the noradrenergic nerves to the same limb produces a decrease in blood flow of about 75%. Interestingly, simple somatic motor denervation, in the presence of an intact sympathetic innervation of striated muscle, will increase blood flow by 25%. This is thought to be the result of overcoming resting somatic muscle tone which causes relative decompression of the blood supply to the muscle, thus opening up flow.[54]

Compared with the local mechanisms regulating muscle blood flow, the noradrenergic nerves control relatively small portions of the maximal flow available to the muscle bed. Nevertheless, because of the great muscle mass within the body, small amounts of variation in flow resistance may permit major changes in total body vascular resistance.[61]

Constriction of the muscle resistance vessels occurs solely by activation of the sympathetic noradrenergic nerves or muscle compression itself. On the other hand, neurogenic vasodilation can occur either by withdrawal of noradrenergic activity or by release of substances that lead to relaxation of vascular smooth muscle. The most important effectors of this type are sympathetic, cholinergic, and histaminergic systems.

The arteriolar resistance vessels within the muscle vascular bed contain receptors of the β_2 subtype. Activation of these receptors causes relaxation of the smooth muscle which can be prevented by β-adrenergic antagonists. Via this system, adrenaline dilates skeletal resistance muscles. The β_2-adrenoceptors in blood vessels within the muscle respond primarily to adrenaline released from the adrenal medulla rather than to any noradrenaline released from adrenergic nerves. The β_2 activation is an additional mechanism to induce large scale vasodilation in the working muscle.

Histamine is found in relatively high concentration in the walls of arteries and veins of the muscle bed. Activation of these histamine receptors causes marked vasodilation of the resistance arterioles similar to that seen with potassium and adenosine. Although resting tone is modulated by endothelial derived NO (EDNO), its role in hyperaemia and exercise is controversial.[62] Factors such as shear stress in the vessel wall, acetylcholine, free Ca^{2+}, and circulating insulin all play a role in inducing NO synthase (NOS) and local NO production. PGI_2 has also been shown to affect muscle arteriolar conductance during low flow states.[63] Other metabolic vasodilators include potassium, histamine, hypoxaemia, and increased osmolality.

There are several factors that modify the amount of noradrenaline from sympathetic nerve endings. Metabolic acidosis, in addition to relaxing active smooth muscles, depresses the contractile response of blood vessels to sympathomimetic amines and nerve stimulation. Potassium ions in large concentrations cause small vessel vasodilation via inhibitory effects on neurotransmission and a direct depressant effect on the vascular smooth muscle cell. Hyperosmolarity causes vasodilation of many vascular beds because of a reduced release of noradrenaline in the sympathetic nerve endings. Adenosine has a relaxing action on the muscle arterioles by a direct effect on vascular smooth muscle and, indirectly, by an inhibitory effect on noradrenergic neurotransmission.

A number of prejunctional receptors have been demonstrated, the activation of which depresses noradrenaline release from sympathetic nerve endings as well. These include specific α_2-adrenoceptors, muscarinic receptors activated by acetylcholine, histamine, and 5-HT receptors. In most animals, and most probably in humans, there is a cholinergic vasodilator pathway that originates in the motor cortex. The descending pathway has discrete relays in the hypothalamus and continues through the mesencephalon descending via the lateral spinothalamic tract. These cholinergic nerves run in the sympathetic nerves to the muscle vessels and they innervate almost exclusively the small arteries and arterioles. The acetylcholine released on activation of these fibres causes an instant dilatation by activating prejunctional muscarinic receptors, thereby reducing the noradrenaline release from the sympathetic nerve endings. They act on postjunctional muscarinic receptors in the vascular smooth muscle cells, which results in dilatation. Cholinergic nerves are generally quiescent. Stimulation of specific hypothalamic areas that produce defence reactions (in times of rage or fear) will, however, increase muscle blood flow mediated by this indirect action without actual muscle activity. In isolated blood vessels from many species, removal of the endothelium abolishes this relaxation induced cholinergic transmitter. Consequently, it is felt that most of this cholinergic reaction may come by way of NO release.[64] Teleologically the resting vasodilation caused by this cholinergic mechanism "primes the pump" for subsequent physical activity. Two excellent reviews of muscle blood flow and its regulation during exercise have been published recently.[63 65]

Reflex regulation

Changes in the activity of both the carotid and aortic high pressure mechanoreceptors result in inverse changes in blood flow to the limb muscles via the sympathetic nervous system. Activation of carotid and aortic chemoreflexes leads to constriction of arteriolar resistance vessels which is most pronounced in the skeletal muscle bed. Recent work has shown that the low pressure mechanoreceptors (atriopulmonary receptors) are much less important than previously thought in causing reflex sympathetic activation and vasoconstriction in the human skeletal muscle circulation during stress.[61] Indeed, the high pressure system predominantly controls the resting tone for these resistance arterioles.

Reflexes originate also from receptors in the skeletal muscle. This reflex, via activation of the adrenergic system, may be a prime cause for the rise in blood pressure in an isolated exercising limb. This suggests that intra-muscular mechanoreceptors generate part of the reflex drive during induced contractions of the skeletal muscle.[66] A summary of factors that influence blood flow in the muscle circulation is illustrated in Figure 8.5.

Effects of anaesthetic drugs on the muscle blood flow

As mentioned before, somatic motor denervation of the muscle leads to a 25% decrease in resting vascular tone in the muscle circulation. Similarly, the use of neuromuscular relaxants in supine, anaesthetised patients shows a fall in calculated vascular resistance compared with the unrelaxed state.

A dual effect by propofol occurs in the muscle bed of humans. An initial increase in blood flow occurs after infusion of propofol which may result, in part, from the direct vasodilating effect of the drug. A sustained fall in calculated muscle bed vascular resistance may, however, continue there-after because of depressed cardiac and muscle sympathetic baroreflex sensitivities. When propofol is used to control the stress response during surgery, the vasodilating effects of the drug override the neural vasocon-striction induced by baroreflex from the surgical stimulation.[67]

Opioids also have a dual effect on vascular tone in the muscular bed. The direct action of morphine is that of venoconstriction, whereas the centrally mediated effects include withdrawal of venous tone in the muscle bed. The short acting synthetic opioids have produced graded, dose related decreases in calculated vascular resistance across the muscle bed in animal studies. Certainly large doses of opioids given acutely may cause marked hypoten-sion through a decrease in calculated vascular resistance.[68] Much of this vascular resistance change occurs in the muscle circulation.

The potent inhalational anaesthetic drugs have a direct vasodilating effect on most skeletal muscle beds. Reflex vasoconstriction from humoral factors, such as vasopressin released during the relative hypotension induced by the potent inhalational agents, however, causes an overriding

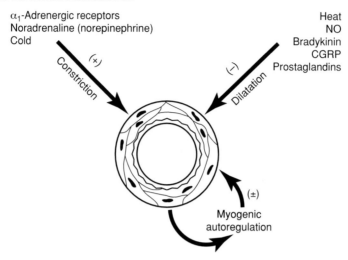

Fig 8.4 Control mechanisms in the cutaneous circulation.

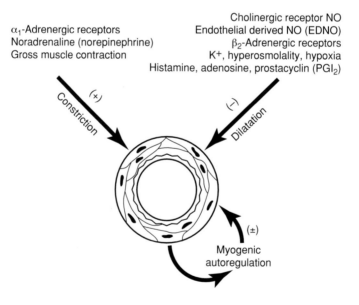

Fig 8.5 Control mechanisms for circulation through skeletal muscle.

vasoconstriction in many of the beds as well. On the whole there is little change in the skeletal muscle blood flow during most inhaled anaesthesia.

With regional blockade, particularly in segments that involve the sympathetic outflow tract to the lower extremities, blood flow to the muscle beds of the lower limbs increases. This is brought about by a reduction in the resting sympathetic tone to the blood vessels. Active vasodilation does not take place, but rather myogenic autoregulation limits the amount of dilatation that evolves.

In summary, control of the skeletal muscle vascular resistance involves complex interactions among neurogenic, autoregulatory, and metabolic systems. From the anaesthetic standpoint, resting control by sympathetic innervation, vasopressin levels, and autoregulatory mechanisms make a significant contribution towards total vascular resistance. The redistribution of cardiac output seen in haemorrhage and mild hypothermia, and with anaesthetic drugs is influenced markedly by the striated muscle circulation.

1 Kanwar YS, Venkatachalam MA. Ultrastructure of glomerulus and juxtaglomerular apparatus. In: *Renal physiology*, Vol 1, Windhager EE, ed, *Handbook of physiology*, Section 8. New York: Oxford University Press, 1992:3–40.

2 Tisher CC, Madsen KM. Anatomy of the kidney. In: Brenner, BM, Rector FC Jr, eds, *The kidney*, vol I. Philadelphia: WB Saunders, 1991:1–75.

3 Dworkin LD, Brenner BM. The renal circulations. In: Brenner BM, Rector FC Jr, eds, *The kidney*, vol I. Philadelphia: WB Saunders, 1991:164–204.

4 Venkatachalam MA, Kriz W. Anatomy. In: Heptinstall RH, ed, *Pathology of the kidney*, vol I. Boston: Little, Brown & Co., 1992:1–92.

5 Jones RD, Berne RM. Intrinsic regulation of skeletal muscle blood flow. *Circ Res* 1964;**14**:126–38.

6 Bayliss WM. On the local reactions of the arterial wall to changes in internal pressure. *J Physiol (Lond)* 1902;**28**:220–6.

7 Navar LG. Integrating multiple paracrine regulators of renal microvascular dynamics. *Am J Physiol* 1998;**274**(3 Part 2):F433–44.

8 Hall JE, Brands MW. The renin–angiotensin–aldosterone systems. Renal mechanisms and circulatory homeostasis. In: Seldin DW, Giebisch B, eds, *The kidney. Physiology and pathophysiology*, vol 2. New York: Raven Press, 1992:1455–1504.

9 Kon V. Neural control of renal circulation. *Mineral Electrolyte Metab* 1989;**15**:33–43.

10 Kien ND, Moore PG, Jaffe RS. Cardiovascular function during induced hypotension by fenoldopam or sodium nitroprusside in anesthetized dogs. *Anesth Analg* 1992;**74**:72–8.

11 Bischoff A, Michel MC. Renal effects of neuropeptide Y. *Pflügers Arch – Eur J Physiol* 1998;**435**:443–53.

12 Keeton TK, Campbell WB. The pharmacologic alteration of renin release. *Pharmacol Rev* 1980;**32**:81–227.

13 Navar LG, Inscho EW, Majid DSA, Imig JD, Harrison-Bernard LM, Mitchell KD. Paracrine regulation of the renal microcirculation. *Physiol Rev* 1996;**76**:425–536.

14 Venuto R, O'Dorisio CT, Ferris TF, Stein JH. Prostaglandins and renal function II. The effects of prostaglandin inhibition on autoregulation of blood flow in the intact kidney of the dog. *Prostaglandins* 1975;**9**:817–28.

15 Pallone TL, Silldorff EP, Turner MR. Intrarenal blood flow: Microvascular anatomy and the regulation of medullary perfusion. *Clin Exp Pharmacol Physiol* 1998;**25**:383–92.

16 Spielman WS, Thompson CI. A proposed role for adenosine in the regulation of renal hemodynamics and renin release. *Am J Physiol* 1982;**242**:F423–35.

17 Terada Y, Tomita K, Nonogushi H, Marumo F. Polymerase chain reaction localization of constitutive nitric oxide synthase and soluble guanylate cyclase messenger RNA_s in microdissected rat nephron segments. *J Clin Invest* 1992;**90**:659–65

18 Mattson DL, Roman RJ, Cowley AW Jr. Role of nitric oxide in renal papillary blood flow and sodium excretion. *Hypertension* 1992;**19**:766–70.

19 Tollins JP, Palmer RMJ, Mondala S, Raij L. Role of endothelium-derived relaxing factor in the hemodynamic response to acetylcholine in vivo. *Am J Physiol* 1990;**258**:665–72.

20 Lüscher TF, Bock HA. The endothelial L-arginine/nitric oxide pathway and the renal circulation. *Klin Wochenschr* 1991;**69**:603–9.

21 Reilly PM, Bulkley GB. Vasoactive mediators and splanchnic perfusion. *Crit Care Med* 1993;**21**:S55–68

22 Rosenblum JD, CM Boyle, LB Schwartz. The mesentric circulation. Anatomy and physiology. *Surg Clin North Am* 1997;**77**:289–306.

23 Takala J. Determinants of splanchnic blood flow. *Br J Anaesth* 1996;**77**:50–8.

24 Nishida O, Moriyasu F, Nakamura R, et al. Relationship between splenic and superior mesenteric venous circulation. *Gastroenterology* 1990;**98**:721–5.

25 Guyton AC. *Textbook of medical physiology*, 9th edn. Philadelphia: WB Saunders, 1996:179–80.

26 Parks DA, Jacobson ED. Physiology of the splanchnic circulation. *Arch Intern Med* 1985;**145**:1278–81.

27 Escourrou P, Raffestin B, Papelier Y, Pussard E, Rowell LB. Cardiopulmonary and carotid baroreflex control of splanchnic and forearm circulations. *Am J Physiol* 1993;**264**:H777–82.

28 Stadeager C, Hesse B, Henriksen O, et al. Effects of angiotensin blockade on the splanchnic circulation in normotensive humans. *J Appl Physiol* 1989;**67**:786–91.

29 Jacobson ED, Pawlik WW. Adenosine mediation of mesenteric blood flow. *J Physiol Pharmacol* 1992;**43**:3–19.

30 Holzer P. Peptidergic sensory neurons in the control of vascular functions: mechanisms and significance in the cutaneous and splanchnic vascular beds. *Rev Physiol Biochem Pharmacol* 1992;**121**:49–146.

31 Gatta A, Merkel C. Clinical pharmacology of splanchnic circulation in cirrhosis. *Pharmacol Res* 1990;**22**:235–52.

32 Ahlborg G, Weitzberg E, Lundberg JM. Circulating endothelin-1 reduces splanchnic and renal blood flow and splanchnic glucose production in humans. *J Appl Physiol* 1995;**79**:141–5.

33 Ahlborg G, Lundberg JM. Nitric oxide-endothelin-1 interaction in humans. *J Appl Physiol* 1997;**82**:1593–600.

34 Tokics L, Brismar B, Hedenstierna G. Splanchnic blood flow during halothane-relaxant anaesthesia in elderly patients. *Acta Anaesthesiol Scand* 1986;**30**:556–61.

35 Tverskoy M, Gelman S, Fowler KC, Bradley EL. Influence of fentanyl and morphine on intestinal circulation. *Anesth Analg* 1985;**64**:577–84.

36 Gelman S. Effects of anesthetics on splanchnic circulation. In: Altura BM, Halevy S, eds, *Cardiovascular actions of anesthetics and drugs used in anesthesia*, vol 2. Basel: Karger, 1986:126–61.

37 Aneman A, Pontén J, Fändriks L, Eisenhofer G, Friberg P, Biber B. Hemodynamic, sympathetic and angiotensin II responses to PEEP ventilation before and during administration of isoflurane. *Acta Anaesthesiol Scand* 1997;**41**:41–8.

38 Love R, Choe E, Lippton H, Flint L, Steinberg S. Positive end-expiratory pressure decreases mesenteric blood flow despite normalization of cardiac output. *J Trauma* 1995;**39**:195–9.

39 Tan OT, Stafford TJ. Cutaneous circulation. In: Fitzpatrick TB, Eisen AZ, Wolff K, Freedberg IM, Austin KF, eds. *Dermatology and general medicine*, 3rd edn. New York: McGraw-Hill, 1987:357–67.

40 Swerlick RA. The structure and function of the cutaneous vasculature. *J Dermatol* 1997;**24**:734–8.

41 Pavletic MM. Anatomy and circulation of the canine skin. *Microsurgery* 1991;**12**:103–12.

42 Midttun M, Sejrsen P. Cutaneous blood flow rate in areas with and without arteriovenous anastomoses during exercise. *Scand J Med Sci Sports* 1998;**8**:84–90.

43 Tripathi A, Mack GW, Nadel ER. Cutaneous vascular reflexes during exercise in the heat. *Med Sci Sports Exerc* 1990;**22**:796–803.

44 Sessler DI, Rubinstein EH. Letter to the editor. *Anesthesiology* 1989;**70**:371–2.

45 Johnson JM. Exercise and the cutaneous circulation. *Exerc Sport Sci Rev* 1992;20:59–97.

46 Jager K, Muench R, Seifert H, Beglinger C, Bollinger A, Fischer JA. Calcitonin gene-related peptide (CGRP) causes redistribution of blood flow in humans. *Eur J Clin Pharmacol* 1990;**39**:491–4.

47 Edfeldt H, Lundvall J. Sympathetic baroreflex control of vascular resistance in comfortably warm man. Analyses of neurogenic constrictor responses in the resting forearm and in its separate skeletal muscle and skin tissue compartments. *Acta Physiol Scand* 1993;**147**:437–47.

48 Johnson JM, Brengelmann GL, Hales JRS, Vanhoutte PM, Wenger CB. Regulation of the cutaneous circulation. *Fed Proc* 1986;**45**:2841–50.

49 Kellogg DL Jr, Johnson JM, Kenney WL, Pergola PE, Koshiba WA. Mechanisms of control of skin blood flow during prolonged exercise in humans. *Am J Physiol* 1993;**265**:H562–8.

50 Holzer P. Neurogenic vasodilation and plasma leakage in the skin. *Gen Pharmacol* 1998;**30**:5–11.

51 Joyner MJ, Dietz NM. Nitric oxide and vasodilation in human limbs. *J Appl Physiol* 1997;**83**:1785–96.

52 Fruhstorfer H, Wagener G. Effects of intradermal lignocaine and mepivacaine on human cutaneous circulation in areas with histamine-induced neurogenic inflammation. *Br J Anaesth* 1993;**70**:167–72.

53 Lundin S, Kirnö K, Wallin BG, Elam M. Effects of epidural anaesthesia on sympathetic nerve discharge to the skin. *Acta Anaesthesiol Scand* 1990;**34**:492–7.

54 Shepherd JT. Circulation to skeletal muscle. In: Shepherd JT, Abboud FM, eds. *Handbook of physiology*, Section 2, *The cardiovascular system*, Vol 3, *Peripheral circulation and blood flow*, Part 1. Baltimore: Williams & Wilkins, 1983:319–70.

55 Carù B, Colombo E, Santoro F, Laporta A, Maslowsky F. Regional flow responses to exercise. *Chest* 1992;**101**:S223–5.

56 Sheriff DD, Rowell LB, Scher AM. Is rapid rise of vascular conductance at onset of dynamic exercise due to muscle pump? *Am J Physiol* 1993;**265**:H1227–34.

57 Smith JJ, Porth CJM. Posture and the circulation: the age effect. *Exp Gerontol* 1991;**26**:141–62.

58 Bevan JA, Laher I. Pressure and flow-dependent vascular tone. *FASEB J* 1991;**5**:2267–73.

59 Grände PO. Myogenic mechanisms in the skeletal muscle circulation. *J Hypertens* 1989;7:S47–53.

60 Mellander S. Functional aspects of myogenic vascular control. *J Hypertens* 1989;7:S21–30.

61 Jacobsen TN, Morgan BJ, Scherrer U, et al. Relative contributions of cardiopulmonary and sinoaortic baroreflexes in causing sympathetic activation in the human skeletal muscle circulation during orthostatic stress. *Circ Res* 1993;**73**:367–78.

62 Reid MB. Role of nitric oxide in skeletal muscle: synthesis, distribution and functional importance. *Acta Physiol Scand* 1998;**162**:401–9.

63 Delp MD, Lauglin MH. Regulation of skeletal muscle perfusion during exercise. *Acta Physiol Scand* 1998;**162**:411–19.

64 Vane JR, Botting RM. Endothelium-derived vasoactive factors and the control of the circulation. *Semin Perinatol* 1991;**15**(1):4–10.

65 Saltin B, Radegran MD, Koskolou, Roach RC. Skeletal muscle blood flow in humans and its regulation during exercise. *Acta Physiol Scand* 1998;**162**:421–36.

66 Longhurst JC, Mitchell JH. Reflex control of the circulation by afferents from skeletal muscle. In: Guyton AC, Young DB, eds, *Cardiovascular physiology III*, vol 18. Baltimore: University Park Press, 1979:125–48.

67 Sellgren J, Ejnell H, Elam M, Ponten J, Wallin BG. Sympathetic muscle nerve activity, peripheral blood flows, and baroreceptor reflexes in humans during propofol anesthesia and surgery. *Anesthesiology* 1994;**80**:534–44.

68 White DA, Reitan JA, Kien ND, Thorup SJ. Decrease in vascular resistance in the isolated canine hindlimb after graded doses of alfentanil, fentanyl, and sufentanil. *Anesth Analg* 1990;**71**:29–34.

9: Microcirculation

JAMES E BAUMGARDNER, ALEX L LOEB,
DAVID E LONGNECKER

A major concern of modern anaesthesia and critical care practice involves optimal preservation of organs and tissues that are at risk for ischaemia. The effects of anaesthetic agents on the preservation of vital organ function influences the selection of anaesthetic drugs and techniques. Anaesthetic drugs have been shown, in animal models, to influence outcome in several abnormal circulatory conditions that compromise perfusion and tissue delivery of nutrients such as oxygen and glucose. These circulatory abnormalities include local organ ischaemia, haemorrhagic shock, and septic shock.

Partial or complete tissue ischaemia presents an obvious compromise of nutrient delivery to tissue. Several anaesthetic drugs have been shown to provide drug specific protective effects for partial ischaemia, or for complete ischaemia followed by reperfusion. Anaesthetic drugs have been shown to differ in their effects on biochemical consequences and histological outcome for incomplete liver ischaemia,[1] for complete liver ischaemia and reperfusion,[2 3] after repeated complete cerebral ischaemic episodes,[4] and after incomplete cerebral ischaemia.[5-7]

Haemorrhagic shock results in selectively reduced blood flow and nutrient delivery to several organs, including the splanchnic, renal, skin, and muscle circulations. Anaesthetic drugs have a drug specific effect on outcome in animal models of haemorrhagic shock (induced by controlled haemorrhage for a fixed period of time, followed by reperfusion). Ketamine provided a markedly better survival than halothane or pentobarbital (pentobarbitone) anaesthesia in haemorrhaged rats.[8] This study also reported a reduction in intestinal mucosal lesions with ketamine anaesthesia. More recently, high epidural anaesthesia combined with general anaesthesia in haemorrhaged dogs improved survival compared with general anaesthesia alone,[9] again suggesting that anaesthetic techniques alter outcome from compromised organ perfusion. Anaesthetic specific differences in bacterial translocation and intestinal histological damage have also been demonstrated in haemorrhaged rats.[10]

The circulatory defects in sepsis and septic shock include a hyper-dynamic circulation with high cardiac output, low systemic resistance, and increased oxygen uptake, with proportionally greater increases in oxygen delivery. The resulting decreased oxygen extraction may represent either inadequate nutrient delivery from blood to tissue or impaired biochemical use of oxygen. Anaesthetics have specific effects on oxygen delivery ($\dot{D}o_2$), oxygen uptake ($\dot{V}o_2$), and serum lactate in dogs infused with endotoxin. In a dog model of septic shock, ketamine caused less lactate accumulation than enflurane,[11] and ketamine preserved cardiovascular function better than halothane, isoflurane, or alfentanil.[12] In contrast, enflurane anaes-thesia in endotoxaemic rats resulted in significantly less intestinal pathology than ketamine anaesthesia,[13] and halothane improved survival compared with ketamine after reperfusion of ischaemic bowel.[14]

Several mechanisms have been suggested to explain these protective effects of anaesthetic drugs:

- they can suppress tissue metabolic requirements and thereby increase tolerance to reduced nutrient delivery
- they can modulate biochemical and cellular mediators of ischaemic tissue damage, and thereby reduce permanent damage after an ischaemic insult
- they are known to have drug specific and dose dependent effects on tissue perfusion, which can increase tissue oxygenation during an ischaemic insult.

Anaesthetic drugs decrease tissue metabolism in several organs; the extent of this metabolic suppression depends on the specific anaesthetic and the specific organ. For example, halothane produces more suppression of metabolism in the myocardium than isoflurane, but isoflurane produces greater inhibition of metabolism in cerebral tissue. Decreased metabolic requirements may ameliorate the effects of reductions in tissue nutrients, but these are specific effects of anaesthetic drugs at the local tissue level and not a uniform consequence of the general anaesthetic state.

Anaesthetic drugs can also modify the biochemical consequences of tissue hypoxia. The past 15–20 years have witnessed a tremendous growth in our knowledge of the role of mediators involved with tissue hypoxia, particularly in the brain. Release of various excitatory neurotransmitters, such as glutamate, increases in intracellular calcium, and generation of free radicals and lipid peroxidation are all thought to play a role in the permanent tissue damage that follows tissue hypoxia. Anaesthetic drugs can have important effects in modulating these changes after ischaemia. For example, ketamine is an antagonist of the N-methyl-D-aspartate (NMDA) subtype of the glutamate receptor, and excessive activation of the glutamate receptor pathway is associated with excitotoxicity and cell death.[15] In addition, anaesthetic drugs have drug specific and organ specific effects on tissue microcirculation, and these actions can modify organ perfusion and cell viability in response to circulatory insults such as shock, ischaemia, or hypoxaemia.

The primary function of the circulatory system is the delivery of nutrients such as oxygen and glucose and the removal of waste such as carbon dioxide. The efficient accomplishment of this task depends on the distribution of blood flow within organs, which is regulated primarily by the resistance vessels in the microcirculation. The microcirculatory effects of anaesthetic drugs can influence nutrient delivery and the distribution of blood flow in the following:

• in cases of globally impaired perfusion and/or oxygenation, as occurs in haemorrhagic and septic shock
• in cases of incomplete tissue ischaemia as might occur in peripheral vascular disease
• during reperfusion after complete ischaemia, such as that after arterial occlusion during certain surgical procedures.

This chapter provides an introduction and overview of the micro-circulation; it covers anatomy and terminology, the normal function of the microcirculation, physiological control mechanisms, and the effects of anaesthetic and other drugs on the microcirculation and microcirculatory control mechanisms. The microcirculation has many biological functions, including immune functions, endocrine functions, and solute and water exchange, but the major focus in this chapter is on the primary tasks of distribution of blood flow, exchange of nutrients, and regulation of vascular capacitance. Wherever possible, the effects of anaesthetic drugs will be related to probable roles in improving outcome in abnormal circulatory conditions.

Anatomy

The microvasculature is described as a series of successive branchings of arterioles, with a decrease in diameter with each branching generation. This arteriolar branching structure culminates in the capillaries, which then coalesce into successively larger branches of venules, finally merging into larger veins. Terminology in the microvasculature follows this branching scheme, with the largest arterioles and venules in a given vital microscopy preparation (a living tissue examined directly under the microscope) designated as first order vessels (for example, 1A arterioles and 1V venules) and the next largest integer assigned to each successively smaller generation of vessels (2A, 3A, etc) down to the capillary level. The assignment of typical vessels in a given preparation is somewhat arbitrary, but it is a useful scheme for comparison between preparations, so that a given vessel of a numbered generation may share some features with the same generation of a different sized animal, even though the absolute vessel diameters may not be the same.

The distinction between large arterioles and small arteries is not definitive, but generally arterioles cover a range of sizes from 10 to 150 μm in diameter. Typically, a microvascular network includes three to five branching orders spanning this size range. The walls of arterioles contain relatively large amounts of vascular smooth muscle, which participate in active circulatory regulation; the smallest arterioles – meta-arterioles – contain intermittent bands of vascular smooth muscle.

Capillaries are long thin tubes of endothelium, typically 5–10 μm in diameter and 50–1000 μm in length. They are devoid of vascular smooth muscle except for special bands of muscle at the arteriolar end of the capillary, the precapillary sphincters, which participate in regulation of capillary density. Precapillary sphincters are present only in some tissues, but most small arterioles appear to exhibit sphincter-like activity, and thus act as functional sphincters. In addition to active regulation of capillary density in a given tissue, different organs and tissues vary widely in their maximal perfused capillary density, with highly metabolically active tissues generally having a denser capillary network.

Venules of a given branching order are larger than their equivalent arterioles and have thinner and more distensible walls. As a result, the cross sectional area of a venular generation is larger, and blood flow is slower, than for the equivalent arteriolar generation. Larger venules tend to pair with adjacent arterioles of the same branch order (Fig 9.1). The parallel arrangement of arterioles and venules may provide an opportunity for countercurrent exchange of gases and solutes, most notably in intestinal mucosa.[16]

Quantitative description of even a simple microcirculatory network would require an enormous number of branch lengths, branch diameters, numbers of branches at bifurcations, and branching angles at each bifurcation. Progress has been made recently in fractal descriptions of these networks, reducing the entire description to a single fractal equation with a small number of parameters.[17]

Function

Resistance

Distribution of cardiac output to individual organs is regulated locally by changes in vascular resistance, which is controlled by regulation of vascular diameters. Resistance (defined as blood flow divided by pressure decrease across a vascular bed) in a cylindrical vessel varies approximately with the

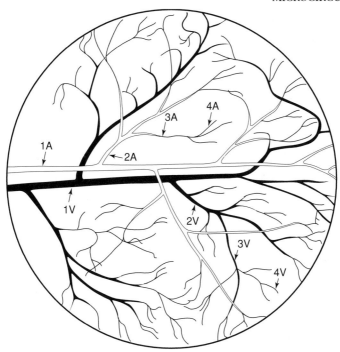

Fig 9.1 Drawing of a typical microvascular network in rat cremaster muscle, with numbering system for vessel generations based on order in branching hierarchy. (Adapted with permission from Hutchins PM, Goldstone J, Wells R. Effects of haemorrhagic shock on the microvasculature of skeletal muscle. *Microvasc Res* 1973;5:131.)

fourth power of the diameter, with the result that small changes in vascular diameter effect large changes in resistance. In skeletal muscle and intestinal circulations, small arterioles (< 100 μm in diameter in the cat) are responsible for nearly all of the vascular resistance to blood flow. Small arterioles make a major contribution to resistance in other circulations as well, but recently it has been recognised that larger arterioles and small arteries make a significant contribution to resistance in the coronary circulation, and even larger arteries make a significant contribution in the cerebral circulation (Fig 9.2).[18][19]

Many organs and tissues can regulate local blood flow to meet tissue metabolic needs. Autoregulation refers specifically to maintenance of constant tissue blood flow over a range of perfusing pressures, when all other variables (for example, tissue metabolic rate, arterial P_{CO_2} or P_{aCO_2}, arterial P_{O_2} or P_{aO_2}, neurohumoral inputs) are constant. This regulation may be mediated by response of vascular smooth muscle to changes in distending pressure (the myogenic hypothesis) or by feedback regulation of

311

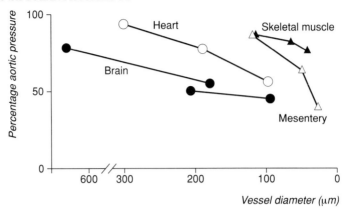

Fig 9.2 Pressure, as percentage of aortic pressure, measured in several sizes of arteries and arterioles of the cat; for brain, heart, mesentery, and skeletal muscle. (Reproduced with permission from Faraci FM, Heistad DD. Regulation of large cerebral arteries and cerebral microvascular pressure. *Circ Res* 1990;**66**:9.)

local metabolic mediators (the metabolic hypothesis). Although the exact mechanism is unknown, it is evident from microvascular studies that the vessels responsible for autoregulation are the small arterioles, with increasingly less contribution as vessel diameter increases and branching order decreases.[19] Many tissues also vary local blood flow in proportion to tissue metabolic rate (again with other variables such as perfusing pressure held constant), a phenomenon known as metabolic regulation. Small arterioles are also primarily responsible for this local regulatory response. The mechanism of metabolic regulation is unknown, but recent studies of the cerebral circulation in particular suggest a prominent role for regulation by increased production of nitric oxide (NO) from specific neurons in response to surrounding neuronal activity.[20]

Microvascular studies have led to a growing appreciation that alterations in vascular diameters are usually not uniform and tend to be very site specific. For example, autoregulatory responses do not change all vessel diameters or vessel resistances proportionately, but tend to affect the most distal arterioles. In contrast, changes in vascular diameter from systemic neural inputs alter the larger arterioles and small arteries. Vasoactive and anaesthetic drugs also affect specific branching orders or sizes of arterioles. For example, nitroglycerine produces dose dependent dilatation of coronary arterioles and arteries more than 200 μm in diameter, but causes little change in smaller arteriolar diameters; in contrast, nifedipine causes homogeneous dilatation of all coronary microvessels.[19] The functional implications of the specificity of microvascular responses are not yet clear, but may in part explain why a group of vasodilators that produce seemingly equivalent decreases in total vascular resistance can have drug specific differences in preventing tissue ischaemia.

Capacitance

Vascular capacitance refers to the ability of the circulatory system to store variable amounts of blood with minimal changes in central filling pressures. Regulation of vascular capacitance by neurohumoral mechanisms plays an important role in cardiovascular responses to haemorrhage and other acute changes in blood volume. About 70% of the blood volume resides in the venous circulation, with most of it contained in venules in the micro-circulation. Neurohumoral regulation controls the diameter of these microcirculatory venules, especially in the splanchnic circulation, whereas large veins function primarily as conduits.[21]

Exchange

The primary function of the microcirculation is the delivery of oxygen and the removal of carbon dioxide from tissue. Adequate gas exchange depends on tissue blood flow and diffusion characteristics between the blood and tissues. It is therefore possible to have adequate overall perfusion but deficient gas exchange. In septic shock, for example, many tissues receive increased blood flow, but the decreased extraction of oxygen may produce tissue hypoxia from inefficient use of this blood flow.[22]

Capillaries have been classically regarded as the only vessels that exchange significant amounts of oxygen between blood and tissue, with regulation of capillary density playing the major role in the regulation of the efficiency of gas exchange. As capillary density increases, the area available for diffusion of gases to tissue increases proportionately. As the cross sectional area available for blood flow also increases, the flow velocity in each capillary decreases, and consequently the time available for diffusion (the capillary transit time) also increases with increasing capillary density. The regulation of capillary density by means of the vascular smooth muscle at the precapillary sphincters therefore represents a potential site for anaesthetic effects on vascular smooth muscle to alter the efficiency of gas exchange. Precapillary sphincters may also play a role in regulating the efficiency of gas exchange by matching individual capillary perfusion to local metabolism, thereby reducing the flow/metabolism heterogeneity that can reduce the efficiency of gas exchange.[23]

In addition to the classic role of capillaries in tissue gas exchange, it is now recognised that other vessels in a microcirculatory vessel network can exchange gases with tissues and with each other.[24] Diffusional interactions between blood vessels function essentially as arteriovenous shunting and thereby impair the efficiency of gas exchange. These diffusional vessel interactions are sensitive to the time available for diffusion (vessel transit time), which is increased by arteriolar or venular dilatation.[25] The vascular smooth muscle of the arterioles and venules therefore represents another potential site for anaesthetic effects to influence the efficiency of tissue gas exchange.

Efficient tissue gas exchange depends on the total number of open vessels in a microvascular network, and on the distribution of blood flow within those vessels. Anaesthetic and other vasoactive drugs that act on vascular smooth muscle probably influence the efficiency of gas exchange by these mechanisms, although experimental studies at this level have been limited. In normal tissue, gas exchange is very efficient and blood flow can be reduced dramatically (by anaesthetic drugs or other mechanisms) in most organs before the onset of cellular hypoxia. When tissue oxygenation is impaired as a result of trauma or disease, however, the microvascular effects of anaesthetic drugs may have an important influence on tissue oxygenation.

Control of the microcirculation

The contractile activity of smooth muscle in the walls of arteries, arterioles, venules, and veins is controlled by many mechanisms. Vascular smooth muscle tone is influenced by remote (for example, centrally mediated) control mechanisms, and by local control mechanisms. Remote control mechanisms can be further subdivided into neural control and humoral control. Alterations in arteriolar smooth muscle contraction that result from these influences are responsible for the changes in resistance that determine the distribution of cardiac output. There is a remarkable variation in basal vascular tone and resistance from organ to organ. Renal arterioles, for example, have a very low resting vascular tone and can constrict markedly in response to stimuli such as hypovolaemia, but they have little capacity to dilate. In contrast, arterioles in the skin have a high resting tone and can both dilate and constrict in response to thermoregulatory stimuli.

Neural control

Arteries and arterioles are innervated by sympathetic fibres terminating in the blood vessel walls. The extent of sympathetic innervation varies from organ to organ. For example, renal vessels and mesenteric vessels receive dense innervation by adrenergic neurons, but the cerebral and coronary vessels receive fairly sparse adrenergic innervation. Accordingly, organs with a rich supply of adrenergic neurons exhibit a much greater constrictor response to sympathetic neural stimulation than occurs in the cerebral and coronary circulations. Similarly, neuronal supply along the generations of the vascular tree is not uniform, but generally tends to be more dense in the larger vessels with a decreasing neuronal supply in the more distal generations. Consequently, vasoconstrictor fibre stimulation results not only in a change in organ vascular resistance, but also in a change in the distribution of organ vascular resistance, with an increased contribution by larger arterioles and arteries.[18][19] Autonomic innervation plays an important regulatory role in coordination of the vascular response to any stimuli that activate the sympathoadrenal axis, such as hypovolaemia, hypoxia, hypercapnia, tissue trauma, and pain. Sympathetic innervation probably plays a minimal role in more local control, such as local regulation of blood flow in response to increased organ metabolism.

Systemic humoral control

Numerous endogenously produced mediators have been shown to constrict or dilate vascular smooth muscle. Intravascularly administered adrenaline (epinephrine), noradrenaline (norepinephrine), angiotensin II, vasopressin, endothelin, prostaglandin $PGF_{2\alpha}$, and thromboxane cause dose dependent, organ specific, and site specific vasoconstriction. Intravascularly administered acetylcholine, atrial natriuretic peptide (ANP), bradykinin, serotonin, adenosine, prostacyclin (PGI_2), and PGE_2 cause dose dependent, organ specific, and site specific vasodilation.[19][26][27] There is no doubt that many of these substances play a role in local humoral regulation of vascular smooth muscle tone. Although our knowledge of the complexities of endogenous mediators in vascular control is growing rapidly, the role of endogenous mediators in remote humoral control remains uncertain.

Local control: vascular endothelium

Over the past two decades there has been a tremendous growth in our understanding of the role of vascular endothelium in mediating effects of vasoactive drugs. For example, endogenous compounds such as acetylcholine, bradykinin, ATP, histamine, and many others dilate arterioles by stimulating the release of multiple endothelium derived relaxing factors (EDRFs), which include nitric oxide (NO), endothelium derived hyperpolarising factor (EDHF), and eicosanoids. These different EDRFs can act independently or in concert to influence microvascular diameters and blood flows.[28-31]

This new understanding of the role of the endothelium in vascular control was initiated by the discovery[32] that NO (then called EDRF) functioned as an important mediator of vasodilation. EDRF, subsequently identified as NO, is produced by the conversion of arginine and oxygen into NO and citrulline, a reaction that is catalysed by the enzyme NO synthase

(NOS).[33][34] Although many forms of NOS have been identified, they may be classified into constitutive forms (that is, always expressed), those found in endothelial cells and neurons, and inducible forms that can be expressed in response to stimuli such as inflammation.

The multiple locations of these isoforms of NOS imply multiple functions for the gaseous transmitter, and it is now evident that NO is involved in a variety of biological functions, including local cardiovascular control, neuronal transmission, immune function, and the control of pathogens (for example, bacteria). This discussion focuses only on microvascular control functions of NO, but concise reviews are available that describe its other biological functions.[35]

The actions of NO on the peripheral circulation can be evaluated by the infusion of an arginine analogue inhibitor of NOS into intact animals, and recording the resultant changes in cardiovascular function. We have used this approach to determine the actions of NO on blood pressure, cardiac output, and regional blood flows in conscious rats, by injecting radio-labelled microspheres into the circulation before and during the infusion of the NOS inhibitor N^G-monomethyl-L-arginine (L-NMMA), and again after the infusion of L-arginine, to demonstrate that the changes observed during response to L-NMMA were reversible by providing more substrate for NO production.[36] Inhibition of NO produced major changes in blood pressure regulation and peripheral circulatory control. The general circulatory effects are summarised in Table 9.1.

In brief, inhibition of NO caused a doubling of systemic vascular resistance and increased arterial pressure, accompanied by decreases in heart rate and cardiac output.

Inhibition of NO by L-NMMA decreased local blood flow in the cerebrum, heart, kidneys, spleen, gastrointestinal tract, portal vein, liver (total flow), skin, ear, and white fat, whereas flow increased in the hepatic artery (presumably in response to the decrease in portal and total hepatic

Table 9.1 *Effects of EDRF/NO inhibition by L-NMMA and reversal of inhibition by L-arginine on systemic haemodynamics*

Parameter	Treatment		
	Control	L-NMMA	L-Arginine
CO (ml/min)	90±5	52±5	68±6
HR (beats/min)	441±13	404±17	430±16
MAP (mm Hg)	129±5	145±5	134±4
SVR (mm Hg × min × g/ml)	1·5±0·1	3·0±0·3	2·1±0·2

CO, cardiac output; HR, heart rate; MAP, mean arterial pressure; SVR, systemic vascular resistance.
(Reproduced with permission from Greenblatt et al.[28][36])

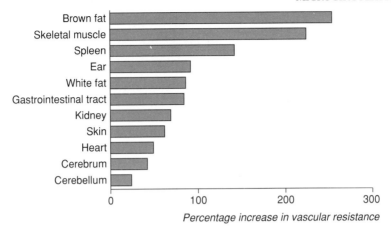

Fig 9.3 The percentage increase in mean regional vascular resistances induced by L-NMMA in conscious rats, reflecting the heterogeneity of the contribution of EDRF/NO to regional vascular control. (Reproduced with permission from Greenblatt EP, Loeb AL, Longnecker DE. Marked regional heterogeneity in the magnitude of EDRF/NO-mediated vascular tone in awake rats. *J Cardiovasc Pharmacol* 1993;**21**:237.)

blood flow). Vascular resistances were increased in virtually every tissue studied, although the magnitude of the response was variable among organs and tissues, indicating that the relative importance of this system depends on local factors (Fig 9.3).

Similar results have been observed in numerous studies in isolated blood vessels or local microvascular networks, suggesting that the results obtained above can be attributed to inhibition of NO in the vascular endothelium, although the possibility of remote effects cannot be ruled out whenever inhibitors of NO are administered systemically. These studies provide clear evidence that NO is a profound and ubiquitous controller of the peripheral circulation. It is clear, however, that NO is not the only controller of the peripheral circulation, and it is impossible to attribute either physiological or pharmacological effects in the microcirculation to a single mechanism, because multiple mechanisms are involved in the control of vascular tone.

Effects of anaesthetic drugs on the microcirculation

This section does not present a comprehensive review of the effects of each anaesthetic on each individual tissue, but focuses instead on a few illustrative studies of the differences in peripheral circulatory effects of anaesthetic drugs. Wherever possible, comparison is made between the effects of two anaesthetic drugs in the same study, using the same protocol.

Isoflurane versus halothane

Comparison of the effects of isoflurane against those of halothane emphatically illustrates that two anaesthetic drugs that appear to be similar on a superficial level can be quite distinctive on more detailed investigation. When delivered in equipotent concentrations (minimum alveolar concentration or MAC), these two agents produce approximately equal decreases in mean arterial blood pressure. However, when cardiac output and systemic vascular resistance are also measured, it becomes apparent that halothane lowers blood pressure primarily by decreases in cardiac output, whereas isoflurane primarily decreases systemic vascular resistance.[37-39] Further differences between these two agents are evident on more detailed investigation of individual organ blood flow and microcirculatory vascular diameters. In general, isoflurane is the more potent vasodilator, but the relative decreases in vascular resistance for these agents are organ specific, and the extent of dilatation also tends to be specific for vessel branching order within a tissue.

Organ resistances and blood flows

Anaesthetic drugs mediate changes in organ blood flow by changes in vascular diameter and resistance. Resistance is a quotient of pressure divided by flow, and therefore measurements of systemic pressure and local (organ or tissue) blood flow can be used to calculate changes in local resistance. Several techniques are available to measure organ blood flow in laboratory and clinical studies. Radioactive microspheres, which distribute to organs in proportion to blood flow, provide a quantitative and absolute measure of tissue blood flow, but require destruction of the tissue sample for counting and weighing to achieve the most accuracy, and therefore are limited to laboratory studies. Indicator dilution techniques (for example, thermal or indocyanine green dilution) also provide absolute and quantitative blood flow measurements. These techniques require venous outflow sampling, but are applicable in some clinical studies when an appropriate venous catheter can be placed. Large vessel flow probes (for example, electromagnetic or Doppler ultrasonic probes) require invasive placement, but can be implanted for chronic use. Some thermal and inert tracer clearance methods are invasive (for example, hydrogen clearance techniques that require implantation of hydrogen microelectrodes), whereas others are non-invasive and are used clinically, for example, radioactive xenon (^{133}Xe) wash-out. More recently, laser Doppler velocimetry (LDV) has been used in both laboratory and clinical studies. This technique measures relative changes in blood flow quantitatively and continuously.

In dogs receiving an opiate general anaesthestic, either halothane or isoflurane was added and titrated to decrease mean arterial pressure to 60 mm Hg.[40] Inspired isoflurane of 1·5% maintained myocardial blood flow (measured by radioactive microspheres) and decreased coronary vascular resistance by 40%. In contrast, 1·1% inspired halothane decreased myocardial blood flow by 35% and decreased coronary resistance by 13%.

Debaene et al[41] induced cirrhosis in rats by bile duct ligation and then compared the influence of anaesthetic drugs on liver blood flow during mild haemorrhage (removal of 20% of estimated blood volume). One MAC (1·3% inspired in rats) isoflurane anaesthesia maintained hepatic arterial flow (measured by radioactive microspheres) at prehaemorrhage values. One MAC (1·0% inspired in rats) halothane anaesthesia caused a significant decrease in hepatic arterial flow during haemorrhage.

Frink et al[1] studied portal venous and hepatic arterial blood flows by means of chronically implanted probes in healthy dogs. They measured the effects of four different anaesthetic drugs on portal venous and hepatic arterial blood flow, compared with conscious controls, for three different doses of anaesthetic drugs (1·0, 1·5, and 2·0 MAC). Halothane reduced hepatic arterial blood flow in a dose dependent fashion and increased hepatic arterial vascular resistance. In contrast, isoflurane maintained hepatic arterial flow at all doses. Isoflurane reduced portal venous flow at the higher doses. Halothane caused greater decreases in portal venous flow at all doses.

Vollmar et al[42] studied liver and pancreatic blood flows (by microspheres) and tissue oxygen tensions (by multiwire surface electrodes) in rats. Isoflurane and halothane were titrated to reduce mean arterial pressure to 50 mm Hg (2·3% inspired isoflurane, and 1·0% inspired halothane). Isoflurane and halothane both caused similar reductions in portal venous and hepatic arterial blood flows (by radioactive microspheres) compared with chloralose anaesthetised controls, but isoflurane reduced mean tissue Po_2 from 4·08 kPa to 2·33 kPa, whereas halothane caused greater reductions to a mean tissue Po_2 of 1·53 kPa. Halothane maintained pancreatic blood flow and tissue oxygen tension compared with controls. In contrast, isoflurane increased pancreatic blood flow and tissue oxygen tension.

Jacob et al[43] studied arterial blood flow (by means of implanted Doppler probes) supplying an ileocolic graft after oesophageal reconstruction in humans.[43] Fentanyl infusions of 300 μg/h that were established intra-operatively were maintained immediately postoperatively and then 0·65 MAC isoflurane or halothane was administered in a crossover design. Halothane did not change mesenteric blood flow and isoflurane increased mesenteric blood flow by 38%.

Hansen et al[44] studied the distribution of cerebral blood flow in rats at 1 MAC of either isoflurane or halothane.[44] Blood flows to the subcortex were not significantly different between halothane and isoflurane, but halothane caused significantly greater blood flows in the neocortex.

Vessel diameters

Vessel diameters can be studied in intact tissue under direct microscopic visualisation (vital microscopy) by means of either transillumination (for a suitably thin tissue) or epi-illumination of a tissue surface. This invasive technique has been applied primarily in anaesthetised animals. Some vascular networks have been examined microscopically in humans (for example, the nail fold),[45] but these are fairly specialised circulations and it is difficult to extrapolate results to other organs of interest. Direct microscopic visualisation has the unique advantage of providing information about the specific vessels and branching orders that are influenced by anaesthetic drugs. The studies are, however, technically demanding and there have been fewer reports of the comparative effects of anaesthetic drugs using these techniques.

Conzen et al[40] studied the microcirculation of the epicardial surface of the left ventricle in intact, beating dog hearts by means of epi-illumination.[40] The dogs were anaesthetised with opiate infusions and then received isoflurane or halothane titrated to reduce mean arterial pressure to 60 mmHg (1·1% inspired halothane, 1·5% inspired isoflurane). Isoflurane caused larger increases in arteriolar diameters than halothane. Both agents dilated 20–200 μm vessels specifically, and had no effects on larger arterioles or on precapillary sphincters.

Leon et al[46] studied rat diaphragm arteriolar diameters and functional capillary density by vital microscopy. All rats received pentobarbital anaesthesia, followed by three concentrations (0·50, 0·75, and 1·0 MAC) of either halothane or isoflurane. Halothane administration caused dose dependent constriction specifically in the A4 arterioles of diaphragm muscle, leaving A2 and A3 arterioles unchanged, and also decreased capillary density in a dose dependent manner. Administration of isoflurane caused no significant changes in arteriolar diameter or capillary density.

Summary of isoflurane versus halothane

This brief and selective review of recent studies of organ resistances and blood flows demonstrates the different effects of isoflurane and halothane for heart, liver, pancreas, mesentery, and brain, and also different effects on specific regions within an organ. In the case of the liver and pancreas, these agent specific microcirculatory effects have been associated with changes in tissue oxygen tension. The vital microscopy studies in cardiac and skeletal muscle demonstrate the specificity of the circulatory effects of anaesthetic drugs for vessels of a particular size and branching order. Further studies will be required to connect the specificity of these changes to the specific influence of anaesthetic drugs on the delivery of nutrients to tissue. In general, isoflurane tends to be a more potent vasodilator than halothane, and as a result tends to maintain tissue blood flow, although there are exceptions for selected tissues and for specific pathologies. The clinical importance is that, in patients with circulatory pathology and compromised tissue oxygenation, the microcirculatory effects of anaesthetic drugs have the potential to influence tissue preservation in the perioperative period.

Parenteral anaesthetic drugs

Compared with the inhalational anaesthetic drugs, considerably fewer studies of the effects of parenteral anaesthetic drugs on organ blood flows and microvascular diameters have been reported. Data are particularly scarce for direct comparisons of two or more parenteral anaesthetic techniques, for example high dose opiate anaesthesia compared with propofol infusion. There have, however, been several microvascular studies comparing ketamine with other anaesthetic techniques, and a selective review of these reports further supports the concept of drug specific effects on organ blood flows and branching generations. Interest in ketamine arises in part because it is used in laboratory animals as well as in humans, and also because of its unique beneficial properties in haemorrhagic shock.[8 47] Ketamine may also be uniquely beneficial in septic shock,[12 48] although the data in this area are more conflicting.[13 14]

Organ resistances and blood flows

Debaene et al[41] compared the effects of several anaesthetic drugs, including ketamine and enflurane, on portal venous blood flow and hepatic arterial blood flow during mild haemorrhage (removal of 20% of estimated blood volume) in cirrhotic rats. During haemorrhage, enflurane (2·2% inspired) decreased portal venous flow more than ketamine (1·5 mg/kg/per min i.v.), but after reinfusion of the shed blood the portal venous blood flows were similar. During haemorrhage, enflurane decreased hepatic arterial blood flow and ketamine resulted in an unchanged hepatic arterial blood flow.

In isolated intestinal loops in dogs, Tverskoy et al[49] found that ketamine (both 8 and 16 mg/kg i.v.) caused increased vascular resistance and decreased blood flow compared with pentobarbital.

Seyde and Longnecker[50] studied the effects of four anaesthetic drugs (ketamine 1 mg/kg/per min i.v., halothane 1·2% inspired, isoflurane 1·4% inspired, and enflurane 2·2% inspired) on organ blood flows (measured by microspheres) and organ vascular resistances in rats. Results were compared with the effects in conscious controls, during both normo-volaemia and moderate hypovolaemia (removal of 30% of estimated blood volume).[50] Before haemorrhage, ketamine maintained cerebral blood flow at conscious values, whereas the inhaled agents increased cerebral blood flow. After haemorrhage, ketamine, enflurane, and halothane reduced cerebral blood flow significantly compared with conscious animals, but isoflurane did not. At baseline, isoflurane maintained myocardial blood flow at conscious values, and ketamine, enflurane, and halothane progressively reduced myocardial blood flow. After haemorrhage, myocardial blood flow increased in conscious animals, did not change under isoflurane or halothane anaesthesia, and decreased under ketamine or enflurane anaesthesia. Before haemorrhage, portal venous flow was increased, compared with conscious animals, by ketamine anaesthesia and was reduced compared with controls by halothane anaesthesia; portal flow was decreased in all groups after haemorrhage. Hepatic arterial blood flow after haemorrhage was greatest in animals receiving isoflurane anaesthesia, although ketamine resulted in an increase in hepatic arterial blood flow, compared with normovolaemia. Several other organ blood flows were studied, and the study demonstrates the drug specific effects of the anaesthetic drugs on organ vascular resistances, as well as the unique properties of ketamine.

Miller et al[51] compared the distribution of cardiac output in conscious rats with that during halothane, enflurane, or ketamine anaesthesia.[51] Halothane (1·3% inspired) decreased cardiac output and increased the percentage of cardiac output going to the brain, kidney, liver, and large intestine. Enflurane (2·2% inspired) also increased the percentage of cardiac output going to the liver, spleen, and large intestine, but the cardiac output did not decrease compared with the conscious state. Ketamine 125 mg/kg i.m., tended to decrease cardiac output (although not significantly), and the percentage of the cardiac output going to the brain increased, whereas the percentage of the cardiac output going to muscle decreased, and that going to the heart, intestine, liver, and kidneys did not change.

In rats haemorrhaged to a mean arterial pressure of 60 mm Hg, ketamine anaesthesia (1·5 mg/kg per min i.v.) resulted in increased blood flow to the brain, heart, kidneys, intestine, and liver, compared with pentobarbital anaesthesia (6 mg/kg per h i.v.)[52]

Gaab et al[53] used multiwire microelectrodes on the surface of rat cerebral cortex to measure tissue Po_2 profiles, local blood flow profiles (by means of hydrogen clearance), and local metabolism (for example, the rate of oxygen depletion during carotid occlusion). Ketamine 320 mg/kg i.p., or pentobarbital, 65 mg/kg i.p. resulted in almost identical tissue Po_2 profiles, but very different local blood flow profiles. Ketamine anaesthesia resulted in greater mean blood flows compared with pentobarbital anaesthesia. Ketamine also resulted in greater tissue metabolism compared with pentobarbitone anaesthesia.

Dempsey et al[54] measured cerebral blood flow in cats after the release of middle cerebral artery occlusion. In cats anaesthetised by pentobarbital, pre-treatment with indometacin (indomethacin) resulted in increased postischaemic cerebral blood flow compared with cats that did not receive indometacin pre-treatment. In cats anaesthetised by ketamine, pre-treatment with indometacin did not affect postischaemic cerebral blood flow.

Vessel diameters

Longnecker et al[55] measured arteriolar diameters microscopically in rat cremaster muscle during haemorrhage, and compared the effects of enflurane anaesthesia and ketamine anaesthesia. They also measured tissue Po_2 with oxygen microelectrodes. Severe haemorrhage (removal of blood to decrease mean arterial pressure to 35 mm Hg for 30 min) during enflurane anaesthesia (2·2 vol% inspired) resulted in constriction in 1A, 3A, and 4A arterioles and decreased tissue Po_2 in skeletal muscle. Haemorrhage during ketamine anaesthesia (125 mg/kg i.m. with supplements of 30 mg/kg i.m. as needed) resulted in less constriction of the larger arterioles and increases in diameter in the 4A arterioles, and no significant decreases in tissue Po_2.

Longnecker and Harris[56 57] reported changes in arteriolar and venular diameters in bat wing, a mammalian skin microvasculature, and compared values with those during ketamine or halothane anaesthesia. Ketamine anaesthesia (120 mg/kg i.m.) produced dilatation of the small arterioles (30–65 μm) and no change in venular diameters, compared with conscious controls. A smaller dose of ketamine, 40 mg/kg i.m., did not change arteriolar or venular diameters. In contrast, 0·71 MAC of halothane (0·81% inspired) caused arteriolar dilatation and no change in venular diameters, whereas 1·25 MAC of halothane (1·42% inspired) caused more dilatation of arterioles and dilatation of the venules as well.

Summary of parenteral anaesthetic drugs

There have been relatively few studies of the microcirculatory effects of parenteral anaesthetic drugs, and generalisations about their effects are therefore difficult. It is clear, however, from the studies on organ blood flows and vessel diameters reviewed here, that the effects of parenteral anaesthetic drugs are agent specific, organ specific, pathology specific (that is, haemorrhage vs normovolaemia) and vessel generation specific (that is, fourth order arterioles versus first and second order arterioles). Further studies will be required to connect the specificity of these changes to the specific influence of anaesthetic drugs on delivery of nutrients to tissue.

Mechanisms of anaesthetic effects on the microcirculation

The microcirculation is controlled by a number of remote (neural, humoral, and hormonal) and local (metabolic, endothelial, and myogenic) regulatory mechanisms, and it is the summation of these actions that result in overall microcirculatory control. Similarly, the anaesthetic drugs alter numerous biological functions, including cellular metabolism, neuronal activity and transmission, humoral and hormonal control, and direct actions on vascular smooth muscle. It is possible, however, to demonstrate the effects of anaesthetic drugs on specific microvascular control systems in some situations, and these at least enhance the logic of the argument that the peripheral vascular actions of the anaesthetic drugs can be explained by actions on physiological systems that control the microcirculation. The actions of nitrous oxide (N_2O), halothane, and isoflurane are used as examples here.

Nitrous oxide has been shown to activate the sympathetic nervous system, as evidenced by increased splanchnic nerve activity when N_2O was administered to cats receiving halothane anaesthesia.[58] We studied the peripheral circulatory actions of N_2O, when added to a halothane anaesthesia in rats, in order to determine whether the reported changes in sympathetic activity in the splanchnic nerve were associated with changes in blood flow and vascular resistance in the splanchnic viscera.[59] Blood flows were measured using radiolabelled microspheres. N_2O, when substituted for nitrogen in the breathing mixture, caused increased vascular resistance in the kidneys, small bowel, and spleen, and decreased blood flow in the kidneys, small bowel, spleen, and liver. Cardiac output decreased in response to N_2O and the cerebral blood flow increased subsequent to cerebral vasodilation. The increase in vascular resistance and the decrease in blood flow to the splanchnic viscera are consistent with the increase in sympathetic nerve activity seen in the splanchnic nerve of cats, and suggests that the effects of N_2O in the splanchnic viscera can be attributed to an action of sympathetic nerves. (This mechanism does not, of course, explain the actions of N_2O on the cerebral circulation, and serves to emphasise the diverse actions of anaesthetic drugs on various peripheral vascular circulations.)

Although both halothane and isoflurane produce arterial hypotension in humans and animals, the mechanism(s) of this effect differ considerably. Halothane decreases blood pressure primarily by decreasing cardiac output,[38 50] whereas isoflurane acts primarily as a peripheral vasodilator.[39 51] We reasoned that the peripheral vascular actions of isoflurane might result from its actions on the NO system, and tested this hypothesis by administering L-NMMA, a blocker of NO synthesis, in the presence of either halothane or isoflurane anaesthesia.[60] Systemic and regional haemodynamics were measured with the radiolabelled microsphere technique.

Blockade of NO by L-NMMA produced greater increases in arterial blood pressure and systemic vascular resistance in animals anaesthetised with isoflurane, indicating that the NO pathway was more prominent under isoflurane anaesthesia (Fig 9.4).

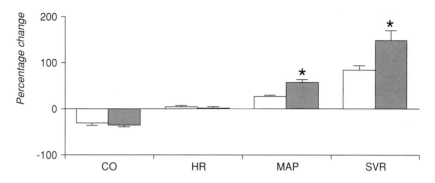

Fig 9.4 Comparison of changes in systemic haemodynamics induced by L-NMMA during 1 MAC of halothane anaesthesia (open columns) versus 1 MAC of isoflurane anaesthesia (filled columns) in rats. CO, cardiac output; HR, heart rate; MAP, mean arterial pressure; SVR, systemic vascular resistance. (Reproduced with permission from Greenblatt and Loeb.[60])

Similarly, blockade of the NO system produced greater increases in vascular resistance in the heart, kidneys, gastrointestinal tract, hepatic artery, and skin in those receiving isoflurane anaesthesia (Fig 9.5).

These results provide evidence that the NO pathway acts during both halothane and isoflurane anaesthesia to produce vasodilation, but the system is much more active during isoflurane anaesthesia and this mechanism contributes at least in part to the vasodilation that is observed during isoflurane anaesthesia.

More recent studies demonstrated that the contribution of NO to agonist-stimulated microvascular responses was greater during isoflurane than during halothane anaesthesia.[61] Acetylcholine and bradykinin induced vasodilation in fourth order rat cremaster muscle arterioles in a NO dependent manner during isoflurane anaesthesia, because vasodilation was attenuated by pre-treatment of the NOS inhibitor L-NMMA. In contrast, responses to these agonists were unaltered by L-NMMA during halothane or ketamine anaesthesia. The NO independent vasodilation seen in the presence of halothane or ketamine was the result of EDHF release from vascular endothelium, because combining NOS inhibition with an increase in K^+ in the muscle superfusate to inhibit EDHF action prevented the dilatation.[61 62] These data indicated that both EDHF and NO contribute to microvascular responsiveness during anaesthesia, and that the relative contributions of the different vasodilators to vascular control can be altered by specific anaesthetic drugs.

The responses to agonists during isoflurane anaesthesia were similar to those observed in the presence of inhibitors of EDHF action, and suggested that anaesthesia could modify vascular cell membrane potential, one of the primary controls over the vascular smooth muscle contractile state. Evidence to support the concept that isoflurane and other anaesthetic drugs may influence vascular smooth muscle membrane potential and EDHF action has been provided by a number of investigators. Lischke and co-workers[63 64] have shown that isoflurane, halothane, enflurane, sevoflurane, desflurane, etomidate, and thiopental can inhibit EDHF activity, with isoflurane being the most potent of the volatile anaesthetic drugs. Yamazaki et al[65] have shown that halothane, isoflurane, and sevoflurane can directly hyperpolarise vascular smooth muscle cells in the rat mesenteric micro-circulation. Hyperpolarisation of the vascular smooth muscle would be expected to induce relaxation and vasodilation.

Hyperpolarisation of vascular smooth muscle by the anaesthetic drug may reduce the sensitivity of the muscle to the additional influences of EDHF, while at the same time inducing vasodilation directly. This mechanism may be responsible for both the direct vasodilator activities of anaesthetic drugs such as isoflurane and modification of the relative contribution of different EDRFs to microvascular control.

Together, these results indicate that the anaesthetic drugs act on at least some of the known peripheral circulatory control mechanisms to produce

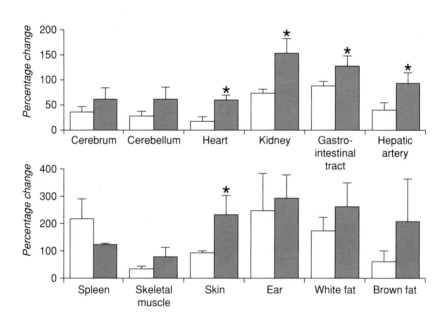

Fig 9.5 Comparison of changes in regional vascular resistances induced by L-NMMA during 1 MAC of halothane (open columns) versus 1 MAC of isoflurane (filled columns) in rats. (Reproduced with permission from Greenblatt and Loeb.[60])

their effects on organ blood flows and vascular resistances. They do not, however, imply that the mechanisms described here are the only mechanisms that may be active during anaesthesia. For example, peripheral vasoconstriction may occur during hypovolaemia under anaesthesia[50] and presumably other remote or local factors may predominate under other circumstances. The results with the inhalational anaesthetic drugs illustrate, however, that an understanding of microcirculatory control mechanisms, combined with an understanding of the actions of the anaesthetic drugs, allows one to make reasonable assumptions about the mechanisms that may explain the peripheral circulatory actions of the anaesthetic drugs.

1 Frink EJ, Morgan SE, Coetzee A, Conzen PF, Brown BR. The effects of sevoflurane, halothane, enflurane, and isoflurane on hepatic blood flow and oxygenation in chronically instrumented greyhound dogs. *Anesthesiology* 1992;**76**:85–90.

2 Nordstrom G, Winso O, Biber B, Hasselgren PO. Influence of pentobarbital and chloralose on metabolic and hemodynamic changes in liver ischaemia. *Ann Surg* 1990;**212**:23–9.

3 Nagano K, Gelman S, Parks D, Bradley EL. Hepatic circulation and oxygen supply–uptake relationships after hepatic ischemic insult during anesthesia with volatile anesthetics and fentanyl in miniature pigs. *Anesth Analg* 1990;**70**:53–62.

4 Holder DS. Effects of urethane, alphaxolone/alphadolone, or halothane with or without neuromuscular blockade on survival during repeated episodes of global cerebral ischemia in the rat. *Lab Anim* 1992;**26**:107–13.

5 Rasool N, Faroqui M, Rubenstein EH. Lidocaine accelerates neuroelectrical recovery after incomplete global ischemia in rabbits. *Stroke* 1990;**21**:929–35.

6 Helfaer MA, Kirsch JR, Traystman RJ. Anesthetic modulation of cerebral hemodynamic and evoked responses to transient middle cerebral artery occlusion in cats. *Stroke* 1990;**21**:795–800.

7 Sano T, Patel PM, Drummond JC, Cole DJ. A comparison of the cerebral protective effects of etomidate, thiopental, and isoflurane in a model of forebrain ischemia in the rat. *Anesth Analg* 1993;**76**:990–7.

8 Longnecker DE, Sturgill BC. Influence of anesthetic agent on survival following hemorrhage. *Anesthesiology* 1976;**45**:516–21.

9 Shibata K, Yamamoto Y, Murakami S. Effects of epidural anesthesia on cardiovascular response and survival in experimental haemorrhagic shock in dogs. *Anesthesiology* 1989;**71**:953–9.

10 LaRocco MT, Rodriguez LF, Chen CY, et al. Reevaluation of the linkage between acute hemorrhagic shock and bacterial translocation in the rat. *Circ Shock* 1993;**40**:212–20.

11 VanderLinden P, Gilbart E, Engleman E, deRood M, Vincent JL. Adrenergic support during anaesthesia in experimental endotoxin shock: norepinephrine versus dobutamine. *Acta Anaesthesiol Scand* 1991;**35**:134–40.

12 VanderLinden P, Gilbart E, Engelman E, Schmartz D, deRood M, Vincent JL. Comparison of halothane, isoflurane, alfentanil, and ketamine in experimental septic shock. *Anesth Analg* 1990;**70**:608–17.

13 Schaefer CF, Brackett DJ, Tompkins P, Wilson MF. Choice of anaesthetic alters the circulatory shock pattern as gauged by conscious rat endotoxemia. *Acta Anaesthesiol Scand* 1987;**31**:550–6.

14 Bavister PH, Longnecker DE. Influence of anaesthetic agents on the survival of rats following acute ischaemia of the bowel. *Br J Anaesth* 1979;**51**:921–5.

15 Lipton SA, Rosenberg PA. Excitatory amino acids as a final common pathway for neurologic disorders. *N Engl J Med* 1994;**330**:613–22.

16 Lundgren O, Haglund U. The pathophysiology of the intestinal countercurrent exchanger. *Life Sci* 1978;**23**:1411–22.

17 Glenny RW, Robertson HT, Yamashiro S, Bassingthwaighte JB. Applications of fractal analysis to physiology. *J Appl Physiol* 1991;**70**:2351–67.

18 Faraci FM, Heistad DD. Regulation of large cerebral arteries and cerebral microvascular pressure. *Circ Res* 1990;**66**:8–17.

19 Marcus ML, Chilian WM, Kanatsuka H, Dellsperger KC, Eastham CL, Lamping KG. Understanding the coronary circulation through studies at the microvascular level. *Circulation* 1990;**82**:1–7.

20 Iadecola C. Regulation of the cerebral microcirculation during neural activity: is nitric oxide the missing link? *Trends Neurol Sci* 1993;**16**:206–14.

21 Hainsworth R. The importance of vascular capacitance in cardiovascular control. *News Physiol Sci* 1990;**5**:250–4.

22 Nelson DP, King CE, Dodd SL, Schumacker PT, Cain SM. Systemic and intestinal limits of O_2 extraction in the dog. *J Appl Physiol* 1987;**63**:387–94.

23 Piiper J, Pendergast DR, Marconi C, Meyer M, Heisler N, Cerretelli P. Blood flow distribution in dog gastrocnemius muscle at rest and during stimulation. *J Appl Physiol* 1985;**586**:2068–74.

24 Ellsworth M, Ellis C, Popel A, Pittman R. Role of microvessels in oxygen supply to tissue. *News Physiol Sci* 1994;**9**:119–23.

25 Secomb TW, Hsu R. Simulation of O_2 transport in skeletal muscle: diffusive exchange between arterioles and capillaries. *Am J Physiol* 1994;**267**:H1214–21.

26 Carmines PK, Fleming JT. Control of the renal microvasculature by vasoactive peptides. *FASEB J* 1990;**4**:3300–9.

27 Vanlersberghe C, Lauwers MH, Camu F. Prostaglandin synthetase inhibitor treatment and the regulatory role of prostaglandins on organ perfusion. *Acta Anaesth Belg* 1992;**43**:211–25.

28 Saito Y, Eraslan A, Lockard V, Hester RL. Role of venular endothelium in control of arteriolar diameter during functional hyperemia. *Am J Physiol* 1994;**267**:H1227–31.

29 Nagao T, Vanhoutte PM. Endothelium-derived hyperpolarizing factor and endothelium-dependent relaxations. *Am J Respir Cell Mol Biol* 1993;**8**:1–6.

30 Koller A, Sun D, Huang A, Kaley G. Corelease of nitric oxide and prostaglandins mediates flow-dependent dilatation of rat gracilis muscle arterioles. *Am J Physiol* 1994;**267**: H326–32.

31 Garland CJ, Plane F, Kemp BK, Cocks TM. Endothelium-dependent hyperpolarization: a role in the control of vascular tone. *Trends Pharmacol Sci* 1995;**16**:23–30.

32 Furchgott RF, Zawadzki JV. The obligatory role of endothelial cells in the relaxation of arterial smooth muscle by acetylcholine. *Nature* 1980;**288**:373–6.

33 Ignarro LJ, Buga GM, Wood KS, Byrns RE, and Chaudhuri G. Endothelium-derived relaxing factor produced and released from artery and vein is nitric oxide. *Proc Natl Acad Sci USA* 1987;**84**:9265–9.

34 Palmer RMJ, Ferridge AG, and Moncada S. Nitric oxide release accounts for the biological activity of endothelium-derived relaxing factor. *Nature* 1987;**327**:524–6

35 Lowenstein CJ, Dinerman JL, Snyder SH. Nitric oxide: a physiologic messenger. *Ann Intern Med* 1994;**120**:227–37.

36 Greenblatt EP, Loeb AL, Longnecker DE. Marked regional heterogeneity in the magnitude of EDRF/NO-mediated vascular tone in awake rats. *J Cardiovasc Pharmacol* 1993;**21**:235–40.

37 Longnecker DE. Effects of general anaesthetic drugs on the microcirculation. *Microcirc Endothel Lymph* 1984;**1**:129–50.

38 Eger EI II, Smith NT, Cullen DJ, Cullen BF, Gregory GA. A comparison of the cardiovascular effects of halothane, fluroxene, ether, and cyclopropane in man: a resumé. *Anesthesiology* 1971;**34**:25–41.

39 Stevens WC, Cromwell TH, Halsey MJ, Eger EI II, Shakespeare TF, Bahlman SH. The cardiovascular effects of a new inhalation anaesthetic, Forane, in human volunteers at arterial carbon dioxide tension. *Anesthesiology* 1971;**35**:8–16.

40 Conzen PF, Habazettl H, Vollmar B, Christ M, Baier H, Peter K. Coronary micro-circulation during halothane, enflurane, isoflurane, and adenosine in dogs. *Anesthesiology* 1992;**76**:261–70.

328

41 Debaene B, Goldfarb G, Braillon A, Jolis P, Lebrec D. Effects of ketamine, halothane, enflurane, and isoflurane on systemic and splanchnic hemodynamics in normovolemic and hypovolemic cirrhotic rats. *Anesthesiology* 1990;**73**:118–24.

42 Vollmar B, Conzen PF, Kerner T, et al. Blood flow and tissue oxygen pressures of liver and pancreas in rats: Effects of volatile anesthetics and of haemorrhage. *Anesth Analg* 1992;**75**:421–30.

43 Jacob L, Boudaoud S, Payen D, et al. Isoflurane, and not halothane, increases mesenteric blood flow supplying esophageal ileocoloplasty. *Anesthesiology* 1991;**74**:699–704.

44 Hansen TD, Warner DS, Todd MM, Vust LJ, Trawick DC. Distribution of cerebral blood flow during halothane versus isoflurane anaesthesia in rats. *Anesthesiology* 1988;**69**:332–7.

45 Fagrell B, Fronek A, Intaglietta M. A microscope–television system for studying flow velocity in human skin capillaries. *Am J Physiol* 1977;**233**:H318–21.

46 Leon A, Boczkowski J, Dureuil B, Vicaut E, Aubier M, Desmonts J. Diaphragmatic microcirculation during halothane and isoflurane exposure in pentobarbital-anesthetized rats. *J Appl Physiol* 1992;**73**:1614–18.

47 Longnecker DE, McCoy S, Drucker WR. Anesthetic influence on response to haemorrhage in rats. *Circ Shock* 1979;**6**:55–60.

48 Worek FS, Blumel G, Zeravik J, Zimmermann GJ, Pfeiffer UJ. Comparison of ketamine and pentobarbital anaesthesia with the conscious state in a porcine model of Pseudomonas aeruginosa septicaemia. *Acta Anaesthesiol Scand* 1988;**32**:509–15.

49 Tverskoy M, Gelman S, Fowler KC, Bradley EL. Effects of anaesthesia induction drugs on circulation in denervated intestinal loop preparation. *Can Anaesth Soc J* 1985;**32**:516–24.

50 Seyde WC, Longnecker DE. Anesthetic influences on regional hemodynamics in normal and haemorrhaged rats. *Anesthesiology* 1984;**61**:686–98.

51 Miller ED, Kistner JR, Epstein RM. Whole-body distribution of radioactively labelled microspheres in the rat during anesthesia with halothane, enflurane, or ketamine. *Anesthesiology* 1980;**52**:296–302.

52 Idvall J. Influence of ketamine anesthesia on cardiac output and tissue perfusion in rats subjected to haemorrhage. *Anesthesiology* 1981;**55**:297–304.

53 Gaab MR, Poch B, Heller V. Oxygen tension, oxygen metabolism, and microcirculation in vasogenic brain edema. *Adv Neurol* 1990;**52**:247–56.

54 Dempsey RJ, Roy MW, Meyer KL, Donaldson DL. Indomethacin-mediated improvement following middle cerebral artery occlusion in cats. *J Neurosurg* 1985;**62**:874–81.

55 Longnecker DE, Ross DC, Silver IA. Anesthetic influence on arteriolar diameters and tissue oxygen tension in hemorrhaged rats. *Anesthesiology* 1982;**57**:177–82.

56 Longnecker DE, Miller FN, Harris PD. Small artery and vein response to ketamine HCl in the bat wing. *Anesth Analg* 1974;**53**:64–8.

57 Longnecker DE, Harris PD. Dilatation of small arteries and veins in the bat during halothane anesthesia. *Anesthesiology* 1972;**37**:423–9.

58 Fukunaga AF, Epstein RM. Sympathetic excitation during nitrous oxide–halothane anesthesia in the cat. *Anesthesiology* 1973;**39**:23–36.

59 Seyde WC, Ellis JE, Longnecker DE. The addition of nitrous oxide to halothane decreases renal and splanchnic flow and increases cerebral blood flow in rats. *Br J Anaesth* 1986;**58**:63–8.

60 Greenblatt EP, Loeb AL, Longnecker DE. Endothelium-dependent circulatory control – a mechanism for the differing peripheral vascular effects of isoflurane versus halothane. *Anesthesiology* 1992;**77**:1178–85.

61 Loeb AL, Godeny I, Longnecker DE. Anesthetics alter the relative contributions of NO and EDHF in the rat cremaster muscle microcirculation. *Am J Physiol* 1997;**273**:H618–27.

62 Adeagbo AS, Triggle CR. Varying extracellular [K+]: A functional approach to separating EDHF- and EDNO-related mechanisms in perfused rat mesenteric arterial bed. *J Cardiovasc Pharmacol* 1993;**21**:423–9.

63 Lischke V, Busse R, Hecker M. Inhalation anesthetics inhibit the release of endothelium-derived hyperpolarizing factor in the rabbit carotid artery. *Anesthesiology* 1995;**83**:574–82.

64 Lischke V, Busse R, Hecker M. Volatile and intravenous anesthetics selectively attenuate the release of endothelium-derived hyperpolarizing factor elicited by bradykinin in the

coronary microcirculation. *Naunyn-Schmiedeberg's Arch Pharmacol* 1995; **352**: 346–9.

65 Yamazaki M, Stekiel TA, Bosnjak ZJ, Kampine JP, Stekiel WJ. Effects of volatile anesthetic agents on *in situ* vascular smooth muscle transmembrane potential in resistance- and capacitance-regulating blood vessels. *Anesthesiology* 1998;**88**:1085–95.

10: Anaesthesia and the cardiovascular system

WOLFGANG BUHRE, ANDREAS HOEFT

The objective of anaesthesia is to provide analgesia, unconsciousness, suppression of reflex responses to surgical stimuli, and muscle relaxation, if required. In general, this goal is achieved by administering a combination of various agents, such as volatile and intravenous anaesthetic drugs, opioids, benzodiazepines, and muscle relaxants. In principle, all drugs used in anaesthetic practice affect the performance of the cardiovascular system, either by direct effects on the heart and the vascular system or indirectly by altering neurohumoral control of the circulation. It is very difficult to obtain a clear pharmacodynamic profile of an anaesthetic drug under in vivo conditions because both direct and indirect effects interact. Moreover, most anaesthetic drugs alter vascular tone and myocardial performance simultaneously. Thus, it is difficult to distinguish whether a decrease in blood pressure and/or stroke volume is the result of changes in myocardial loading conditions or of a direct negative inotropic effect of the anaesthetic agent itself. In vitro studies using isolated heart and vessel preparations, in which loading conditions can be carefully controlled, are therefore a rational approach to investigate the cardiovascular effects of anaesthetic drugs. Such studies have shown that most of the volatile and many of the intravenous anaesthetic drugs exert direct negative inotropic effects on the myocardium, and some of them cause systemic vasodilation. The isolated models are, however, relatively artificial, and the experimental results are not always in accordance with clinical observations. For instance, opioids as well as benzodiazepines are thought to be more or less haemodynamically inert, that is, to elicit no negative inotropic effects on the myocardium or cause significant vasodilation.[1-5] However, in some patients induction of anaesthesia with these drugs leads to dramatic hypotension, even if small doses are given.[6] Conversely, patients with compromised myocardial function and documented low ejection fraction often tolerate anaesthetic drugs with known negative inotropic properties surprisingly well. Thus, clinical experience suggests that, at least in some patients, centrally mediated indirect effects of anaesthesia (in particular the depression of the sympathetic drive) may be as important as the direct effects of the anaesthetic drug on the myocardium or vascular smooth muscle.

In fact, the interaction of anaesthesia with central control mechanisms of the circulation seems to be an intrinsic dilemma of anaesthesia. Even if the ideal anaesthetic drug with no adverse effects on the myocardium or vascular smooth muscle could be found, it is questionable whether the centrally mediated effects of anaesthesia on autonomic control of the cardiovascular system could be separated from the desired goals of anaesthesia. Basically (with the possible exception of ketamine), centrally mediated depression of cardiovascular performance is more or less common to all anaesthetic techniques, regardless of whether volatile anaesthetic or intravenous anaesthetic agents are employed.

In the clinical setting, it is unlikely that loading conditions (that is, preload, afterload) remain unchanged during the study of the effects of anaesthetic drugs on the cardiovascular system. At the same time, most parameters of myocardial function are clearly load dependent. The clinical application of echocardiography and specific indicator dilution techniques may overcome these problems, because calculation of load independent parameters may become possible in clinical practice.

Effects of anaesthesia on the sympathetic system

Cardiovascular homoeostasis is largely regulated by the autonomic nervous system, which controls heart rate, myocardial contractility, vascular resistance, and the tone of the venous capacitance vessels. Anaesthesia alters basic sympathetic tone as well as the sympathetic response to painful (surgical) stimuli. It is essential for the anaesthetist to be familiar with the interaction of anaesthesia with the autonomous nervous system in order to evaluate and treat haemodynamic disorders that may occur during anaesthesia. Current knowledge about the interaction of anaesthetic agents with the sympathetic nervous system is based mainly on studies of plasma catecholamine levels, assessment of baroreceptor reflex response, and direct recordings of sympathetic nerve activity.[7–12]

Sympathetic nerve activity

Muscle sympathetic nerve activity can be recorded from the peroneal nerve. A very thin epoxy coated needle (0·2 mm) with a small tip (5 μm) is placed within the peroneal nerve below the bony prominence at the head of the fibula. Using a reference electrode and a special set-up with a differential preamplifier and a bandpass filter, identification of characteristic muscle sympathetic nerve activity is possible (Fig 10.1). Sympathetic nerve activity is quantified by the number of bursts per minute or number of bursts per 100 cardiac cycles, or as total activity calculated from the

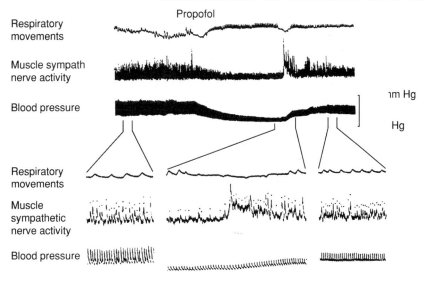

Fig 10.1 Respiratory movements, muscle sympathetic nerve activity, and blood pressure in a patient undergoing induction of anaesthesia with propofol. The upper panel shows condensed recordings, the lower panel depicts selected periods in an enlarged time scale. Induction of anaesthesia with propofol decreases muscle sympathetic nerve activity and blood pressure (upper panel). Tracheal intubation causes a dramatic increase in muscle sympathetic nerve activity. (Modified from Sellgren et al.[11])

product of bursts per minute and mean burst amplitude. Efferent bursts frequently occur in pulse synchronous groupings and are often phase locked to late expiration and early inspiration efforts.[7] This pattern is thought to be caused by baroreceptor modulation.[10]

Effects of induction of anaesthesia on sympathetic nerve activity

There are a number of investigations on the effects of induction of anaesthesia, tracheal intubation, and surgical stimulation on muscle sympathetic nerve activity. Most of the work has been performed by the groups of Ebert et al. and Sellgren et al.[7 9–15] Induction of anaesthesia decreased sympathetic outflow (Fig 10.2). Propofol and thiopentone (thiopentone) had the most pronounced effects,[7 10–11] whereas etomidate preserved muscle sympathetic nerve activity[7](Fig 10.2). Moreover, the decrease of muscle sympathetic nerve activity after propofol is more pronounced in unpremedicated patients than in those who received benzodiazepine premedication[7 11]. Obviously, baseline sympathetic drive seems to be an important determinant of the impact of anaesthesia on

333

sympathetic outflow and the resulting haemodynamic effects. These findings are in accordance with the clinical observation that propofol occasionally causes severe hypotension, particularly in patients who presumably are under an increased sympathetic drive in the conscious state, for example. patients with borderline hypovolaemia or compensated myocardial failure. Induction of anaesthesia with methohexital (methohexitone) has also been reported to decrease muscle sympathetic nervous activity.[10] These experimental data would support the clinical impression that etomidate is the induction anaesthetic agent of choice for patients with compromised cardiovascular performance and compensatory increased sympathetic drive. Laryngoscopy as well as surgical stimulation are associated with an immediate and often dramatic increase of sympathetic activity (Fig 10.1). Under such conditions, the pulse synchronous

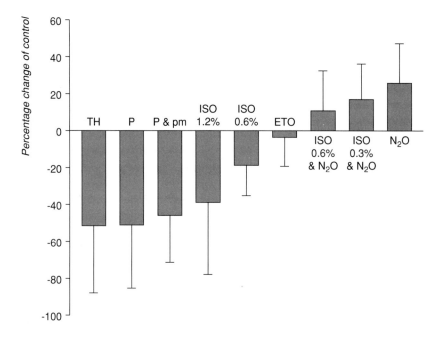

Fig 10.2 Effect of various anaesthetics on muscle sympathetic nerve activity. Muscle sympathetic nerve activity is given as bursts per minute and percent change of baseline values. Induction of anaesthesia with thiopentone (TH, 4 mg/kg), propofol (P, 2·5 mg/kg), and propofol after premedication with diazepam (P & pm, 2–2·5 mg/kg and 0·25 mg/kg, respectively), is associated with a significant decrease in muscle sympathetic nerve activity, whereas etomidate (ETO, 0·3 mg/kg) exerts only minor effects. Isoflurane alone (ISO 1·2 vol% and ISO 0·6 vol%) also inhibits muscle sympathetic nerve activity. In contrast, nitrous oxide (N_2O, 70%) causes sympathetic hyperactivity, which is counterbalanced by combination with isoflurane (ISO 0·6 vol% & N_2O 70%, ISO 0·3 vol% and N_2O 70%). (Data from Ebert et al.[7][12] and Sellgren et al.[10])

rhythmicity is lost and a more continuous activity pattern is observed in some patients.[11]

Effects of maintenance of anaesthesia on sympathetic nerve activity

As maintenance of anaesthesia is inevitably associated with suppression of cerebral activity, it is to be expected that all maintenance anaesthetic agents, that non-specifically inhibit neuronal activity, will also decrease sympathetic outflow. This has been demonstrated for propofol and halothane.[10 11] In contrast to other volatile anaesthetic agents, larger concentrations of desflurane are associated with increasing sympathetic outflow, and sympathetic activation is amplified during rapid increase in the inspired desflurane concentration.[14] There is evidence that this effect is caused by effector sites within the lungs.[15] Desflurane caused marked increases in heart rate and blood pressure. These haemodynamic responses may pose a risk for myocardial ischaemia to patients with ischaemic heart disease (Fig 10.3).[15] Isoflurane and sevoflurane were not associated with increases in muscle sympathetic nerve activity, even when the concentration was rapidly increased.[16 17] Nitrous oxide (N_2O) is also known to enhance sympathetic drive under certain circumstances. In healthy volunteers, a progressive increase in muscle sympathetic nerve activity was observed when low doses of N_2O (25% and 40%) are inhaled via a facemask.[9] These changes are associated with a significant increase in blood pressure. Sellgren et al[11] also observed that sympathetic nerve activity is enhanced by N_2O in comparison to the conscious state and that the combination of isoflurane and N_2O increases sympathetic nervous activity compared with isoflurane alone[11] (see Fig 10.2). Fentanyl 3 μg/kg given before induction of anaesthesia to a spontaneously breathing patient induces a temporary slight increase in muscle sympathetic nerve activity,[10] possibly because of associated hypercapnia. Data for sufentanil or alfentanil are currently not available.

Plasma catecholamines

Several authors have measured plasma catecholamine concentrations during induction and maintenance of anaesthesia.[18] Noradrenaline (nor-epinephrine) is thought to correlate more or less with overall sympathetic nervous activity,[19] whereas adrenaline (epinephrine) concentrations vary with adrenal release.[20] Interpretation of circulating plasma catecholamine concentrations is, however, hampered by the fact that measurable circulating noradrenaline is the result of an "overspill" phenomenon at the nerve ending, that is, the net effect of release and reuptake mechanisms.[20 21] Furthermore, data on plasma catecholamines from earlier studies have to be interpreted cautiously because baseline levels of adrenaline and noradrenaline were barely in the range of detection.[20] Despite these

a)

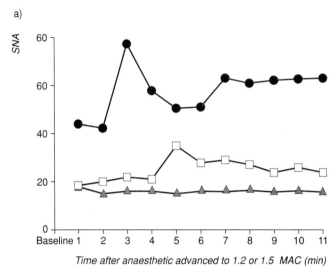

Time after anaesthetic advanced to 1.2 or 1.5 MAC (min)

b)

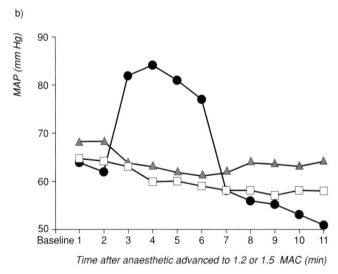

Time after anaesthetic advanced to 1.2 or 1.5 MAC (min)

Fig 10.3 Effects of rapid advancement in the anaesthetic concentration of volatile anaesthetic agents in human volunteers. The rapid increase in the inspired concentration was performed after a 30 min stabilisation period at 0·8 (sevoflurane) or 1·0 MAC (isoflurane, desflurane) concentration. In contrast to all other anaesthetic agents, an increase in the inspired concentration of desflurane leads to a significant increase in sympathetic nerve activity (SNA), resulting in an increase in mean arterial pressure (MAP) and heart rate (not shown). SNA is measured as burst frequency per 100 heart beats. ●, desflurane; ▲, isoflurane; □, sevoflurane. (Data from Ebert et al.[14][16] Reproduced with permission from Lippincott, Williams and Wilkins. *Anesthesiology* 1993;**79**:444–53 and *Anesthesia Analgesia* 1995;**81**:11–22.)

limitations, changes in plasma noradrenaline levels seem to correlate well with muscle sympathetic nerve activity in healthy volunteers.[22]

Induction of anaesthesia is usually associated with a decrease in plasma catecholamine concentrations.[23] A complete suppression of noxious stimuli is, however, difficult to achieve, even with very high doses of opioids. Neither very high doses of fentanyl (50 μg or 100 μg/kg) nor high doses of sufentanil (10, 20, or 30 μg/kg) prevented increases in plasma catecholamines during sternotomy.[24] This study confirmed earlier results of Sonntag et al.[25] who showed that neither high doses of sufentanil (10 μg/kg bolus followed by continuous infusion of 0·15 μg/kg min) nor moderate doses of sufentanil (1 μg/kg bolus followed by continuous infusion of 0·015 μg/kg per min) in combination with N_2O (30% O_2/70% N_2O) prevented a response to surgical stimuli as judged by increases in blood pressure and noradrenaline plasma concentrations (Fig 10.4). Interestingly, despite significant increases in circulating noradrenaline concentrations no concomitant change in the adrenaline concentration levels was observed.[25]

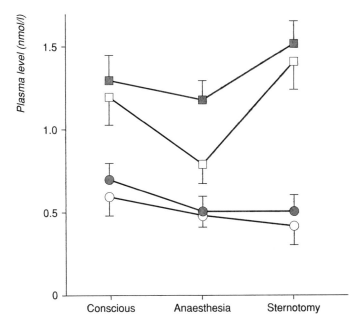

Fig 10.4 Plasma levels of adrenaline (epinephrine) and noradrenaline (norepinephrine) in patients undergoing cardiac surgery with sufentanil anaesthesia. Neither high dose sufentanil (10 μg/kg + 0·10 μg/kg per min) nor sufentanil–nitrous oxide anaesthesia (1 μg/kg + 0·015 μg/kg per min in 30% O_2/70% N_2O) are able to prevent the noradrenaline response to surgical stimulation (sternotomy). No additional hypnotics were used in this study. ■, Noradrenaline: sufentanil-nitrous oxide; □, noradrenaline: high dose sufentanil; ●, adrenaline: sufentanil-nitrous oxide; ○, adrenaline: high dose sufentanil. (Data from Sonntag et al.[25])

Similarly, in patients anaesthetised with sufentanil and midazolam, a significant increase in noradrenaline concentrations occurred during sternotomy but adrenaline concentrations remained unchanged.[26] In the same study, thoracic epidural anaesthesia in combination with light general anaesthesia (N_2O and midazolam) blocked the haemodynamic and humoral (noradrenaline) response to sternotomy. Moreover, compared with general anaesthesia, lower concentrations of noradrenaline and adrenaline were observed during bypass. Possibly, thoracic epidural anaesthesia is an appropriate method to block the sympathetic response to surgical stimuli.[26] In contrast, desflurane increases plasma noradrenaline concentrations dose dependently in healthy volunteers.[17 27]

In summary, induction and maintenance of anaesthesia with volatile and intravenous anaesthetic drugs are generally associated with depression of the sympathetic drive and decreased catecholamine concentrations. Pure opioid anaesthesia is not able to block the sympathetic response to intense surgical stimulation. In contrast to other volatile anaesthetic drugs, desflurane can cause sympathetic hyperactivity, most probably mediated by airway receptor sites, resulting in tachycardia, hypertension and increased muscle sympathetic nerve activity.[16] Another exception is ketamine, which produces increases in heart rate and arterial pressure. This effect can be attributed to the central sympathomimetic effects of ketamine which include the block of reuptake of monoamines into adrenergic nerves.

Baroreceptor reflex

Baroreflex control of heart rate can be studied in conscious and anaesthetised subjects by intravenous administration of vasoactive drugs, such as phenylephrine (pressor test) and sodium nitroprusside (depressor test). A bolus of phenylephrine (approximately 150 μg) is administered, preferably via a central venous catheter. As a result of the baroreceptor reflex, the increase in blood pressure results in a reflex slowing of heart rate. Baroreceptor sensitivity is defined as the slope of arterial pressure change divided by the R–R interval change in the ECG. In a similar way, baroreceptor reflex, after an abrupt decline in blood pressure, can be determined. Usually boli of sodium nitroprusside (100 μg) are used. Pressor and depressor tests are affected by anaesthetic drugs to various degrees.[28]

Of the three induction anaesthetic drugs, propofol, etomidate, and thiopentone, etomidate has the least effect on baroreceptor reflex function, followed by propofol and thiopental (Fig 10.5).[7] The latter almost abolished the baroreceptor response when given in equipotent doses. Methohexital also inhibits the baroreceptor reflex in experimental animals.[28] A significant decrease in pressor baroreceptor response after administration has also been observed for midazolam and diazepam.[29]

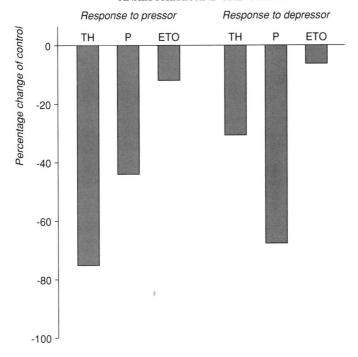

Fig 10.5 Effects of intravenous induction anaesthetic agents on baroreceptor response. Baroreceptor response to pressor (phenylephrine 150 μg) and depressor stimulus (sodium nitroprusside 100 μg) is assessed by cardiac baroslopes, that is, the ratios of R–R interval change to systolic blood pressure changes. Induction of anaesthesia with thiopentone (TH, 4 mg kg⁻¹) and propofol (P, 2·5 mg/kg) significantly inhibits baroreceptor response whereas etomidate (ETO, 0·3 mg/kg) preserves the activity of the baroreceptor reflex. (Data from Ebert et al.[7 12])

Inhaled anaesthetic agents depress the arterial baroreceptor reflex in both humans and animals.[30 31] Early studies had demonstrated that both isoflurane and halothane attenuate the cardiac baroreflex.[31] It was, however, hypothesised that isoflurane and enflurane preserve cardiac baroreflex function because a dose dependent increase in heart rate was observed with both anaesthetic agents.[32] The depression of the baroreflex response caused by isoflurane is less pronounced than with equipotent doses of halothane or enflurane.[26] Recent data clearly demonstrate that halothane, isoflurane, and enflurane do not differ with respect to reflex heart rate response to both increasing and decreasing blood pressure[32] (Fig 10.6). As the effects of desflurane and sevoflurane seem to be very similar to those obtained with isoflurane, it can be concluded that there are no clinically relevant differences between inhaled anaesthetic agents with respect to baroreflex control.[32]

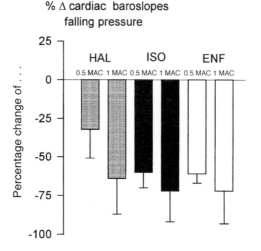

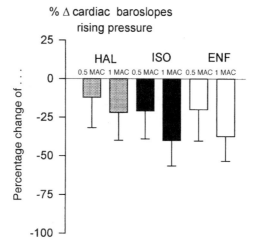

Fig 10.6 Changes in cardiac baroreflex response associated with isoflurane (ISO), halothane (HAL), and enflurane (ENF). Percentage change (from conscious baseline) in cardiac baroreflex slope during sodium nitroprusside (falling pressure response, top) and phenylephrine (rising pressure response, bottom). Slope was calculated as the linear relationship between mean arterial presure and R–R interval. No significant differences between isoflurane, halothane, and enflurane were observed. Thus, the results suggest that reflex heart rate response to both decreasing and increasing blood pressure does not differ between isoflurane, halothane, and enflurane in this experimental setting. (Modified from Muzi and Ebert.[32] Reproduced by permission of Academic Press, Inc. *Advances in Pharmacology* 1994;**31**:379–87.)

Heart rate variability

Analysis of small oscillations in heart rate, termed "heart rate variability" (HRV), provides a non-invasive estimate of autonomic reflex function.[33 34] Typically, two major components are seen in a heart rate spectrum. The high frequency component (0·15–0·5 Hz) is said to be mediated by the parasympathetic nervous system. The low frequency component (0·04–0·15 Hz) is influenced by both the sympathetic and the para-sympathetic nervous system, and is related to waves in arterial pressure mediated by the baroreceptor reflex. The ratio between low and high frequency (LF/HF) is considered to be a useful indicator of cardiac sympathetic nerve activity.[35] The LF/HF ratio has been used as an estimate of autonomic reflex activity in several clinical studies comparing different anaesthetic or premedication regimens.[36–43] In practice, analogue ECG recordings are digitised and the spectral power distribution is calculated using fast Fourier transformation.[33–35] The total power spectrum is divided into the LF and HF component, and the ratio between LF and HF (LF/HF) as well as the total power (LF + HF) of HRV is then calculated.

The LF/HF ratio increased in elderly unpremedicated patients, but not in young patients after arrival in the operating room.[36] Both midazolam 0·06 µg/kg i.m. and diazepam 0·2 µg/kg orally decreased the LF/HF ratio, suggesting that both drugs are equally effective in attenuating sympathetic nerve activity. The route of administration (that is, intramuscularly or orally) is apparently of no clinical relevance.[36] A significant reduction in total power, the LF and the HF component of HRV in elderly compared with young patients was observed, consistent with a decline in para-sympathetic nerve activity with age.[36] Recently, Michaloudis et al.[37] studied the effects of midazolam 0·08 µg/kg, morphine 0·15 µg/kg and clonidine 2 µg/kg as premedication, on total HRV and the LF and HF components of HRV.[37] In accordance with previous results,[36] they observed that midazolam reduces both the LF and the HF component of HRV. Although the ratio between both remained unchanged, however, morphine and clonidine decreased the LF more than the HF component, suggesting parasympathetic dominance.[37] Latson and O'Flaherty[42] studied the effects of surgical stimulation and different anaesthetic regimens on changes in total heart rate variability. They compared two groups of patients receiving either isoflurane–N_2O or continuous propofol infusion for laparoscopic tubal ligation. In both groups, total HRV decreased significantly after induction of anaesthesia. After skin incision, HRV recovered in patients receiving propofol, but it remained depressed in patients receiving isoflurane–N_2O.[42] These results suggest that a shift in autonomic balance towards sympathetic dominance took place only in patients receiving propofol.[42] These results are somewhat surprising because it is well documented that propofol blunts the sympathetic response when compared with other anaesthetic regimens. In the study by Latson and O'Flaherty, however, only small doses of fentanyl were given to patients receiving propofol.[42] Thus, the observed increase in HRV after surgical stimulation may be the result of inappropriate analgesia or insufficient anaesthetic depth.[42] The effects of fentanyl 7·5 μg/kg and different dosages of midazolam (0·075, 0·1, 0·2 mg/kg) on HRV were studied by Zickman et al[43] in patients scheduled for coronary bypass surgery. A significant decrease in the LF component was observed, whereas the HF component was only slightly decreased. The authors concluded that this anaesthetic induction technique decreases sympathetic, but not parasympathetic autonomous nervous activity.[43] As expected, the use of ketamine results in an increase in sympathetic activity reflected by an increase in the LF component.[40]

A number of studies investigated the effects of volatile anaesthetic agents on changes in HRV during surgery and recovery from anaesthesia.[38 41] Comparing isoflurane and desflurane, total power of HRV was back to control values by 60 min after the end of surgery in desflurane treated patients, but remained suppressed in patients who underwent isoflurane anaesthesia.[38] These findings suggest that neural reflex control is restored earlier after desflurane anaesthesia. In contrast, no significant differences were observed between halothane or isoflurane.[41] When comparing the effects of induction of anaesthesia with thiopentone 4 mg/kg and etomidate 0·3 mg/kg, Latson et al[44] found that both induction agents decrease total HRV by 89% and 58%, respectively. The decrease was, however, more pronounced with thiopentone than with etomidate.[44]

In summary, it seems that determination of HRV allows characterisation of the effects of anaesthesia on autonomic control.

Effects of anaesthesia on the heart

The effect of anaesthetic drugs on the myocardium has been the subject of numerous experimental and clinical investigations. As outlined above, it is very difficult to differentiate, under in vivo conditions, between direct myocardial effects of anaesthetic agents, direct vascular effects, and indirect effects mediated via the autonomic nervous system. A reasonable approach is to investigate the influence of anaesthetic agents on myocardial contractility in isolated in vitro models, such as cultured myocytes, papillary muscles, or isolated working heart preparations. Preload and afterload can be well controlled in these preparations, and any interference with sympathetic or parasympathetic innervation is avoided. For the same reasons, it is, however, very difficult to apply results obtained in vitro to the clinical situation. Basically, the more isolated a preparation is, the more artificial the physiological environment. For instance, isolated working heart preparations are deprived of any basic sympathetic drive, and coronary oxygen supply is often limited because of asanguineous crystalloid perfusion. Papillary muscle preparations are devoid of a blood supply, and the experiments are often performed at room temperature in order to decrease metabolic rate and to facilitate sufficient oxygen supply by diffusion. Cultured myocytes or skinned muscle fibres are obviously very artificial models and far from clinical reality.

Myocardial contractility

Nevertheless, isolated models can be useful to identify the pure effect of substances on the myocardium itself. Several induction agents have been shown to elicit negative inotropic properties in papillary muscle preparations or isolated working heart models.[45-56] Most recently, for example, Stowe and co-workers[50] investigated the effects of etomidate, ketamine, midazolam, propofol, and thiopental on cardiac function and metabolism in an isolated guinea pig heart model at equimolar doses. In principle, all induction agents (including midazolam and etomidate) produce a dose dependent decrease in myocardial contractility (Fig 10.7) On a molar basis, propofol (less so midazolam and etomidate) depresses cardiac function moderately more than thiopentone and ketamine. The peak concentrations required for induction of anaesthesia are, however, quite different between agents. Peak plasma concentrations during induction of anaesthesia have been reported to be approximately 0.5 μmol/l for midazolam, 3 μmol/l for etomidate, 60 μmol/l for ketamine, 50 μmol/l for propofol, and 100 μmol/l for thiopentone (Fig 10.7). Thus, under clinical conditions midazolam and etomidate are basically not cardiodepressive, whereas thiopental and propofol exert significant direct negative inotropic action.

In contrast to volatile anaesthetic agents,[52] only little is known about the molecular mechanisms responsible for the direct negative inotropic properties of intravenous induction agents. Initial contradictory results about the direct action of ketamine on the myocardium prompted some more detailed investigations. Ketamine is a myocardial depressant in intact dogs, isolated dog heart preparations, and isolated rabbit hearts.[53 54] Riou et al[65] have demonstrated that ketamine has a dual opposing effect on the myocardium:

1 A positive inotropic effect associated with increased Ca^{2+} influx.
2 A negative inotropic effect possibly because of an impaired function of the sarcoplasmic reticulum.[55]

In an isolated ventricular papillary muscle model of a ferret, the positive inotropic effects of ketamine could be blocked by bupranolol, indicating involvement of β-receptors.[56] Moreover, depletion of noradrenaline stores by reserpine also abolished the positive inotropic action of ketamine. It was concluded that inhibition of neuronal catecholamine uptake is the predominant mechanism of the positive inotropic effect of ketamine.[56] The negative inotropic effect of ketamine was elucidated by Kongsayreepong et al.[31] using measurements of intracellular Ca^{2+} transients with aequorin.

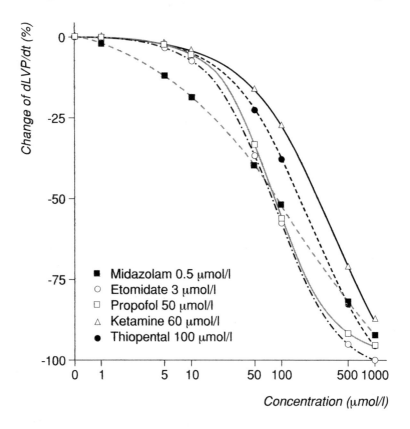

Fig 10.7 Comparison of the direct negative inotropic effects of common intravenous induction anaesthetic agents in an isolated working heart model. The effects of etomidate, ketamine, midazolam, propofol, and thiopental were studied in an isolated working heart model. Percent change in the peak positive derivative of left ventricular pressure ($+dLVP/dt_{max}$) are shown. A wide range of concentrations from 0·5 to 1000 µmol/l was investigated (symbols). All induction anaesthetic agents (including midazolam and etomidate) produce a concentration dependent depression of myocardial contractility. In concentrations that are equivalent to peak plasma levels during induction of anaesthesia (marked by symbols, name, and equivalent anaesthetic concentration for each agent), however, propofol and thiopentone appear to depress cardiac function more than ketamine, etomidate, and midazolam. ■, midazolam; ○, etomidate; △, ketamine; □, propofol; ●, thiopentone. (Data from Stowe et al.[64])

Ketamine decreased intracellular calcium availability, which also occurred when the sarcoplasmic reticulum was blocked by ryanodine.

Gelissen et al[58] were the first to compare the direct effects of different intravenous hypnotics on the intrinsic contractility of isolated human myocardium. They recorded force development during isometric contraction of atrial myocytes exposed to various concentrations of etomidate, propofol, ketamine, and thiopental.[58] All anaesthetic agents produced dose dependent inhibition of isometric contraction. At clinically relevant concentrations, however, the effects of thiopental and ketamine were pronounced, whereas propofol and etomidate had no direct negative inotropic effect on the atrial myocyte. There are some methodological limitations to this study. First, some patients were under chronic therapy with β-adrenoceptor blocking agents or Ca^{2+} channel antagonists. Second, experiments were performed under hypothermic conditions (30°C). Third, no control experiments with the solvent alone were carried out. Moreover, as atrial but no ventricular myocytes were studied, it remains unclear whether the results can be extrapolated to ventricular preparations.[58] In contrast to earlier work, propofol produced no direct negative inotropic effect, suggesting that the clinically observed cardiovascular depression is predominantly the result of changes in cardiac loading conditions and sympathetic drive.[58]

The influence of volatile anaesthetic agents on myocardial contractility has been extensively investigated in papillary muscle experiments, working heart models, and intact animals.[52] All volatile anaesthetic agents decrease myocardial contractility in a dose dependent manner.[59-64] Isoflurane seems to be less negative inotropic than enflurane and halothane[59] (Fig 10.8). Desflurane and sevoflurane also decrease developed contractile force in different in vitro models.[65 66] The decreases are comparable to those caused by isoflurane. The cardiodepressive effect of volatile anaesthetic agents is caused by an alteration of calcium transients involving sarcolemmal calcium exchange processes, as well as uptake and release of calcium by the sarcoplasmic reticulum.[63] It has been suggested that halothane and isoflurane depress cardiac function by different mechanisms.[63] In papillary muscle preparations, N_2O exerted moderate negative inotropic effects (that is, 5–15% depression of contractility by 50% N_2O).[67]

The effects of opioids on cardiac muscle have been studied in only a very few isolated papillary muscle experiments. Negative inotropy has been demonstrated for morphine, meperidine, fentanyl, and alfentanil. These effects occurred, however, at concentrations one hundred to several thousand times above those expected clinically.[5 68]

Assessment of myocardial contractility in intact animals or in patients requires considerable methodological efforts. The crucial question is whether an observed decline in blood pressure or stroke volume after application of an anaesthetic drug is the result of decreased contractility or merely of changes in loading conditions. Several contractility indices have been suggested in the literature (see Chapter 2). The end systolic elastance index[69] and the preload recruitable stroke work are considered relatively load independent (see Chapter 2). There is, however, a paucity of clinical studies in which the effects of anaesthetic agents on myocardial function are characterised based on end systolic elastance or preload recruitable stroke work. A reason might be that transoesophageal echocardiography has only recently become available as a research tool in anaesthesiology. A very interesting clinical study of this type has been performed by Mulier et al,[70] in which the haemodynamic effects of thiopental and propofol were compared. In contrast to previous studies, propofol significantly decreased myocardial contractility, and (in accordance with the in vitro results of Stowe et al[50]) was at least as negative inotropic in vivo as thiopental. The authors even suggested that the negative inotropic properties of propofol are more pronounced and more prolonged than those of equipotent doses of thiopental.[70] The differences were, however, only marginal and statistically barely significant. It is questionable whether the observation of Mulier et al is the result of direct negative inotropic effects of propofol alone. An alternative explanation could be a marked decrease in sympathetic outflow,

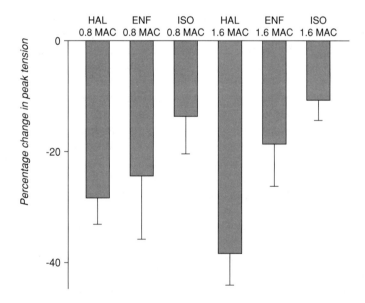

Fig 10.8 Effects of halothane (HAL), enflurane (ENF), and isoflurane (ISO) on myocardial contractility in isolated papillary muscles. All volatile anaesthetic agents exert a dose dependent negative inotropic effect shown as percentage depression of peak developed tension. Halothane was found to be significantly more depressant than isoflurane at 1·6 MAC, wheras enflurane caused intermediate depression. (Data from Lynch and Frazer.[59])

which has been demonstrated during propofol anaesthesia[7] (see Fig 10.2). As in other studies, the induction anaesthetic agent with the least negative inotropic effects seemed to be etomidate.

As expected from results in isolated models, volatile anaesthetic agents are cardiodepressants in intact animals and patients[67 71 72] during systole and early diastole mainly via alterations of intracellular Ca^{2+} homoeostasis. In general, the inward Ca^{2+} current is diminished by inhibiting the function or reducing the number of Ca^{2+} channels in the sarcolemmal membrane. Thus, both the availability of Ca^{2+} for contraction and the amount of Ca^{2+} stored in the sarcoplasmic reticulum are decreased. In addition, the concentration of intracellular Ca^{2+} is decreased by direct anaesthetic induced alteration of the sarcoplasmic reticulum, combined with partial inhibition of Ca^{2+} uptake and enhanced Ca^{2+} leakage. Whether inhalational anaesthetic agents modify the responsiveness of contractile proteins to Ca^{2+} remains controversial. Pagel et al[73] demonstrated, in chronically instrumented dogs with and without autonomic blockade, that isoflurane and desflurane produce less depression of myocardial contractility than halothane or enflurane. Without autonomic blockade, however, desflurane preserved mean arterial pressure and cardiac output to a greater degree than equipotent doses of isoflurane, especially at higher concentrations.[73] This finding can be explained by the enhanced sympathetic drive caused by desflurane. Sevoflurane decreases contractility dose dependently by up to 40–45% of baseline values in animal experiments with and without autonomic blockade. This magnitude of contractile depression is comparable to that observed with isoflurane.[74]

The in vivo effects of N_2O are very complex. As outlined above, N_2O increases sympathetic activity and in some patients increases blood pressure.[9 11 12] The weight of currently available evidence suggests, however, that N_2O is a myocardial depressant[75] when used as supplement during anaesthesia. Pagel et al[75] investigated N_2O in chronically instrumented dogs in the presence of pharmacological blockade of the autonomic nervous system. Based on preload recruitable stroke work, myocardial contractility decreased when N_2O was added to a baseline anaesthesia with isoflurane or sufentanil (Fig 10.9). The evidence for a myocardial depressant effect of N_2O is strong in patients with compromised myocardial function, that is, in those patients in whom the cardiovascular properties of anaesthetic agents are clinically relevant. In summary, N_2O has a weak direct myocardial depressant effect, which may be counterbalanced by an increase in sympathetic activity by N_2O in intact animals and healthy patients.[75]

Myocardial oxygen consumption

Measurements of myocardial blood flow and myocardial oxygen consumption in patients are very cumbersome and can, therefore, be performed only for investigational purposes (see Chapter 4). An estimate of myocardial oxygen demand from haemodynamic parameters would therefore be desirable. The major determinant of myocardial oxygen demand is the energy required for development and maintenance of systolic wall tension. As reliable measures of wall tension are difficult to obtain, several derived indices of myocardial oxygen demand have been suggested.[76] Intuitively, most clinicians believe that an increase in both heart rate and blood pressure will increase myocardial oxygen demand. This belief forms the rationale for using the rate pressure product (RPP), which was first suggested by Rhode,[77] and which is still widely used as an index of myocardial oxygen demand. In animals as well as in patients, however, only a poor correlation is found between RPP and myocardial oxygen uptake.[78 79] Similarly, the tension time index (TTI) does not correlate very well with

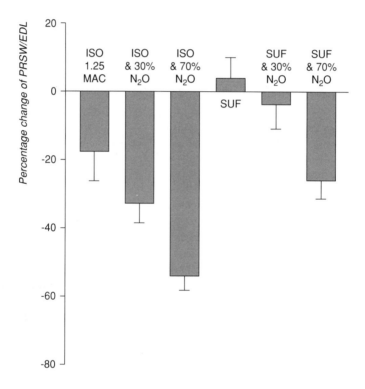

Fig 10.9 Influence of nitrous oxide (N_2O) on myocardial contractility in chronically instrumented dogs. Two sets of experiments were performed in chronically instrumented dogs with pharmacological blockade of the autonomic nervous system. Basic anaesthesia was performed with isoflurane (ISO, 1·25 MAC) or sufentanil (SUF, 100–150 $\mu g/kg^{-1}h^{-1}$). Myocardial contractility was evaluated by the relationship of preload recruitable stroke work (PRSW) to end diastolic length (EDL). The addition of nitrous oxide (N_2O 30% and N_2O 70%) results in a decrease in myocardial contractility in both groups. (Data from Pagel et al.[75])

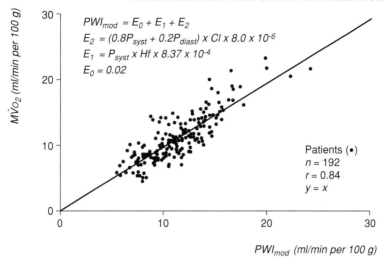

Fig 10.10 Correlation of myocardial oxygen uptake (M$\dot{V}o_2$) and modified pressure work index (PWI$_{mod}$) as an estimate of myocardial oxygen consumption. PWI$_{mod}$ and M$\dot{V}o_2$ showed a correlation coefficient of 0.84 in patients undergoing coronary artery bypass surgery. Haemodynamic variables required for calculation of myocardial oxygen demand by PWI$_{mod}$ are heart rate (Hf), arterial blood pressure (P$_{syst}$, P$_{diast}$) and cardiac index (CI: ml/m^2). The modified pressure work index is currently the most reliable index for estimation of myocardial oxygen demand derived from haemodynamic variables in patients. (Data from Hoeft et al.[76])

measured myocardial oxygen uptake.[76 78] A clinically useful alternative is the pressure work index, which was first suggested by Rooke and Feigl.[79 80] In addition to blood pressure and heart rate, this index requires measurement of cardiac output, which is routinely performed in many critically ill patients. But (as with all other haemodynamic indices of myocardial oxygen demand) species specific differences exist between animals and humans. The empirical constants derived by Rooke and Feigl for dogs cannot be used for estimation of myocardial oxygen demand in humans.[79] A modification of the pressure work index was therefore developed and validated by Hoeft et al.[76] It is based on data derived from measurements of myocardial blood flow and myocardial oxygen uptake in patients using a modified Kety–Schmidt technique (Fig 10.10). Currently, this modified pressure work index seems to be the best alternative for the clinical estimation of myocardial oxygen demand. This estimate seems to be applicable during the conscious state as well as during anaesthesia.[76 79]

Effects of anaesthetic agents on myocardial oxygen consumption

Theoretically, it is possible that anaesthesia is associated with specific metabolic effects, such as uncoupling of oxidative phosphorylation or

349

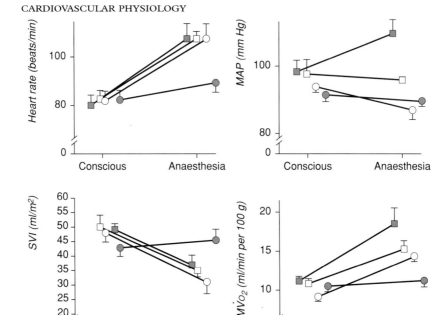

Fig 10.11 Influence of thiopentone, methohexital, etomidate, and ketamine on heart rate, mean arterial blood pressure, stroke volume index, and myocardial oxygen consumption. Induction of anaesthesia with thiopental (○), and methohexitone (□) is associated with a decrease in blood pressure (MAP) and stroke volume index (SVI), while heart rate (HR) and myocardial oxygen consumption (M$\dot{V}O_2$) are increased. Ketamine (■) exerts the most pronounced effect on myocardial oxygen consumption because sympathetic activation leads to an increase in heart rate and blood pressure. Stroke volume index is, however, decreased by ketamine, too. The haemodynamic effects of etomidate (●) are almost negligible and myocardial oxygen consumption remains unchanged. (Data from Kettler and Sonntag.[81])

uncoupling of myocardial energy turnover from myocardial haemodynamic performance. Myocardial oxygen demand (estimated by the modified pressure work index) and measured myocardial oxygen uptake do not, however, in general differ between the conscious state and anaesthesia.[76] Therefore, a specific metabolic effect of anaesthesia, for example uncoupling of myocardial energy conversion, is very unlikely.

Under resting conditions, myocardial oxygen uptake is approximately 10–11 ml/min per 100 g (Figs 10.11, 10.12, and 10.13). As most anaesthetic agents are cardiodepressive either by their direct negative inotropic effects or indirectly by decreasing sympathetic drive, induction with virtually any anaesthetic agent leads to a decrease in arterial blood

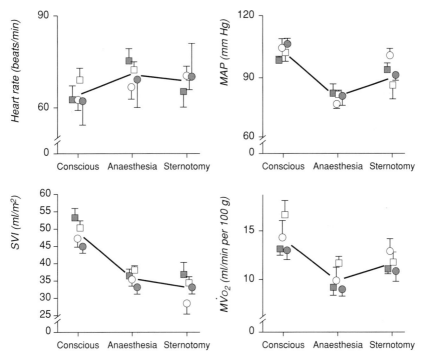

Fig 10.12 Effects of volatile anaesthetic agents and propofol on heart rate, mean arterial pressure, stroke volume index, and myocardial oxygen consumption in patients undergoing coronary artery bypass surgery. Induction of anaesthesia with volatile anaesthetic agents or propofol is associated with a decrease of blood pressure and stroke volume index, and only minor changes of heart rate. As a result, myocardial oxygen consumption is decreased as well. ○, enflurane; ■, propofol; □, halothane; ●, isoflurane; —, pooled data. (Data from Hoeft et al.[82])

pressure and stroke volume index (Figs 10.11, 10.12, and 10.13). Ketamine (without supplemental benzodiazepines) might be an exception (Fig 10.11); it causes sympathetic stimulation, and increases in arterial blood pressure and heart rate, whereas stroke volume is decreased (Fig 10.11). In general, a reflex increase in heart rate is seen with barbiturates, but only a slight increase with etomidate (Fig 10.11). Heart rate, on the one hand, and arterial pressure and stroke volume, on the other, have opposing effects on myocardial oxygen demand. The net effect is an increase in myocardial oxygen consumption with methohexital and thiopental, more so with ketamine, and mostly unchanged haemodynamics and myocardial metabolic rate with etomidate[81] (Fig 10.11).

Induction of anaesthesia with volatile anaesthetic agents as well as with propofol leads to a decrease in blood pressure and stroke volume. As a result of inhibition of the baroreceptor reflex, the increase in heart rate is

351

less blunted. Myocardial oxygen consumption therefore decreases by almost one third, which is more than seen with classic induction agents (Fig 10.12). Induction of anaesthesia with high doses of opioids is associated with a decrease in blood pressure and stroke volume, and also a considerable reduction in myocardial oxygen consumption[82] (Fig 10.13).

Intense surgical stimulation (for example sternotomy) results in sympathetic activation, which is difficult to block by anaesthesia. Blood pressure control is usually easier to achieve with volatile anaesthetic agents than with high dose opioids (Fig 10.12 and 10.13).[82] The poor control of blood pressure during opioid based anaesthesia can lead to up to a twofold increase in myocardial oxygen consumption. Adjuvant measures (such as vasodilators, β blockade, and other antihypertensive drugs) and supple-

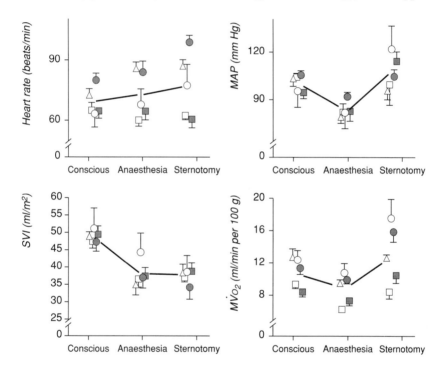

Fig 10.13 The effects of opioid based anaesthesia on heart rate, mean arterial pressure, stroke volume index, and myocardial oxygen consumption in patients undergoing coronary artery bypass surgery. As with volatile anaesthetic agents (see Fig 10.12), induction of anaesthesia is associated with a decrease in blood pressure and stroke volume index, whereas heart rate remains unchanged. Myocardial oxygen consumption is therefore also decreased. Blood pressure control is more difficult to achieve during sternotomy. On average, an increase in myocardial oxygen consumption is observed. $\triangle$, fentanyl–midazolam; $\bullet$, high dose fentanyl; $\bigcirc$, high dose morphine; $\square$, high dose sufentanil; $\blacksquare$, sufentanil–nitrous oxide; —, pooled data. (Data from Hoeft et al.[82])

mentation with volatile anaesthetic agents are therefore often employed during opioid based anaesthesia in order to maintain arterial pressure within normal limits.

Very high rates of myocardial oxygen consumption can develop during the recovery period. A dramatic sympathetic activation occurs during this phase, and noradrenaline (norepinephrine) levels by far exceed levels observed during anaesthesia and surgery (Fig 10.14).[83] Although measurements of myocardial blood flow and myocardial oxygen consumption are not available for this critical period, an estimation of myocardial oxygen demand can be made based on the modified pressure work index and on data from the literature. Shivering patients in particular may have an extremely high myocardial oxygen demand,[83] because the very high systemic metabolic rates will increase cardiac work load. During anaesthesia, total body oxygen consumption is in the range of 80–120 ml/min per m^2. Thus, with a haemoglobin of 12 g% and an arteriovenous oxygen extraction of 25% the required cardiac index is 1·5–2·3 l/min per m^2. For a normal blood pressure (120/80 mm Hg) and heart rate (80 beats/min), myocardial oxygen demand calculated by the modified pressure work index

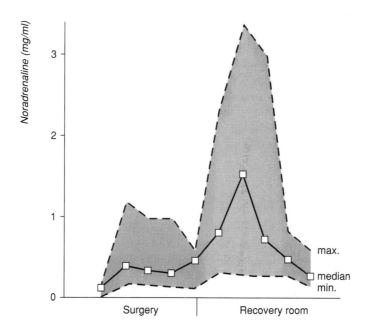

Fig 10.14 Noradrenaline (norepinephrine) levels during major abdominal surgery and during recovery from surgery. Median and range (min., max.) of noradrenaline plasma levels during and after major abdominal surgery are shown. The most pronounced sympathetic activation occurs during recovery from surgery. (Data from Turner.[83])

is in the range of 10·4–10·9 ml/min per 100 g, which is consistent with values measured in patients. Myocardial oxygen demand also depends on the haemoglobin content of the blood. The lower the haemoglobin content, the higher the required cardiac output. During the recovery period, systemic metabolic rates can be extremely high. On average, a systemic metabolic rate of 260 ml/min per m^2 is observed during this period in patients after major abdominal surgery. Corresponding myocardial oxygen demand is 13·5 ml/min per m^2 at a haemoglobin of 12 g%, which increases to more than 19.2 ml/min per 100 g at a haemoglobin of 8 g%. Values of up to 480 ml/min per m^2 have been observed in shivering patients.[83] Thus, a decrease in haemoglobin content, as often observed after surgery in the recovery room, would further increase myocardial oxygen demand and may cause problems in patients with limited coronary blood supply.

Effect of anaesthesia on myocardial efficiency

In technical terms, efficiency is the ratio of work performed to energy required. In a similar way efficiency of myocardial oxygen utilisation can be defined as the ratio of external pressure–volume work to myocardial oxygen consumption. Pressure–volume work is by definition the area under the left ventricular pressure–volume loop, which is unfortunately difficult to assess in patients. For clinical purposes, however, a good estimate of external pressure–volume work can be obtained from the product of stroke volume and mean systolic pressure during the ejection phase.

It has been known for a long time that myocardial efficiency is not constant but varies with preload, afterload, and contractility. Evans and Matsuoka[84] demonstrated as early as 1915 that an increase in cardiac work caused by an increase in blood pressure requires a higher increase in oxygen consumption than the same increase in cardiac work caused by an increase in stroke volume.[84] Recently, theoretical models have been developed that try to relate the efficiency of myocardial oxygen utilisation to haemo-dynamics, that is, to indices of preload, afterload, and contractility.[85–87] Although the approaches for estimation of myocardial efficiency differ in the way that myocardial oxygen demand is estimated from haemodynamic indices, comparable results have been obtained. In general, myocardial efficiency is improved by an increase in preload and/or by a decrease in afterload. The most notable implication of the theoretical models is the hypothesis that myocardial performance can be optimised with respect to myocardial efficiency: for a given preload and afterload a maximal efficiency is achieved when contractility is neither too low nor too high, that is, when contractility is ideally tuned to an optimal value. In fact, there is a growing body of evidence that preload, afterload, and contractility are optimised under resting conditions at the point of maximal efficiency.[85 87] Induction of anaesthesia is associated with a decrease in myocardial oxygen utilisation efficiency (Fig 10.15). Myocardial oxygen consumption is not, however, decreased in proportion to the decrease of external myocardial work (Fig 10.15). As a result, efficiency is decreased, regardless of the type of anaesthesia[87] (Fig 10.15). Theoretically, an increase in efficiency would be possible because of a decrease in afterload (blood pressure). The decrease in contractility and stroke volume outweigh the former effect, that is, contractility and afterload do not match preload conditions after induction of anaesthesia. In terms of "ventricular–vascular matching" (see Chapter 2), stroke volumes and contractility are too low. It is somewhat

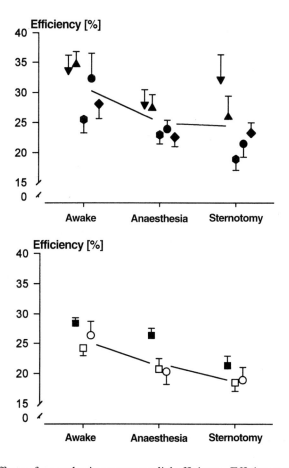

Fig 10.15 Effects of anaesthesia on myocardial efficiency. Efficiency of myocardial oxygen use is calculated from the ratio of external myocardial work (mean systolic pressure × cardiac index) to myocardial oxygen consumption. Induction and maintenance of anaesthesia with any anaesthetic agent is associated with decreased myocardial efficiency. Upper: ◆, fentanyl-midazolam; ●, high dose fentanyl; ◆, high dose morphine; ▼, high dose sufentanil; ▲, sufentanil – N₂O; —; pooled data. Lower: ○, enflurane; □, halothane; ■, propofol; —, pooled data. (Data from Hoeft et al.[87])

355

surprising that this effect is seen not only with anaesthetic agents that are well known to have direct negative inotropic properties (that is, halothane and enflurane), but also to the same extent with anaesthetic agents that supposedly have no direct negative inotropic effects (that is, opioids).[87] This finding indicates that under in vivo conditions even opioid anaesthesia is associated with a decrease in contractility, presumably because of decreased or inadequate sympathetic drive.

There is evidence that sympathetic activation during anaesthesia is of a different quality than that during conscious conditions. Usually, increases in heart rate are not very pronounced, and sometimes heart rate even decreases (because of the attempt to block the cardiovascular response by deepening anaesthesia). At times, however, significant increases in blood pressure can be observed, in particular during opioid based anaesthesia. Although sympathetic activation should enhance myocardial contractility, stroke volume indices and myocardial efficiency of oxygen utilisation remain decreased. These findings also suggest that anaesthesia significantly interferes with cardiovascular control mechanisms because optimal tuning of the system is obviously not achieved during volatile as well as opioid anaesthesia. Thus, there is substantial evidence that, under in vivo conditions, the direct negative inotropic effects of anaesthetic agents might be of minor importance compared with the central effects of anaesthesia on cardiovascular control mechanisms.

Another approach to quantify the interaction between the mechanical state of the left ventricle and the vascular bed is based on sequential pressure–volume measurements and a series of elastic chamber model of the circulation.[88 89] The ratio of the elastances of the left ventricle (end systolic elastance, E_{es}) and the arterial elastance (E_a) defines coupling between the left ventricle and the arterial tree. This approach enables relatively load independent studies on the effects of ventricular–arterial coupling in vivo. In addition, the pressure–volume analysis permits evaluation of left ventricular efficiency as defined by the ratio of stroke work (SW) to pressure–volume area (PVA). Hettrick and co-workers[90–92] performed a series of experiments in which they studied the effects of isoflurane, desflurane, sevoflurane, and propofol on left ventricular–arterial coupling and mechanical efficiency in the open chest dog model anaesthetised with barbituates. All three inhalational anaesthetic agents caused similar, dose dependent decreases in ventricular contractility and afterload. Isoflurane, sevoflurane, and desflurane preserved optimum left ventricular–arterial coupling at low anaesthetic concentrations (<0.9 MAC) (see Fig 10.18), whereas coupling was impaired at 1.2 MAC. Mechanical efficiency was also altered at higher anaesthetic concentrations (>0.9 MAC for isoflurane and desflurane, >0.6 MAC for sevoflurane) (Fig 10.16). These experimental data demonstrate that ventricular–arterial coupling is impaired at higher anaesthetic concentrations, indicating that the reduction

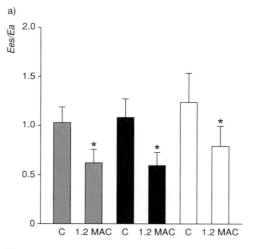

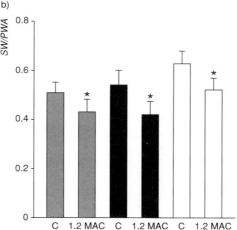

Fig 10.16 Effects of increasing doses of volatile anaesthetic agents on left ventricular–arterial coupling and mechanical efficiency. Ventricular–arterial coupling was assessed by the ratio of left ventricular end systolic elastance (E_{es}) to effective arterial elastance (E_a) (see text for details). Mechanical efficiency was examined by the ratio of left ventricular stroke work (SW) and pressure volume area (PVA). A significant decrease in both variables could be observed at 1·2 MAC of each volatile anaesthetic agent compared with control (C) values. Thus, it can be concluded that left ventricular–arterial coupling and myocardial efficiency were preserved at low concentrations of anaesthetic agents, whereas mechanical matching was impaired at higher end tidal concentrations. No significant differences between the three agents could be observed. These findings support in vivo results showing a dose dependent reduction of cardiac performance by volatile anaesthics. ▨, desflurane; ■, sevoflurane; □, isoflurane. (Modified from Hettrick et al.[90] Reproduced with permission from Lippincott, William and Wilkins. *Anesthesiology* 1996;**85**:403–13.)

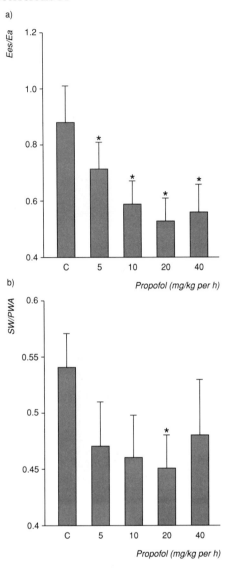

Fig 10.17 Effects of increasing infusion rates of propofol on (a) left ventricular–arterial coupling and (b) mechanical efficiency. A significant dose dependent decrease in left ventricular–arterial coupling (E_{es}/E_a) and mechanical efficiency (SW/PVA) could be observed after infusion of propofol compared with control (C). The effects were most pronounced at a dose of 20 mg/kg per h. Higher infusion rates did not lead to more pronounced effects on either E_{es}/E_a or SW/PVA, demonstrating that the effects of propofol on ventricular–arterial coupling are not strictly dose dependent. (Modified from Hettrick et al.[92] Reproduced with permission from Lippincott, Williams and Wilkins. *Anesthesiology* 1997;**86**:1088–93.)

in myocardial contractility is not appropriately counterbalanced by simultaneous declines in afterload.[91]

Propofol in a dose range of 5–40 mg/kg per h impairs ventricular–arterial coupling significantly[92] (Fig 10.17). The reduction of the ratio E_{es}/E_a is primarily caused by a decrease in end systolic elastance. In contrast to volatile anaesthetics, E_{es}/E_a plateaus at higher doses of propofol (20–40 mg/kg per h) resulting from modest further reductions in arterial elastance, indicating that the impairment of left ventricular–arterial coupling associated with propofol is not strictly dose dependent.[92] Mechanical myocardial efficiency as derived from the SW/PVA ratio was decreased at the intermediate dose of propofol (5–20 mg/kg per h), whereas at the 40 mg/kg per h dose, the decline in SW/PVA ratio was reverted to some degree.

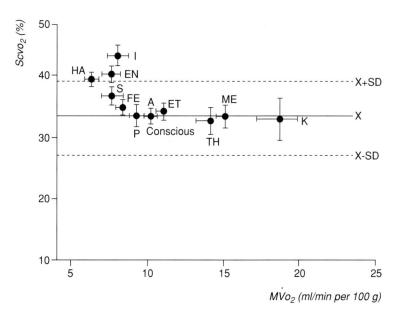

Fig 10.18 Coronary venous oxygen saturation ($Scvo_2$) in conscious patients (A) and after induction of anaesthesia with ketamine (K), methohexitone (ME), thiopental (TH), etomidate (ET), isoflurane (I), halothane (HA), enflurane (EN), propofol (P), sufentanil (S), and fentanyl (FE). With the exception of isoflurane, coronary venous oxygen saturation remains more or less unchanged compared to the conscious state, that is, autoregulatory control of coronary blood flow is not affected by most anaesthetic agents. Halothane, enflurane, and more so isoflurane are coronary vasodilators. (Modified from Hoeft et al.[93])

Effects of anaesthetic drugs on coronary blood flow

With the exception of isoflurane, anaesthetic agents do not effect autoregulation of coronary blood flow. Myocardial blood flow is adjusted to match myocardial oxygen demand. As a result myocardial blood flow decreases with induction of anaesthesia in conjunction with the decrease in myocardial oxygen demand, and coronary sinus oxygen saturation remains practically unchanged[93] (Fig 10.18). In contrast, administration of iso-flurane causes coronary vasodilation, resulting in a concomitant increase in coronary sinus oxygen saturation.[93] Halothane, sevoflurane, and enflurane are coronary vasodilators as well, but to a lesser degree.[93] The coronary vasodilatory effects of volatile anaesthetic agents are probably mediated by ATP sensitive potassium channels located on the surface of vascular smooth muscle.[94 95] A potassium leakage causes hyperpolarisation of vascular smooth muscle cells, resulting in muscle relaxation.[94] For instance, Crystal et al.[94] demonstrated that the coronary vasodilating effects of halothane can be blocked by administration of glibenclamide (a K^+ ATP channel inhibitor). Glibenclamide also inhibits the vasodilatory effects of adenosine which strongly supports the fact that adenosine receptors are involved in mediating vasodilation by K^+ ATP channels.[94]

A variety of studies has been performed to investigate whether the coronary vasodilator properties of isoflurane cause coronary steal.[95] In most studies that demonstrated myocardial ischaemia during isoflurane, how-ever, high doses were used with considerable concomitant arterial hypotension. It is now commonly accepted that isoflurane can be used safely in patients with coronary artery disease as long as high doses and arterial hypotension are avoided.[95] Thus, in cases of a hypertensive response to surgical stimuli, isoflurane can safely be used for blood pressure control.

Effects of anaesthesia on ischaemia–reperfusion injury

In patients undergoing coronary revascularisation procedures, brief periods of ischaemia are regularly observed and result in general or regional ischaemia–reperfusion injury.[96] This injury can cause moderate to severe myocardial dysfunction.[96] Depression of myocardial contractility associated with the use of volatile anaesthetic agents may be advantageous during ischaemic episodes if the decrease in myocardial oxygen consumption is greater than the regional decrease in myocardial perfusion caused by anaesthetic induced hypotension.[97–100] There is growing evidence that volatile anaesthetic agents protect the myocardium by different cellular mechanisms during periods of ischaemia. First, volatile anaesthetic agents alter the Ca^{2+} homoeostasis in the myocardium by inhibiting trans-sarcolemmal calcium influx. This effect can be reversed by an increase in the extracellular calcium concentration. In the presence of isoflurane and halothane, increased leakage of Ca^{2+} from ryanodine sensitive Ca^{2+}

channels was observed,[98] which reduces the available activator Ca^{2+} by depleting the Ca^{2+} content in the sarcoplasmic reticulum. There is experimental evidence that Ca^{2+} myofilament sensitivity is reduced during exposure to volatile anaesthetic agents.[99] Second, isoflurane, enflurane, and halothane decreased the size of the infarct zone after global as well as regional ischaemia, whereas propofol, pentobarbital and ketamine/xylazine do not.[100] P-Sulphophenyl theophylline, an adenosine receptor antagonist, prevents the protective effect of halothane, suggesting involvement of the adenosine receptor cascade in this process.[100]

Second, there is evidence that the inhibition of the protein kinase C also limits the protective effects of halothane. Thus, it can be hypothesised that factors related to protein kinase C activation (for example, generation of inositol trisphosphate and diacylglycerol) may be alternative targets for anaesthetic action in the myocardium.[101] Third, Kersten et al[102] demonstrated that administration of 1 MAC isoflurane is beneficial in restoring segment shortening after a myocardial ischaemic episode in dogs. The selective blockade of the adenosine-1 receptor prevents the protective effects of isoflurane on ischaemia–reperfusion injury. Blockade of K^+_{ATP} channels also inhibits anaesthetic induced myocardial protection.[103] Thus, it is possible that both mechanisms are related, resulting in anaesthetic dependent stimulation of adenosine-1 receptors which, in turn, activate K^+_{ATP} channels. The efflux of K^+ through this sarcolemmal channel hyperpolarises the myocardium. This may be the mechanism by which anaesthetic agents (as well as myocardial preconditioning) limit the extent of myocardial stunning.[99] Halothane increases the potassium conductance and emphasises transmembrane polarity,[104] resulting in a decrease in the duration of systole and a concomitant decrease in Ca^{2+} influx and ATP consumption. These physiological changes preserve energy stores and transmembrane ion gradients. The effects of 1–2·5 MAC sevoflurane seem to be similar to those of halothane. Sevoflurane also decreases the Ca^{2+} influx into myocytes and causes a mild decrease in contractility.[105]

As in other fields of research in anaesthesia, the interaction of drugs and reactive species of oxygen are a matter of interest. Volatile anaesthetic agents may protect the ischaemic myocardium by preventing the generation of reactive species of oxygen. Glantz et al[106] demonstrated that halothane anaesthesia attenuates hydroxyl radical generation during the reperfusion period after regional myocardial ischaemia in dogs.[107] Furthermore, lactate efflux into the coronary sinus was significantly reduced in dogs anaesthetised with halothane compared with control animals.[106]

The exposure of isolated human neutrophils to halothane, enflurane, or sevoflurane results in a decrease in oxygen burst and hydrogen peroxide production in response to the bacterial peptide.[107] In contrast, exposure to desflurane results in an increase in oxygen burst and generation of hydrogen peroxide. Thus, anti-inflammatory effects of some volatile anaesthetic drugs may be beneficial in limiting the extent of ischaemia–reperfusion injury.[107] Halothane, isoflurane, and sevoflurane reduced the postischaemic adhesion of polymorphonuclear neutrophils (PMNs) in the coronary system in an isolated Langendorff preparation.[108] The inhibitory effect of volatile anaesthetic drugs on adhesion of PMNs may be beneficial for the heart under ischaemic conditions.

In contrast to the effects of volatile anaesthetic agents on ischaemia–reperfusion injury, only a little is known about the effects of intravenous drugs. Ketamine/xylazine, pentobarbital or propofol did not reduce the infarct size after ischaemia in rabbit myocardium.[100] In contrast, a marked enhancement of energy metabolism, as well as mechanical function, was observed when propofol was given both pre-ischaemia and during reperfusion.[109] In summary, there is evidence that volatile anaesthetic agents, with the possible exception of desflurane, as well as propofol, protect the myocardium against brief periods of ischaemia by different mechanisms.

Central and peripheral circulation

Anaesthesia exerts direct and indirect effects on the peripheral circulation. As in the case of the heart, it is difficult to differentiate between direct and indirect effects under in vivo conditions. Decreased sympathetic drive, which is associated with virtually any anaesthetic technique, will also affect peripheral vascular tone. This can be expected to alter regional vascular resistances, blood flows, and the distribution of intravascular blood volume. In addition, many anaesthetic agents exert direct effects on vascular smooth muscle, either by direct vasodilation or by altering the response to other factors that modulate vascular tone.

Effects of anaesthetic agents on vascular smooth muscle

Volatile anaesthetic agents are known to cause mild vasodilation under in vivo conditions. This is the result of both diminished vascular smooth muscle sensitivity to circulating catecholamines and diminished neurovascular tone. Halothane selectively attenuates α_2-adrenoceptor mediated vasoconstriction.[110] It was suggested that this is the result of interference with calcium entry through smooth muscle membranes. More recent investigations have demonstrated that volatile anaesthetic drugs might additionally attenuate the response to α_1-adrenoceptor mediated vasoconstriction, and that this effect is not mediated by blockade of calcium influx through voltage dependent channels.[111] The attenuation of α_1- and α_2-responsiveness most probably contributes to in vivo effects of volatile anaesthetic agents because stimulation of α_1- and α_2-adrenoceptors contributes to basal vascular tone. Contractility of vascular smooth muscle is also regulated by intracellular concentration of Ca^{2+}. The effects of halothane and isoflurane/sevoflurane on myoplasmic Ca^{2+} transients of muscle cells from peripheral arteries vary.[112] The administration of halothane inhibits Ca^{2+} loading of the sarcoplasmic reticulum and potentiates Ca^{2+} release from it after caffeine stimulation. In contrast, isoflurane and sevoflurane administration do not lead to caffeine induced Ca^{2+} release which may partly explain the different effects of halothane and isoflurane/sevoflurane on peripheral arterial resistance.[112]

As outlined above, the vasodilator effects of volatile anaesthetic agents can differ within the circulation. For instance, halothane, like nitroglycerine, is a more potent dilator of large coronary arteries, whereas isoflurane is a more potent dilator of small coronary arteries.[113] Only the second will cause a significant increase in coronary blood flow, because, under in vivo conditions, dilatation of large coronary arteries is counteracted by the metabolic control of coronary blood flow at the level of the arterioles and the microcirculation.

Many in vivo studies indicate that propofol has a vasodilating effect. It is, however, still controversial whether this effect is caused by a direct vasodilating action of propofol or by a reduction in sympathetic outflow. Propofol in concentrations of 1·1–4 mmol/l causes vasodilation of isolated vascular rings.[114 115] Since 97–99% of Propofol is bound to plasma proteins, clinically relevant concentrations do not lead to direct vasodilation.[115]

Recently, Robinson et al[116] studied the effects of therapeutic doses of propofol (directly infused into the brachial artery) on forearm vascular resistance (FVR) and forearm vein compliance (FVC) in conscious human volunteers. Infusion of propofol does not lead to a reduction in FVR or an increase in FVC, despite therapeutic plasma concentrations. In contrast, infusion of sodium nitroprusside leads to a reduction in forearm vascular resistance.[116] In a second study, one sided stellate blockade was performed, and subsequently general anaesthesia with propofol was initiated (Fig 10.19). Under these circumstances a significant decrease in FVR and an increase in FVC were observed only in the arm without sympathetic denervation. Changes in resistance and compliance were comparable to those found with stellate blockade. These results suggest that the peripheral vascular actions of propofol can primarily be attributed to the effects on sympathetic nerve activity[116] (Fig 10.19).

Anaesthesia and vascular tone

It is obvious that the mechanical properties of the arterial vascular tree oppose left ventricular ejection. Quantitative evaluation of afterload in vivo remains, however, difficult. In clinical as well as experimental studies, decreases in systemic vascular resistance are most often used to describe reductions in left ventricular afterload after exposure to anaesthetic drugs.[117] It is, however, known that systemic vascular resistance inade-

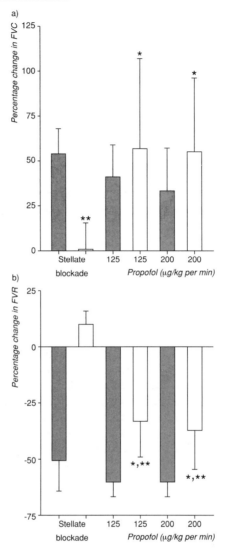

Fig 10.19 Change in vascular resistance after infusion of propofol with and without autonomic blockade, shown as percentage change in (a) compliance (FVC) and (b) forearm vascular resistance (FVR) in the left arm after stellate blockade (■) and in the right arm before and during propofol infusion (□). Stellate blockade increased FVC and decreased FVR on the side of blockade. After infusion of propofol no further changes were observed in the blocked arm, whereas a significant change in FVR and FVC in the unblocked arm was observed, suggesting that the effects of propofol are primarily caused by inhibition of sympathetic vasoconstrictor nerve activity. (Modified from Robinson et al.[116] Reproduced with permission from Lippincott, Williams and Wilkins. *Anesthesiology* 1997;**86**:64–72.)

quately describes afterload, because this calculated index does not take into account the viscoelastic and frequency dependent properties of the arterial wall. Furthermore, the dynamic phase nature of pressure and flow, as well as the effects of wave reflection in the arterial tree, are not included in the clinically used calculation of systemic vascular resistance. Thus, attempts have been made to characterise arterial mechanical properties by the measurement of aortic input impedance spectra (Z_{in}). Z_{in} incorporates the viscoelastic and resistive properties of the arterial system and has become a widely accepted experimental description of left ventricular afterload (see Chapter 2). Many of the characteristics of the aortic impedance spectra are difficult to quantify because of frequency dependence and, therefore, a three element Windkessel model is often used to interpret aortic impedance. This model consists of a resistor (characteristic aortic impedance, Zc) in series with another resistor (total arterial resistance, R) and a capacitor (total arterial compliance, C). Using the three element Windkessel model, Hettrick et al[117] demonstrated that halothane and isoflurane produced different effects on left ventricular afterload in the chronically instrumented dog. Both drugs do not alter characteristic aortic impedance, but halothane at 1·25, 1·5, and 1·75 MAC alters total arterial resistance, a property of arteriolar vessels.

Thus, the effects of volatile anaesthetic agents are primarily located at the level of the resistance vessels. Using the same study design, Lowe et al[118] investigated the effects of propofol on aortic impedance. Propofol alters left ventricular afterload by a decrease in arteriolar tone and an increase in characteristic aortic impedance and total aortic compliance.[116 118] Etomidate increases left ventricular afterload and compromises left ventricular systolic and diastolic performance in chronically instrumented dogs with pre-existing left ventricular failure.[119] These results indicate that the use of etomidate for induction of anaesthesia may impair left ventricular function, especially in patients with preoperative myocardial dysfunction.[119]

Effects of anaesthesia on blood volume distribution

From a physiological point of view, the vascular system can be divided into two parts. One is the low pressure system that comprises all postarteriolar vessels, the right heart, the pulmonary vascular system, and the left heart during diastole. The other is the high pressure system, which includes the left ventricle during systole, systemic arteries, and arterioles. The low pressure system holds about 85% of the total intravascular blood volume, one third of which is in the intrathoracic compartment and two thirds in the extrathoracic low pressure system. According to the definition by Gauer and Henry,[120] the central blood volume, which represents the intravascular blood volume between the pulmonary and the aortic valve, is part of the intrathoracic blood volume. Intrathoracic and central blood volumes hold a key position within the circulation because they serve as a reservoir for the left ventricle.[120] [121] It is common clinical practice to deduce changes in intrathoracic and central blood volumes from simultaneous changes in central venous and pulmonary capillary wedge pressures.[122] [123] There are, however, several problems that limit the applicability of pressure measurements in the low pressure system for evaluation of intravascular volume status during anaesthesia:

1 It was Gauer and Henry who demonstrated a considerable inter-individual variability of low pressure compliance.
2 The compliance of the low pressure system is naturally affected by vascular smooth muscle tone. When adrenergic drive is enhanced by infusion of noradrenaline, the compliance decreases.[124] Consequently, sympathetic tone influences central venous pressure as a result of changes in effective compliance.[125]
3 Mechanical ventilation with positive airway pressure (in particular with positive end expiratory pressure, PEEP) will alter the relationship between central venous pressure, pulmonary capillary wedge pressure, and intrathoracic volume status.[121]
4 It has repeatedly been demonstrated that changes in central venous pressure do not correlate with changes in pulmonary capillary wedge pressure in patients with impaired left ventricular function.[126]

Direct measurements of intrathoracic or central blood volume by indicator dilution techniques appear to be better suited for evaluation of intravascular volume status, particulary in patients undergoing cardiac surgery, in whom myocardial dysfunction and a critical dependence on adequate intra-vascular filling can be anticipated.[127]

Surprisingly, very few studies have been performed on the impact of anaesthesia on intrathoracic blood volume and left ventricular preload. It is common practice to give additional fluids with induction of anaesthesia in order to compensate for decreases in blood pressure. It has not, however, been systematically investigated to what extent the commonly observed decrease in blood pressure results from a volume shift between the intra- and extrathoracic compartment or of a decrease in contractility. In general, both can be expected with decreased sympathetic drive. Hedenstierna et al[128] as well as Krayer et al[129] found that anaesthesia with muscle paralysis and mechanical ventilation leads to a decrease in thoracic blood volume associated with a decrease in functional residual capacity. Both groups, however, presented different results with respect to the intrathoracic blood volume. Krayer et al[129] measured total thoracic cavity volume by three dimensional x ray computed tomography, and functional residual capacity by inert gas clearance techniques. From the difference between both, Krayer derived an increase in intrathoracic blood volume after induction and during maintenance of anaesthesia.[129] In contrast, Hedenstierna et al[128] measured a decrease in intrathoracic blood volume using a double indicator dilution technique. This result seems to be more plausible taking into account the known effects of anaesthesia on the sympathetic system and the impact of mechanical ventilation on intrathoracic pressures. A volume redistribution from the intrathoracic to the extrathoracic compartment with induction of anaesthesia would support the clinical practice in which hypotension after intubation is treated by intravenous fluids. Different anaesthetic techniques could possibly explain the contradictory findings. Krayer et al used fentanyl/thiopentone anaesthesia, whereas Hedenstierna and co-workers used halothane anaesthesia.[128 129] Currently, there are no systematic data available on how different types of anaesthesia affect the expected redistribution of intravascular blood volume from the intra-thoracic to the extrathoracic compartment.

It is well known, that spinal and epidural anaesthesia cause a loss of sympathetic innervation in the corresponding areas. The impact of regional sympathectomy by spinal and epidural anaesthesia has been investigated by Arndt and co-workers[130] in a very elegant way using labelled erythrocytes and whole body scintigraphy.[130] Regional anaesthesia elicits a redistribution of blood to the denervated musculature and skin at the expense of cardiac filling. The capacitance vessels of the remaining innervated muscles and skin areas, usually of the upper extremities, might constrict in a compensatory manner. The data of Arndt and co-workers[130] also suggest that compensatory vasoconstriction might occur in the splanchnic area, the mechanism of which is unknown. In patients with compromised compensa-tory mechanisms, central blood volume might decrease dramatically. On the basis of these findings, Lipfert and Arndt[131] concluded that the poor outcome of resuscitation attempts in cases of cardiac arrest during spinal anaesthesia[132] results largely from insufficient filling of the central vascular system.

In summary, there is evidence that regional as well as general anaesthesia is associated with a redistribution of blood volume from the intrathoracic to the extrathoracic compartment. Little is known about the time course of volume distribution during surgery and especially during recovery from anaesthesia. This, together with the influence of various anaesthetic techniques on intravascular volume distribution, is certainly a subject that merits further investigations.

1 Sebel PS, Bovill JG. Cardiovascular effects of sufentanil anesthesia. *Anesth Analg* 1982;**61**:115–19.
2 Bovill JG, Sebel PS, Stanley TH. Opioid analgesics in anesthesia: With special reference to their use in cardiothoracic anesthesia. *Anesthesiology* 1984;**61**:731–55.
3 Skarvan K, Schwinn W. Haemodynamic interactions between midazolam and alfentanil in patients with coronary disease. *Anaesthesist* 1986;**35**:17–23.
4 Tomicheck RC, Rosow CE, Philbin DM, Moss J, Teplick RS, Schneider RC. Diazepam-fentanyl interaction-hemodynamic and hormonal effects in coronary artery surgery. *Anesth Analg* 1985;**62**:881–4.

5 Strauer BE. Contractile response to morphine, piritramide, meperidine and fentanyl: A comparative study of effects on the isolated ventricular myocardium. *Anesthesiology* 1972;**37**:304–10.

6 Hug CC Jr. Does opioid "anesthesia" exist. *Anesthesiology* 1990;**73**:1–4.

7 Ebert TJ, Muzi M, Berens R, Goff D, Kampine J. Sympathetic responses to induction of anaesthesia in humans with propofol or etomidate. *Anesthesiology* 1992;**76**:725–33.

8 Wallin BG, Fagius J. Peripheral sympathetic neural activity in conscious humans. *Annu Rev Physiol* 1988;**50**:565–76.

9 Ebert TJ, Kampine JP. N$_2$O augments sympathetic outflow: Direct evidence from human peroneal nerve recordings. *Anesth Analg* 1989;**69**:444–9.

10 Sellgren J, Ponten J, Wallin BG. Characteristics of muscle sympathetic nerve activity during general anaesthesia in humans. *Acta Anaesthesiol Scand* 1992;**36**:336–45.

11 Sellgren J, Ponten J, Wallin G. Percutaneous recordings of muscle nerve sympathetic nerve activity during propofol, N$_2$O, and isoflurane anesthesia in humans. *Anesthesiology* 1990;**73**:20–7.

12 Ebert TJ, Kanitz DD, Kampine JP. Inhibition of sympathetic neural outflow during thiopental anesthesia in humans. *Anesth Analg* 1990, 71:319–26.

13 Yli-Hankala A, Randell T, Seppala T, Lindgren L. Increases in hemodynamic variables and catecholamine levels after rapid increase in isoflurane concentration. *Anesthesiology* 1993;**78**:266–71.

14 Ebert TJ, Muzi M. Sympathetic hyperactivity during desflurane anesthesia in healthy volunteers. A comparison with isoflurane. *Anesthesiology*, 1993;**79**:444–53.

15 Muzi M, Ebert TJ, Hope WG, Robinson BJ, Bell LB. Site(s) mediating sympathetic activation with desflurane. *Anesthesiology*. 1996;**85**:737–47.

16 Ebert TJ, Harkin CP, Muzi M. Cardiovascular responses to sevoflurane: a review. *Anesth Analg* 1995;**81**:11–22.

17 Ebert TJ, Muzi M, Lopatka CW. Neurocirculatory responses to sevoflurane in humans. A comparison to desflurane. *Anesthesiology* 1995;**83**:88–95.

18 Griffiths R, Norman RI. Effects of anesthetics on uptake, synthesis and release of transmitters. *Br J Anaesth* 1993;**71**:96–107.

19 Goldstein DS, McCarty R, Polinsky RJ, Kopin IJ. Relationship between plasma norepinephrine and sympathetic nerve activity. *Hypertension*, 1983;**5**:552–9.

20 Honda T, Ninomiya I. Changes in AdSNA and arterial catecholamines to coronary occlusion in cats. *Am J Physiol* 1988;**255**:H704–10.

21 Esler M, Jennings G, Korner P. Assessment of human sympathetic nervous system activity from measurements of norepinephrine turnover. *Hypertension* 1988;**11**:3–20.

22 Wallin B, Sundlf G, Eriksson B. Plasma noradrenaline correlates to sympathetic muscle nerve activity in normotensive man. *Acta Physiol Scand* 1981;**111**:69–73.

23 Pocock G, Richards CD. Cellular mechanisms in general anaesthesia. *Br J Anaesth* 1991;**66**:116–28.

24 Philbin DM, Rosow CE, Schneider RC, Koski G, D'Ambra MN. Fentanyl and sufentanil anesthesia revisited: How much is enough. *Anesthesiology* 1990;**73**:5–11.

25 Sonntag H, Stephan H, Lange H, Rieke H, Kettler D, Martschausky N. Sufentanil does not block sympathetic responses to surgical stimuli in patients having CABG. *Anesth Analg* 1989;**68**:584–92.

26 Liem TH, Booij LHDJ, Gielen MJM, Hasenbos MAWM, van Egmond J. Coronary artery bypass grafting using two different anesthetic techniques: Part 3: Adrenergic responses. *J Cardiothorac Vasc Anesth* 1992;**6**:162–7.

27 Ebert TJ. Sympathetic hyperactivity during desflurane anesthesia in healthy volunteers. *Anesthesiology* 1993;**79**:444–53.

28 Skovstedt P, Price ML, Price HL. The effect of short acting barbiturates on arterial pressure, preganglionic sympathetic activity and barostatic reflexes. *Anesthesiology* 1970;**33**:10–8.

29 Marty J, Gauzit R, Lefevre P, et al. Effects of diazepam and midazolam on baroreflex control of heart rate and on sympathetic activity in humans. *Anesth Analg* 1986;**65**:113–9.

30 Kotrly KJ, Ebert TJ, Vucins EJ, Roerig DL, Stadnicka A, Kampine JP. Effects of fentanyl–diazepam–N_2O anaesthesia on arterial baroreflex control of heart rate in man. *Br J Anaesth* 1986;**58**:406–14.
31 Kotrly KJ, Ebert TJ, Vucins E, Igler FO, Barney JA, Kampine JP. Baroreceptor reflex control of the heart rate during isoflurane anesthesia in humans. *Anesthesiology* 1984;**60**:173–9.
32 Muzi M, Ebert TJ. Randomized, prospective comparison of halothane, isoflurane, and enflurane on baroreflex control of heart rate in humans. *Adv Pharmacol* 1994;**31**:379–87.
33 Akselrod S, Gordon D, Ubel FA, Shannon DC, Barger AC, Cohen RJ. Power spectrum analysis of heart rate fluctuation: a quantitative probe of beat to beat cardiovascular control. *Science* 1981;**213**:220–2.
34 Pomeranz B, Macaulay RJ, Caudill MA, et al. Assessment of autonomic function in humans by heart rate spectral analysis. *Am J Physiol* 1985;**248**:H151–3.
35 Pagani M, Lombardi F, Guzzetti S, et al. Power spectral analysis of heart rate and arterial pressure variabilities as a marker of sympatho-vagal interaction in man and conscious dog. Circ Res 1986;**59**:178–93.
36 Ikeda T, Doi M, Morita K, Ikeda K. Effects of midazolam and diazepam as premedication on heart rate variability in surgical patients. *Br J Anaesth* 1995;**73**:479–83.
37 Michaloudis D, Kochiadakis G, Georgopoulou G, et al. The influence of premedication on heart rate variability. *Anaesthesia* 1998;**53**:446–53.
38 Widmark C, Olaison J, Reftel B, Jonsson LE, Lindecrantz K. Spectral analysis of heart rate variability during desflurane and isoflurane anaesthesia in patients undergoing arthroscopy. *Acta Anaesthesiol Scand* 1998;**42**:204–10.
39 Ireland N, Meagher J, Sleigh JW, Henderson JD. Heart rate variability in patients recovering from general anaesthesia. *Br J Anaesth* 1996;**76**:657–62.
40 Komatsu T, Singh PK, Kimura T, Nishiwaki K, Bando K, Shimada Y. Differential effects of ketamine and midazolam on heart rate variability. *Can J Anaesth* 1995;**42**:1003–9.
41 Galletly DC, Buckley DH, Robinson BJ, Corfiatis T. Heart rate variability during propofol anaesthesia. *Br J Anaesth* 1994;**72**:219–20.
42 Latson TW, OFlaherty D. Effects of surgical stimulation on autonomic reflex function: assessment by changes in heart rate variability. *Br J Anaesth* 1993;**70**:301–5.
43 Zickmann B, Hofmann HC, Potkamper C, Knothe C, Boldt J, Hempelmann G. Changes in heart rate variability during induction of anesthesia with fentanyl and midazolam. *J Cardiothorac Vasc Anesth* 1996;**10**:609–13.
44 Latson TW, McCarroll SM, Mirhej MA, Hyndman VA, Whitten CW, Lipton JM. Effects of three anesthetic induction techniques on heart rate variability. *J Clin Anesth* 1992;**4**:265–76.
45 Komai H, Rusy BF. Differences in the myocardial depressant action of thiopental and halothane. *Anesth Analg* 1984;**63**:313–8.
46 Kissin I, Motomura S, Aultmann DF, Reves JG. Inotropic and anesthetic potencies of etomidate and thiopental in dogs. *Anesth Analg* 1983;**62**:961–5.
47 Roewer N, Proske O, Schulte am Esch J. The effects of midazolam on the mechanical and electrical properties of the isolated ventricular myocardium. *Anaesth Intensivther Notfallmed* 1990;**25**:354–61.
48 Azuma M, Matsumura C, Kemmotsu O. Inotropic and electrophysiological effects of propofol and thiamylal in isolated papillary muscles of the guinea pig and the rat. *Anesth Analg* 1993;**77**:557–63.
49 Mattheusen M, Housmans PR. Mechanisms of the direct, negative inotropic effect of etomidate in isolated ferret ventricular myocardium. *Anesthesiology* 1993;**79**:1284–95.
50 Stowe DF, Bosjnak ZJ, Kampine JP. Comparison of etomidate, ketamine, midazolam, propofol and thiopental on function and metabolism of isolated hearts. *Anesth Analg* 1992;**74**:547–58.
51 Park WK, Lynch C III. Propofol and thiopentone depression of myocardial contractility. A comparative study of mechanical and electrophysiological effects in isolated guinea pig ventricular muscle. *Anesth Analg* 1992;**74**:395–405.

52 Rusy BF, Komai H. Anesthetic depression of myocardial contractility. A review of possible mechanisms. *Anesthesiology* 1987;**67**:745–66.

53 Dowdy EG, Kaya K. Studies of the mechanisms of cardiovascular responses to CI-581. *Anesthesiology* 1968;**29**:931.

54 Urthaler F, Walker AA, James TN. Comparison of the inotropic action of morphine and ketamine studies in canine artery muscle. *J Thorac Cardiovasc Surg* 1976;**72**:142.

55 Riou B, Viars P, Lecarpentier Y. Effects of ketamine on the cardiac papillary muscle of normal hamsters and those with cardiomyopathy. *Anesthesiology* 1990;**73**:910–18.

56 Cook DJ, Carton EG, Housmans PR. Mechanisms of the positive inotropic effect of ketamine in isolated ferret ventricular papillary muscle. *Anesthesiology* 1991;**74**:880–8.

57 Kongsayreepong S, Cook DJ, Housmans PR. Mechanisms of the direct, negative inotropic effect of ketamine in isolated ferret and frog ventricular myocardium. *Anesthesiology* 1993;**79**:313–22.

58 Gelissen HP, Epema AH, Henning RH, Krijnen HJ, Hennis PJ, den Hertog A. Inotropic effects of propofol, thiopental, midazolam, etomidate, and ketamine on isolated human atrial muscle. *Anesthesiology* 1996;**84**:397–403.

59 Lynch C III, Frazer MJ. Depressant effects of volatile anesthetics upon rat and amphibian myocardium: Insights into anesthetic mechanisms of action. *Anesthesiology* 1989;**70**:511–22.

60 Wolf WJ, Neal MB, Mathew BP, Bee DE. Comparison of the in vitro myocardial depressant effects of isoflurane and halothane anesthesia. *Anesthesiology* 1988;**69**:660–6.

61 Kemmotsu O, Hashimoto Y, Shimosato S. Inotropic effects of isoflurane on mechanics of contraction in isolated cat papillary muscles from normal and failing hearts. *Anesthesiology* 1973;**39**:402–15.

62 Kemmotsu O, Hashimoto Y, Shimosato S. The effects of fluroxene and enflurane on contractile performance of isolated papillary muscles from failing hearts. *Anesthesiology* 1974;**40**:253–60.

63 Lynch C III. Differential depression of myocardial contractility by volatile anesthetics in vitro: Comparison with uncouplers of excitation–contraction coupling. *J Cardiovasc Pharmacol* 1990;**15**:655–65.

64 Stowe DF, Monroe SM, Marijic J, Bosnjak ZJ, Kampine JP. Comparison of halothane, enflurane, and isoflurane with nitrous oxide on contractility and oxygen supply and demand in isolated hearts. *Anesthesiology* 1991;**75**:1062–74.

65 Hatakeyama N, Momose Y, Ito Y. Effects of sevoflurane on contractile responses and electrophysiologic properties in canine single cardiac myocytes. *Anesthesiology* 1995;**82**:559–65.

66 Gueugniaud PY, Hanouz JL, Vivien B, Lecarpentier Y, Coriat P, Riou B. Effects of desflurane in rat myocardium: comparison with isoflurane and halothane. *Anesthesiology* 1997;**87**:599–609.

67 Lawson D, Frazer MJ, Lynch C III. Nitrous oxide effects on isolated myocardium: a reexamination in vitro. *Anesthesiology* 1990;**73**:930–43.

68 Bovill JG, Boer F. Opioids in cardiac anesthesia. In: Kaplan J, ed, *Cardiac anesthesia*. 3rd edn. WB Saunders & Co, 1993:467–511.

69 Sagawa K. The ventricular pressure–volume diagram revisited. *Circ Res* 1978;**46**: 677–87.

70 Mulier JP, Wouters P, van Aken H, Vermaut G, Vandermersch M. Cardiodynamic effects of propofol in comparison with thiopental: Assessment with transesophageal echocardiographic approach. *Anesth Analg* 1991;**72**:28–35.

71 Pagel PS, Kampine JP, Schmeling WT, Warltier DC. Reversal of volatile anesthetic induced depression of myocardial contractility by extracellular calcium also enhances left ventricular diastolic function. *Anesthesiology* 1993;**78**:141–54.

72 Heinrich H, Fontaine L, Fösel TH, Spilker D, Winter H, Ahnefeld FW. Echocardiographic assessment of the negative inotropic effects of halothane, enflurane and isoflurane. *Anaesthesist* 1986;**35**:465–72.

73 Pagel PS, Kampine JP, Schmeling WT, Warltier DC. Influence of volatile anesthetics on myocardial contractility in vivo: Desflurane versus Isoflurane. *Anesthesiology* 1991;**74**:900–7.

74 Harkin CP, Pagel PS, Kersten JR, Hettrick DA, Warltier DC. Direct negative inotropic and lusitropic effects of sevoflurane. *Anesthesiology* 1994;**81**:156–67.

75 Pagel PS, Kampine JP, Schmeling WT, Warltier DC. Effects of nitrous oxide on myocardial contractility as evaluated by the preload recruitable stroke work relationship in chronically instrumented dogs. *Anesthesiology* 1990;**73**:1148–57.

76 Hoeft A, Sonntag H, Stephan H, Kettler D. Validation of myocardial oxygen demand indices in patients awake and during anesthesia. *Anesthesiology* 1991;**75**:49–56.

77 Rhode E. Über den Einfluss der mechanischen Bedingungen auf die Tätigkeit und den Sauerstoffverbrauch des Warmblüterherzens. *Archiv für Experimentelle Pathologie und Pharmakologie* 1915;**68**:401–34.

78 Baller D, Bretschneider HJ, Hellige G. Validity of myocardial oxygen consumption parameters. *Clin Cardiol* 1979;**2**:317–27.

79 Rooke GA, Feigl EO. Work as a correlate of canine left ventricular oxygen consumption, and the problem of catecholamine wasting. *Circ Res* 1982;**50**:273–86.

80 Rooke GA. Low dose halothane anesthesia does not affect the hemodynamic estimation of myocardial oxygen consumption in dogs. *Anesthesiology* 1990;**72**:682–93.

81 Kettler D, Sonntag H. Intravenous anaesthetics: Coronary blood flow and myocardial oxygen consumption. *Acta Anaesthesiol Belg* 1974;**25**:384–401.

82 Hoeft A, Sonntag H, Stephan H, Kettler D. The influence of anesthesia on myocardial oxygen utilization efficiency in patients undergoing coronary bypass surgery. *Anesth Analg* 1994;**78**:857–66.

83 Turner E. *Pathophysiologie der Aufwachphase. Anästhesiologie und Intensivmedizin* (Bd 179). 1986, Berlin: Springer Verlag.

84 Evans CL, Matsuoka Y. The effect of various mechanical conditions on the gaseous metabolism and efficiency of the mammalian heart. *J Physiol (Lond)* 1915;**49**:378–405.

85 Burkhoff D, Sagawa K. Ventricular efficiency predicted by an analytical model. *Am J Physiol* 1986;**250**:R1021–7.

86 Suga H, Igarashi Y, Yamada O, Goto Y. Mechanical efficiency of the left ventricle as a function of preload, afterload, and contractility. *Heart Vessels* 1985;**1**:3–8.

87 Hoeft A, Koeb H, Hellige G, Sonntag H. Energetics and efficiency of cardiac pump work. *Anaesthesist* 1991;**40**:465–78.

88 Sunagawa K, Maughan WL, Burkhoff D, Sagawa K. Left ventricular interaction with arterial load studied in isolated canine ventricle. *Am J Physiol* 1983;**245**:H773–80.

89 Sunagawa K, Maughan WL, Sagawa K. Optimal arterial resistance for the maximal stroke work studied in isolated canine left ventricle. *Circ Res* 1985;**56**:586–95.

90 Hettrick DA, Pagel PS, Warltier DC. Desflurane, sevoflurane, and isoflurane impair canine left ventricular–arterial coupling and mechanical efficiency. *Anesthesiology* 1996;**85**:403–13.

91 Hettrick DA, Pagel PS, Warltier DC. Isoflurane and halothane produce similar alterations in aortic distensibility and characteristic aortic impedance. *Anesth Analg* 1996;**83**:1166–72.

92 Hettrick DA, Pagel PS, Warltier DC. Alterations in canine left ventricular–arterial coupling and mechanical efficiency produced by propofol. *Anesthesiology* 1997;**86**:1088–93.

93 Hoeft A, Sonntag H, Stephan H. Coronary flow and myocardial oxygen balance in anaesthesia. *AINS* 1993;**26**:398–407.

94 Crystal GJ, Gurevicius J, Salem MR, Zhou X. Role of adenosine triphosphate sensitive potassium channels in coronary vasodilation by halothane, isoflurane, and enflurane. *Anesthesiology* 1997;**86**:448–58.

95 Priebe HJ. Isoflurane and coronary hemodynamics. *Anesthesiology* 1989;**71**:960–76.

96 Nicklas JM, Becker LC, Bulkley BH. Effects of repeated brief coronary occlusion on regional left ventricular function and dimension in dogs. *Am J Cardiol* 1985;**56**:473–8.

97 Gurevicius J, Holmes CB, Salem MR, Abdel Halim A, Crystal GJ. The direct effects of enflurane on coronary blood flow, myocardial oxygen consumption, and myocardial segmental shortening in in situ canine hearts. *Anesth Analg* 1996;**83**:68–74.

98 DeTraglia MC, Komai H, Redon D, Rusy BF. Isoflurane and halothane inhibit tetanic contractions in rabbit myocardium in vitro. *Anesthesiology*. 1989;**70**:837–42.

99 Nader-Djalal N, Knight PR. Volatile anaesthetic effects on ischaemic myocardium. *Curr Opin Anaesthesiol* 1998;**11**:403–6.

100 Cope DK, Impastato WK, Cohen MV, Downey JM. Volatile anesthetics protect the ischemic rabbit myocardium from infarction. *Anesthesiology* 1997;**86**:699–709.

101 Shah AM, Silverman HS, Griffiths EJ, Spurgeon HA, Lakatta EG. cGMP prevents delayed relaxation at reoxygenation after brief hypoxia in isolated cardiac myocytes. *Am J Physiol* 1995;**268**:H2396–404.

102 Kersten JR, Orth KG, Pagel PS, Mei DA, Gross GJ, Warltier DC. Role of adenosine in isoflurane induced cardioprotection. *Anesthesiology* 1997;**86**:1128–39.

103 Liu Y, Gao WD, O'Rourke B, Marban E. Synergistic modulation of ATP sensitive K^+ currents by protein kinase C and adenosine. Implications for ischemic preconditioning. *Circ Res* 1996;**78**:443–54.

104 Hirota K, Ito Y, Momose Y. Effects of halothane on membrane potentials and membrane ionic currents in single bullfrog atrial cells. *Acta Anaesthesiol Scand* 1988;**32**:333–8.

105 Park WK, Pancrazio JJ, Suh CK, Lynch C III. Myocardial depressant effects of sevoflurane. Mechanical and electrophysiologic actions in vitro. *Anesthesiology* 1996;**84**:1166–76.

106 Glantz L, Ginosar Y, Chevion M, et al. Halothane prevents postischemic production of hydroxyl radicals in the canine heart. *Anesthesiology* 1997;**86**:440–7.

107 Frohlich D, Rothe G, Schwall B, et al. Effects of volatile anaesthetics on human neutrophil oxidative response to the bacterial peptide FMLP. *Br J Anaesth* 1997;**78**:718–23.

108 Kowalski C, Zahler S, Becker BF, et al. Halothane, isoflurane, and sevoflurane reduce postischemic adhesion of neutrophils in the coronary system. *Anesthesiology* 1997;**86**:188–95.

109 Kokita N, Hara A, Abiko Y, Arakawa J, Hashizume H, Namiki A. Propofol improves functional and metabolic recovery in ischemic reperfused isolated rat hearts. *Anesth Analg* 1998;**86**:252–8.

110 Larach DR, Schuler HG, Derr JA, Larach MG, Hensley FA, Zelis R. Halothane selectively attenuates α_2-adrenoceptor mediated vasoconstriction, in vivo and in vitro. *Anesthesiology* 1987;**66**:781–91.

111 Kenny D, Pelch LR, Brooks HL, Kampine JP, Schmeling WT, Warltier DC. Calcium channel modulation of α_1- and α_2-adrenergic pressor responses in conscious and anesthetized dogs. *Anesthesiology* 1990;**72**:874–81.

112 Yamamoto M, Hatano Y, Kakuyama M, et al. Different effects of halothane, isoflurane and sevoflurane on sarcoplasmic reticulum of vascular smooth muscle in dog mesenteric artery. *Acta Anaesthesiol Scand* 1997;**41**:376–80.

113 Nakamura K, Toda H, Hatano Y, Mori K. Comparison of the direct effects of sevoflurane, isoflurane and halothane on isolated canine coronary arteries. *Can J Anaesth* 1993;**40**:257–61.

114 Park WK, Lynch C III, Johns RA. Effects of propofol and thiopental in isolated rat aorta and pulmonary artery. *Anesthesiology* 1992;**77**:956–63.

115 Nakamura K, Hatano Y, Hirakata H, Nishiwada M, Toda H, Mori K. Direct vasoconstrictor and vasodilator effects of propofol in isolated dog arteries. *Br J Anaesth* 1992;**68**:193–7.

116 Robinson BJ, Ebert TJ, O'Brien TJ, Colinco MD, Muzi M. Mechanisms whereby propofol mediates peripheral vasodilation in humans. Sympathoinhibition or direct vascular relaxation? *Anesthesiology*. 1997;**86**:64–72.

117 Hettrick DA, Pagel PS, Warltier DC. Differential effects of isoflurane and halothane on aortic input impedance quantified using a three-element Windkessel model. *Anesthesiology* 1995;**83**:361–73.

118 Lowe D, Hettrick DA, Pagel PS, Warltier DC. Propofol alters left ventricular afterload as evaluated by aortic input impedance in dogs. *Anesthesiology* 1996;**84**:368–76.

119 Pagel PS, Hettrick DA, Kersten JR, Tessmer JP, Lowe D, Warltier DC. Etomidate adversely alters determinants of left ventricular afterload in dogs with dilated cardiomyopathy. *Anesth Analg* 1998;**86**:932–38.

120 Gauer OH, Henry JP. Circulatory basis of fluid volume control. *Physiol Rev* 1963;**43**:423–81.

121 Arndt JO. The low pressure system: the integrated function of veins. *Eur J Anaesth* 1986;**3**:343–70.
122 Henry JP, Gauer OH, Sieker HO. The effects of moderate changes in blood volume on left and right atrial pressure. *Circ Res* 1956;**4**:91–4.
123 Gauer OH, Henry JP, Behn C. Changes in central venous pressure after moderate hemorrhage and transfusion in man. *Circ Res* 1956;**4**:79–90.
124 Echt M, Düweling J, Gauer OH, Lange L. Effective compliance of the total vascular bed and the intrathoracic compartment derived from changes in central venous pressure induced by volume changes in man. *Circ Res* 1974;**34**:61–8.
125 Bonica JJ, Kennedy WF, Nakamatsu TJ, Gerbershagen HU. Circulatory effects of peridural block: III effects of acute blood loss. *Anesthesiology* 1972;**36**:219–27.
126 Mangano DT. Monitoring pulmonary artery pressure in coronary artery disease. *Anesthesiology* 1980;**53**:364–70.
127 Hoeft A, Schorn B, Weyland A, et al. Bedside assessment of intravascular volume status in patients undergoing cardiac surgery. *Anesthesiology* 1994;**81**:76–86.
128 Hedenstierna G, Strandberg A, Brismar B, Lundquist H, Svensson L, Tokics L. Functional residual capacity, thoracoabdominal dimensions and central blood volume during general anesthesia with muscle paralysis and mechanical ventilation. *Anesthesiology* 1985;**62**:247–54.
129 Krayer S, Rehder K, Beck KC, Cameron PD, Didier EP, Hofman EA. Quantification of thoracic volumes by three dimensional imaging. *J Appl Physiol* 1987;**62**:591–8.
130 Arndt JO, Höck A, Stanton-Hicks M, Stühmeier KD. Peridural anesthesia and the distribution of blood in supine humans. *Anesthesiology* 1985;**63**:616–23.
131 Lipfert P, Arndt JO. Major conduction anaesthesia, Pathogenesis, prophylaxis, and therapy of circulatory complications *Anaesthesist* 1993;**42**:773–87.
132 Caplan RA, Ward RJ, Posner K, Cheney FW. Unexpected cardiac arrest during spinal anesthesia: A closed claims analysis of predisposing factors. *Anesthesiology* 1988;**68**:5–11.

Index

379